SOMETHING HIDDEN ∞∞∞∞∞∞

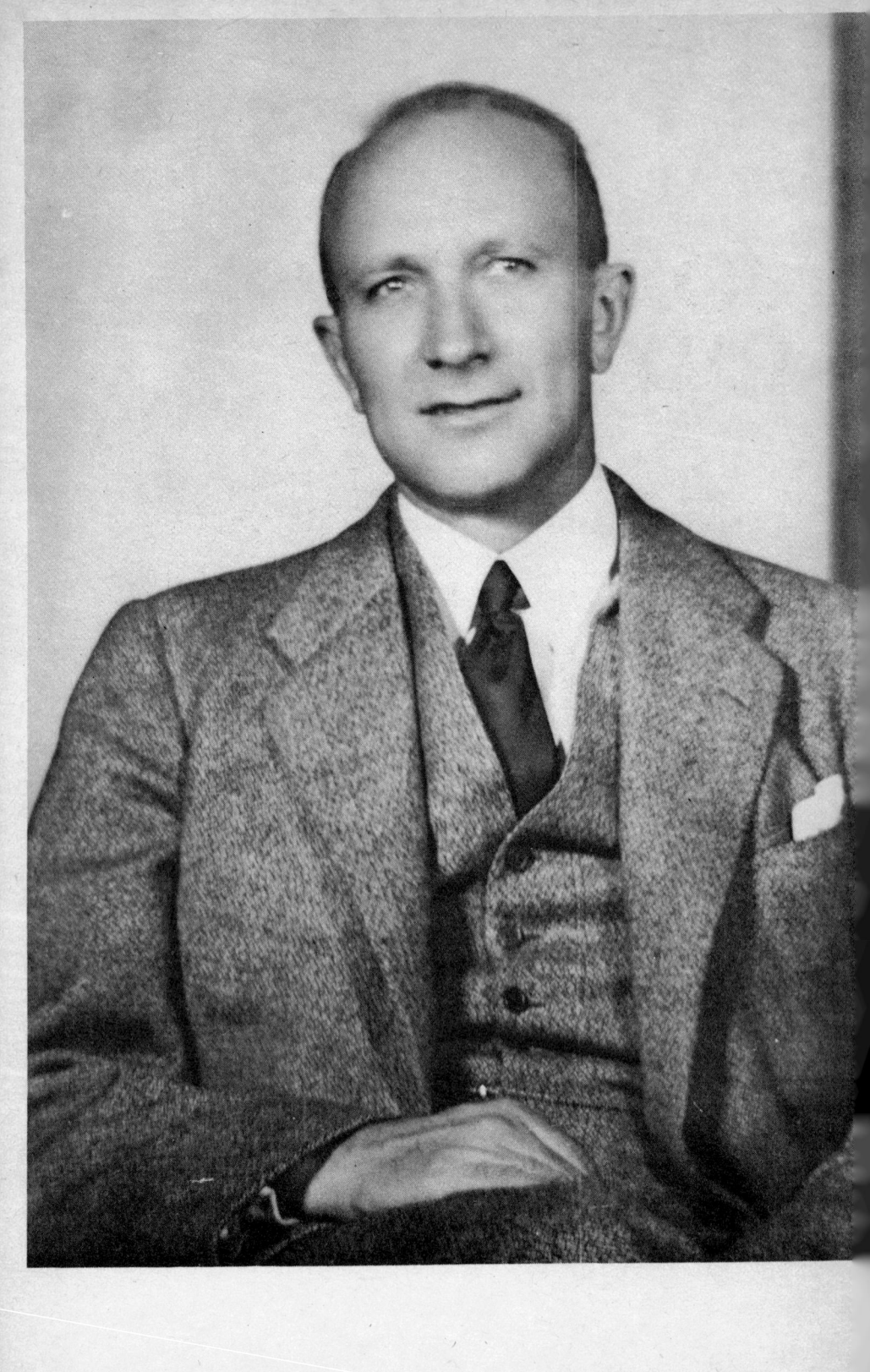

SOMETHING HIDDEN

A Biography of Wilder Penfield

JEFFERSON LEWIS

1981

DOUBLEDAY CANADA LIMITED,
Toronto, Ontario
DOUBLEDAY & COMPANY, INC.,
Garden City, New York

Library of Congress Catalog Card Number 81-43110

Copyright © 1981 by Howard Jefferson Lewis
All rights reserved
FIRST EDITION

Printed in Canada by Webcom Limited
Typesetting by ART-U Graphics
Design by Robert Burgess Garbutt

Canadian Cataloguing in Publication Data

Lewis, H. Jefferson (Howard Jefferson), 1951-
   Something hidden

Includes index.
ISBN 0-385-17696-1

1. Penfield, Wilder, 1891-1976. 2. Neurosurgeons—
Canada—Biography. 3. Brain—Surgery—History—
20th century. I. Title.

R464.P46L48   617'.092'4   C81-094818-4

Author's Note: The sometimes eccentric punctuation, spelling, and grammar in excerpts from Wilder Penfield's unpublished letters and diaries has been retained except where it would cause unnecessary confusion.

The author wishes to thank The Canada Council, The Hannah Institute for the History of Medicine, and the Ontario Arts Council for their generous financial assistance during the writing of this book; the literary executors of Wilder Penfield's estate for access to private papers and permission to quote from them; and Mr. Charles Hodge, head of the Department of Neurophotography at the Montreal Neurological Institute for his assistance in locating and reproducing many of the photographs in this book.

No Man Alone: A Neurosurgeon's Life by Wilder Penfield. Quoted by permission of Little, Brown & Company, Boston, and The Canadian Publishers, McClelland and Stewart Limited and Little, Brown & Company (Canada) Limited, Toronto. Copyright © 1977 by William Feindel, M.D., Wilder Penfield, Jr., and Theodore Rasmussen, M.D., as Literary Executors for the Estate of Wilder Penfield.

The epigraphs to Part Two and Part Three are from "The Love Song of J. Alfred Prufrock" in *Collected Poems 1909-1962* by T. S. Eliot, copyright © 1936 by Harcourt Brace Jovanovich, Inc.; copyright © 1963, 1964 by T. S. Eliot. Reprinted by permission of Harcourt Brace Jovanovich, Inc., and Faber and Faber Limited.

*for my mother and father
Ruthmary and Crosby Lewis*

ACKNOWLEDGEMENTS

My biggest debt is to the friends, family members and editors who, in the four years since I began work on this book, read, listened, encouraged, scolded, advised, or patiently refrained from all of these. In particular, I would like to thank R. W. B. Lewis, Valerie Frith, John Pearce, Timothy Wilson, Matthew Hart, Christina Hartling, Wendy Penfield and Mrs. Margaret Jasper. I owe a special debt of thanks to Dr. Herbert Jasper for taking great pains to steer me around the worst pitfalls in summarizing the scientific material in this book. Any errors of fact and interpretation are, of course, my own.

I would also like to separately thank my aunt and uncle, Wilder and Berry Penfield, and my mother and father, for their constant, unwavering support, and patient correction of my mistakes.

In the latter stages of writing I had the good fortune to work on a documentary film portrait of Wilder Penfield, an experience that confirmed some of my ideas, altered others, and introduced new ones which are reflected in these pages. For many helpful discussions I would like to thank Bob Lower, the director of the film, and Vincent Tovell, executive producer for the CBC.

My thanks also to Rick Archbold, managing editor at Doubleday Canada, for his considerable patience and tact, and to Avanthia Swan, my copyeditor, for a devotion to this book that went well beyond any reasonable expectation.

Finally, there are many individuals—former patients, colleagues, friends and acquaintances of Wilder Penfield—who submitted to being interviewed at various stages; too many to thank here, but my thanks are nonetheless heartfelt.

My greatest debt of all is to Catherine, who read, corrected and improved the manuscript immeasurably at every stage, and still kept her sense of humour.

CONTENTS

ACKNOWLEDGEMENTS vii
PREFACE xi

PART ONE

ONE • *A Stubborn Lot*
        CHARLES AND JENNIE 2
        SPOKANE 10
        CHILDHOOD 12

TWO • *Growing Up*
        HUDSON 17
        THE GALAHAD SCHOOL 22

THREE • *Wilder Penfield, Esq.*
        PRINCETON 29
        DECISIONS 36

FOUR • *An Unusual Apprenticeship*
        OXFORD 49
        JOHNS HOPKINS 63
        PARIS 68
        THE HIGH ROAD 73

FIVE • *A Young Surgeon to Watch*
- NEW YORK 84
- FREDERICO 89
- SPAIN 93
- THE MONTREAL OFFER 99

PART TWO

SIX • *His Own Master*
- MONTREAL 112
- RUTH 118
- EPILEPSY 125
- PUTTING DOWN ROOTS 133
- THE MONTREAL NEUROLOGICAL INSTITUTE 140

SEVEN • *Cursed with Success*
- THE CHIEF 152
- WAR YEARS 162
- AMBASSADOR FOR SCIENCE 176

EIGHT • *In Full Flight*
- GREAT DISCOVERIES 190
- "THE GHOST IN THE MACHINE" 210

PART THREE

NINE • *Other Doors Open*
- A SECRET WRITER 220
- INTERLUDE IN ENGLAND 228
- TROUBLE AT THE INSTITUTE 230

TEN • *An Old Doctor*
- "A HORRID RIVER" 242
- THE WORLD OUTSIDE 247

ELEVEN • *Champion of the Old Order*
- SECOND CAREERS 260
- A CALL 284
- THE MYSTERY OF THE MIND 292

A NOTE ON SOURCES 305
INDEX 306

PREFACE

In the early stages of the research for this book I came across a letter addressed to me in my grandfather's handwriting, stamped, sealed, but never mailed. I found it one morning going through his filing cabinets after his death. I remember I sat there awhile, staring at the familiar, sprawling hand in which he had written my name and address; he had drawn a line through it and penned above "not sent." What, I wondered, did he have to say to me at this late date? What would he have thought of my plans to write about his life?

Eventually I slit the envelope and extracted the letter. It was dated January 11, 1976, and was a reaction to our meeting two weeks earlier. I was to be married in the summer and I had brought my future wife to meet my grandparents. The dinner turned out to be the last time I saw my grandfather before his death in April.

He was approaching 85 then, bald, gaunt, walking with a cane. My grandmother was growing deaf, and seemed to have trouble, occasionally, following the conversation. Because of their age, and because of the formal nature of this visit I was not expecting a meeting of minds and was not disappointed when one did not occur.

His letter revealed a very different reaction to the evening: "It seemed to me, at least, that we did not communicate as we should." Then he went to say what he had wanted to say that evening: "In our 58 years of married life the most wonderful source of security and strength and happiness came to us from the awareness of companionship. At 84, soon to be 85, bodily attraction burns low and love continues. It is a thing of the spirit, as companionship is.... Some women have a mysterious gift of insight that can make a strong man into a creative one. I found such a one. I have a hunch you have."

As I read through the letter I was struck by how much he had cared—in those last months when he knew he hadn't long to live—about the impending marriage of one among his fifteen grandchildren, about the things he knew were true, and, most of all, about telling them. Often, in the four years I spent preparing this book, the gentle Victorian echoes of that letter came into my mind, balancing the sterner Victorian echoes of another letter, the last I received from my grandfather while he was still alive. Its tone was strikingly different and more in keeping with the relationship we had developed over the years. It was a cranky, worried criticism of an article of mine that he had read.

The subject of the article was the ease with which large corporations bend government regulatory agencies to their wills. He and my grandmother had read the article one night before going to bed, he explained and, disturbed by what I had written, "I have left that bed now to write to you." He charged that instead of proposing an effective solution to the problem, the article was "a well-told joke and cynical laughter that turned one's thoughts to the Christian being devoured by the lion." After saying that I had "let the side down," he reminded me: "The Christians won in the end you know, not the emperor nor the Roman citizen with the depraved appetite for amusement."

I needn't describe here my letter back, except to say that it was a brilliant riposte that would have settled once and for all the issue of a journalist's role in society—only I delayed sending it, and meanwhile he died.

He left behind for me to discover over the next four years, an occasionally overpowering record of his passing. It includes whole shelves of scientific summaries and theories, seven non-medical books, including two historical novels and a partial autobiography (*No Man Alone*), fat bundles of speeches, and volume after volume of letters. It wasn't until I was a year into the research that I came across the diaries, which I found to be the most painful and the most illuminating source of all. These diaries, in which he wrote intermittently from the age of thirteen until just a few days before his death, revealed the man I had known, and a different one, a man more ambivalent, self-critical, musing, and troubled than any of us around him would ever have guessed. Aside from all of these sources, there were the memories of everyone who knew him, including memories of my own.

Throughout my childhood, he was a powerful but distant figure; someone to be proud of because he was famous, someone to be wary of because his occasional anger was apocalyptic. In the winter, it was a solemn occasion to make the trek across the city to dinner with them, one that called for a clean face and best behaviour. In the summer we lived in a cottage by the lake, and he lived in a house at the top of the hill, where we would spend Sunday mornings listening to him read from the Bible, and then would speak the family prayer and sing the family hymn. I would sit on the window seat and, on sunny mornings, would sneak anxious looks away from where he sat by the fire, talking, down the hill beyond the pasture where the cows grazed and past the spinneys of trees, to the lake where I wanted to be, sailing or swimming or exploring.

As I grew older, the vague outlines of this man and his views took on a sharper edge. Throughout my adolescence and early adulthood, he was a perfect foil, one who could be relied on to take the diametrically opposite position on any matter touching politics, social issues, public morality or personal ambition. His rebukes, which he passed out willingly, were signs that you, and your current opinions, mattered to him. And if I found his views strait-laced, impossibly conservative and infuriatingly certain, I appreciated nonetheless his willingness to do battle. I don't think I ever *won* a point, but it was fun, and good practice, and his concern was somehow flattering.

Years later, in conducting interviews for this book, I was astonished to discover how many other people had engaged with him in much the same way, and had come away similarly provoked, flattered and puzzled. It did not seem to matter whether I was talking to a distinguished elder scientist or a journalist, a surgeon or a family member, a politician or a social worker. All of them had discovered that the force of his opinions demanded an equally forceful response. Cynicism to him was a contemptible vice—the cheap evasion of a wasted mind. He wore his own prejudices and convictions like a slightly old-fashioned uniform, with a touchy pride.

It was difficult not to come away either fervently admiring him, or fervently disliking him. He was, first and last, a committed man, and one, as I learned through my research, who relished the challenge of an uneven match. He fought a long and lonely battle to make radical surgery of the brain a safe and respectable cure for diseases like epilepsy. He was a pioneer in the study of the human brain, and he launched one revolutionary scientific theory after another that brought him as much criticism as praise and respect. He was a scientist who was not afraid to make bold hypotheses.

When his career in medicine came to an end, he used his fame as a weapon to fight on other fronts for what he believed in. His speeches made headlines, his opinion was sought on a wide variety of issues, and his presence became a certain, special kind of blessing on any gathering. Yet, despite the range of his many interests, he was not so much a Renaissance man, as a Victorian activist: constantly in search of causes, impelled by the urge to intervene, the need to serve a greater good, the conviction that he had something to contribute.

It has not been an easy task to try to present an unvarnished portrait. As strong as the urge, at times, to make this book the final argument with him—one I would win by default—are my admiration for his sense of commitment, and the memories of his deep and genuine loving-kindness. Such are the memories from my childhood: of the gentle stroke of his hands on my side as he probed a bruise from a bad fall, and the dazzling blur of his gaze focussed on me—for a second? a minute? an hour? I don't remember. But I basked in its warmth and I have never forgotten it. I hope that my affection, my admiration, and my critical eye have struck a balance in the pages of this book.

JL
Magog Meadows
July, 1981

SOMETHING HIDDEN

PART ONE

*Thus strangely are our souls constructed,
And by such slight ligaments are we bound to prosperity or ruin.*

MARY SHELLEY

CHAPTER ONE

A Stubborn Lot

∞ CHARLES AND JENNIE

"I gather the only certain virtue that came into the world with me was tenacity of purpose. Some would say this is stubbornness, which, at least when it appears in others, is more of a nuisance than a virtue." With that self-mocking judgment and a few sparse references, Wilder dispensed with his ancestors altogether. He was in his eighties at the time, and grumpily writing a book he'd always sworn he wouldn't, "my pseudo-autobiography." On the pretext that it was to be the "biography of an idea" that led to the creation of the Montreal Neurological Institute, he had allowed himself to be persuaded to tackle the project. It was only later that he discovered how deeply in his life the idea had its roots. With his usual meticulousness, he had traced its source back step by step until he found himself talking about his mother.

She was his first and greatest inspiration. His father, on the other hand, was even at that late date an angry and unhappy memory, and it was with great reluctance that Wilder agreed, when readers objected to the gap in the story, to talk about his father and his ancestors at all.

It is a pity that the shadow of his father loomed so forbiddingly across the line connecting him to his ancestors, because if he had probed a bit deeper he might have understood the restlessness that drove and puzzled and confounded him over and over in his life. As much as the stubbornness which he was quick to note, restlessness was an inherited trait. Neither the Penfields nor his mother's family, the Jeffersons, were sitters and thinkers—they were doers and wanderers.

Middle class almost before there was such a thing as a middle class in America, Penfields and Jeffersons were university-educated at a time when such education was a rarity. Yet they were outsiders, drawing a certain measure of security from their middle class background, but little nourishment or peace. The generations of Penfields and Jeffersons preceding Wilder Penfield moved from place to place, shifting slowly and inexorably westward from their New England roots. They would settle in one town or village for a generation or two, then set off again. They had a gift for making money, and they worked hard. They were not pioneers—they did not have that craving for conquest and open space. Instead, they followed a step behind, bringing their trades—farmer, wheelwright, millwright, eventually doctor—to the settlements and towns that sprang up in the wake of the first explorers and settlers. But if they were missing the qualities that made pioneers, they lacked the qualities that made for settlers. They also lacked the edge of ruthlessness or brilliance that would have turned a small fortune into a large one. They were, in sum, intelligent, obstinate, occasionally inspired but not particularly ambitious, neither stalwart citizens nor great radicals. Although they followed the westward push which was the overriding impulse of the second half of the nineteenth century, they did so for reasons of their own.

The first Penfield to arrive in the New World was a supporter of Oliver Cromwell who had been driven out of his native Cornwall when the monarchy was restored. He left his home just a step ahead of the king's soldiers and made his way to New England. For the next half-dozen generations, Penfields moved around new England, from Rhode Island to Massachusetts to Connecticut, the prototypical Yankee traders: thrifty, devout, industrious, inventive, tough and prolific. Penfield families usually had ten or a dozen children—boys named Abel, Isaac and Zebulon, girls named Silence, Prudence and Submit. When Wilder was born, he became the 1,645th entry in *The Penfield Genealogy*, whose author in a weary moment would confide to a relative, "There are times when I regard an unmarried Penfield as a public benefactor."

The first Penfield born in the New World was named Samuel. Seven generations later there was another Samuel, born in 1804. In him stubbornness became perversity that in turn became a family legend. Perhaps because Wilder felt they had something in common, this Samuel (Wilder's great-grandfather) was the only forebear in whom he showed much interest.

When Samuel was five, his father died and left him, the youngest son, a tract of land in Ohio. At the age of twenty-three Samuel set off on foot to claim his legacy.

Ohio was five hundred miles or more over the Allegheny Mountains, through dense forests and steep, rocky valleys. Indian alarms were "as frequent as fires in Boston," wrote one settler from a little outpost called Pittsburgh on the Ohio River. Pioneers had already begun the trek over the mountains before the Revolution, but after Independence, the trickling streams became a flood.

The trip took Samuel many months, but he arrived at last in Huron County. There he built a small cabin before returning to Connecticut for his widowed mother and two unmarried sisters. They were joined on their return to Ohio by the third sister and her husband.

Like the Penfields before him, Samuel worked hard and prospered. For a while he practised the trade of wagonmaker, and later he took up farming. In 1832 he married a young schoolteacher named Clara Woodworth, who had come to Ohio from Connecticut a year before.

Samuel was a staunch Baptist, one of the first prohibitionists in Ohio and a dedicated abolitionist—quite a feat in those days, since the Baptist Church, with its strong Southern connections, was a steadfast supporter of slavery.

In defiance of community sentiment and the laws against assisting runaway slaves, Samuel's big house in Fairfield became an important link in the underground railroad that spirited runaway slaves across Lake Erie and into Canada. As for his prohibitionism, there is the queer story of a barn-raising Samuel held. When he notified the congregation in the Sunday notices that no liquor would be served, the announcement reportedly raised such a commotion that it ended in his being put out of the church. "Then he quietly went to the other church until it all blew over," so the story goes. Samuel had already given the Baptist church a bell, a presentation that some judged frivolous. After a delegation had been sent to ask him to come back to the church, he presented the church with its first organ. The gift raised a storm of protest and both Samuel and the organ were expelled.

That's family history. Either one of the stories is wrong or we will have to take it on faith that a congregation of Ohio Baptists would expel one of its members for *not* serving liquor at a barn-raising, and a short while later, cast him out again for inviting in the devil disguised as an organ.

In 1833, Wilder's grandfather, Ephraim Penfield, was born. When he reached the age of fourteen, Ephraim was sent from the little hamlet of North Fairfield to the nearby town of Norwalk to be educated. Ephraim was to be the first Penfield doctor. In 1854 he began studying medicine with a practitioner in his native village, and then attended Homeopathic Medical College fifty miles away in Cleveland on the shores of Lake Erie.

The homeopathic system of medicine is based on the principle that diseases can be cured by drugs that produce, in a healthy person, the same pathological effects that are symptomatic of the disease. In other words, a homeopathic doctor would treat a feverish patient, who sweated profusely and was drowsy and delirious, by giving him a dose of opium—which produces essentially the same symptoms. According to homeopathic principle, a very small dose is better than a large one. Whether the village doctor with whom Ephraim studied was a homeopath or whether the choice reflects, once again, Samuel's avant-garde opinions, the rising popularity of the specialty made it a very profitable branch of medicine for a young doctor to enter.

When Ephraim had completed his studies, he returned to Norwalk, practised for a while there, and then moved forty miles away to a bigger town, Bucyrus, Ohio. We don't know much about Ephraim, aside from the brief information that he voted Republican, was fond of music and "intelligent conversation," was beloved by his patients and, despite his father's tilting with the local church authorities, was himself a sober and religious church-goer. There is a picture of him, taken some years later, that shows a formidable figure with an enormously long, flowing beard, bushy eyebrows and a resolute demeanour. And yet he had the Penfield restlessness: at an age when most doctors would be thinking of retiring, Ephraim sold his house and practice in Ohio, moved out to the frontier and started over again.

In 1857, Ephraim had married Delia Louise Smith, a pretty, cheerful young woman of nineteen, and nine months later Charles Samuel Penfield, father of Wilder Penfield, was born. When Charles was eleven, his brother James was born. After an interval of nine years James was followed by a third son named Arthur. They grew up in Bucyrus, in a big brick house surrounded by a wrought-iron fence and facing onto a quiet avenue; there was a long, tree-shaded lawn where plants bloomed and flowers blossomed in carved stone pedestals. The front door opened onto a prim little porch with ornate pillars. A faded daguerreotype of the house shows a moustachioed Ephraim in a long coat standing proudly, hands on hips, beside the separate entrance that led to his medical office and consulting room on the ground floor. As they grew up, the Penfield brothers were forbidden to play cards and engage in other idle pursuits; instead, Charles sang in the church choir, and learned to play the French Horn. At the age of fifteen or sixteen, a slender, rather elegant young man with dark brown hair and a thoughtful air, he was sent to Oberlin College a hundred miles away—the first step on the road to becoming a doctor like his father. It was at Oberlin, in his third or fourth year, that Charles met Jennie Jefferson from Wisconsin.

Jennie had come to Oberlin on her father's instructions—to keep an eye on her wild younger brother Thomas and to recover from a tragic love affair.

Amos Jefferson, her father, was a chief shareholder, cashier and later president of the First National Bank of Hudson, Wisconsin. He was a big, handsome, forceful and humourless man, and he would exert a powerful and not always happy influence on Jennie's youngest son, Wilder. By all accounts, Amos's father was cut from the same cloth. He was the self-styled squire of a small, upstate New York village. He had a small farm, but he was primarily, in his granddaughter's words, "a trader and puller of wires...not dishonestly so, but a mixer in all kinds of affairs. He made money, and spent it on his family. Clean in his living and a despot at home."

Amos had a twin named Alva and there is a story about the twins and their father that Jennie would recite to her young son to help him understand his grandfather's ways. Here is the story in her own words, in a letter to Wilder many years later:

"The twins, Amos and Alva, were as different in character as two brothers could well be. Their father's idea was to educate them to make money. They received good, hard training along that line. The difference in the two was illustrated in a certain story their father loved to tell. The two were given a certain sum of money to go out and buy sheep. They were to go separate ways—and to return on a certain day—and the one who made the best bargain was to receive a certain prize. When they came back, Alva brought in a few fine, fat, clean sheep. Amos brought in a big herd of lean, scrawny looking animals to be fed and brought up to perfection by personal care. They were never told which one had made the best bargain—but each received a prize.

"Alva," Jennie went on, "was a brilliant, erratic man whose mother, perhaps, understood him better than anyone else, as, on her death bed, she extracted a solemn promise from Amos that he would always look out for, and care for Alva." Alva apparently had no enthusiasm for manual work or regular hours, and ended up involved with mines, making a great deal of money at one time.

But then, Jennie explained, "came misfortune—how much he was to blame I know not. He claimed—and I am inclined to believe him—that his partners salted the mine and made him the goat. He believed he was selling a bona fide mine—but the courts decided against him and he lived under an assumed name for many years."

"Thomas Edgar," as Alva called himself thereafter, would spend the rest of his life thinking up schemes to make money, devising patents and relying on his twin brother's generosity to help him over the frequent hard times. In a way he had a right to his brother's help, because it was one of Alva's ideas that gave Amos the capital he needed to go into the banking business. With the outbreak of the Civil War, Alva suggested buying sheep, cattle and mules in the North and driving them to the South to sell them to the armies for enormously inflated prices. Despite the risks, the scheme was successful, and after a couple of trips, they had enough money to quit. Amos never liked to speak of those days: "He felt it was a case of what, today, we call profiteering," his daughter explained.

Nonetheless, the profits allowed Amos to become a partner in the bank, the first to open its doors in the small but promising town of Hudson, Wisconsin.

Hudson was founded in 1840, but the great influx of settlers came in the 1850s and 60s. They were drawn to the Saint Croix Valley by its prosperous lumber business, which grew until the whole valley was dotted with saw mills. Packets, stern- and side-wheelers plied the Saint Croix River until the railroad came through in the 1870s and river traffic dwindled.

Hudson, like many other towns that built their fortunes on the lumber business, had to endure the periodic rampages of lumberjacks released from months of hard work and celibacy in the camps. The lumberjacks would descend on the town's hotel, and for days the main street would be crowded with roistering and drunken men; the good burghers would sniff haughtily and step over the snoring bodies.

In the small world of Hudson, where Jennie grew up, the Jeffersons were society people. The doorways throughout their house on Third Street were extra large so that ladies with fashionably wide skirts could easily pass through them. One wing of the house was constructed as a library, and here the Ladies' Literary Society held its meetings. During the last years of the Civil War, the library boasted five hundred volumes and subscriptions to various newspapers and periodicals, among which anxious wives and mothers would scan the missing-in-action lists for news of their men.

When Jennie was fourteen she was enrolled in Milwaukee Female College, three hundred miles away. Its purpose was to equip young women not only "to adorn the higher circles of society, but to meet the varied and practical responsibilities of life." The school had been founded in 1851, and included in the course of studies calculated to accomplish these desirable results were, "trigonometry, natural and mental philosophy, logic, Evidences of Christianity and Butler's Analogy." By Jennie Jefferson's time the curriculum had acquired a distinctly Calvinist bent, evident in the many courses offered in Biblical History, Church History, History of Religion and Philosophy, etc.

Jennie returned to Hudson in 1875, having developed a rather severe and utilitarian attitude toward literature and the arts generally. Her education now complete, Jennie lived with her parents until a suitable husband could be found. There was no shortage of suitors: Jennie had the Jeffersons' good looks—large blue eyes, a strong profile and long chestnut hair, which she wore severely pulled away from her face and flowing down her back.

To the young men of Hudson who came to court her that summer of 1875, she appeared, I suspect, an intimidatingly mature young woman, strong-willed and secretive and faintly superior in her attitude. To complicate matters still further, just beneath this prepossessing exterior was a highly romantic spirit. One by one, the suitors went away, daunted and discomfited.

After a fire in the new Hudson library, the books that were saved from the blaze were brought to the library wing of her father's big house, and Jennie became the temporary librarian. Then, in the fall, a young minister fresh from Yale Seminary came to town and paid a visit to the library. He and the young librarian fell in love. He became a regular visitor, and all through the winter they sat close by the stove, heads together, reading and discussing the Bible. The couple became engaged, with the Jeffersons' blessings. Just when the future seemed rosy, very suddenly, the young minister died. For months Jennie sat alone in the library. Her parents grew impatient with her grief and decided she should be sent somewhere away from the memories, preferably somewhere with a good supply of eligible young men. On the pretext that her younger brother Tom needed a chaperone, it was decided that she should accompany him to Oberlin College. And there she met Charles Penfield.

The handsome, young doctor's son and his best friend, Wilder

Metcalfe (after whom Charles would name his own son) were considered the "catches" of Oberlin College—primarily because they showed no interest in the college's young ladies. Jennie and Charles met at a picnic one afternoon. That much she told her son many years later—that and the fact that by the end of the afternoon she and Charles had become engaged. The reasons are a mystery: perhaps the campus 'catch' was piqued by her lack of interest.

In any event, three years later, after Charles graduated from Chicago's Hahnemann Homeopathic Medical College, he and Jennie were married. On December 23, 1881, the *St. Paul Pioneer Press* dutifully reported, "the grand social event of the season in Hudson society," the wedding of Miss Jennie Jefferson, "who has long enjoyed the honor of being one of Hudson's most popular and handsome young ladies," and Chas. S. Penfield, M.D., of Chicago.

Charles and Jennie were in Chicago only a few months before Charles was struck with the first of a series of mysterious attacks that nearly killed him. It was appendicitis, but in those days before the first appendectomy, it was called inflammation of the bowels when it was recognized at all and few survived it.

The doctors who examined Charles in Chicago after his first attack diagnosed tuberculosis, or "consumption," and prescribed an immediate move to a dryer climate. So Charles and Jennie packed up and moved to Kansas City. Shortly after they arrived, Charles had another attack, more serious than the first. When he eventually recovered and was well enough to travel, they returned to Chicago for yet another consultation. This time the Chicago doctors told him that the only cure was to go and live "under canvas," meaning out west on the frontier.

It is hard to imagine what mysterious benefits the patient was expected to derive from living in a tent and why he was required to travel into the wilderness for the treatment to have the proper effect. Possibly there was some arcane correlation between discomfort and effectiveness now lost on medical practitioners. In any case, at least on the frontier Charles wouldn't embarrass the Chicago doctors by dying while under their care.

Now twenty-one, Jennie had been married to Charles less than a year. He was twenty-two, an urbane, educated and pampered young man hardly equipped for the rigours of frontier life. But since no alternative was proposed, Charles escorted his now-pregnant wife to his parents' home in Bucyrus, Ohio, said good-bye and boarded the next train heading west. The train left him at a way station in Montana. There, after listening to the advice of the resident trappers and hunters—who must have been dourly amused at this polished, courteous young eastern gentleman—he outfitted himself and set off for Porcupine Creek, Montana, on horseback, with a dog, a rifle and a packhorse laden with supplies.

Charles left no record of what he endured in the year and a half he spent wandering through Montana and into Washington Territory. Aside from the dangers of fierce predators and a harsh climate, his route would have taken him through territory where bands of Crow, Blackfoot and Sioux still roamed, and not far from the Little Big Horn River, where the massacre of Custer's troops had taken place six years before. Perhaps he suffered another attack, alone in some remote campsite. But somehow during this period, his body healed itself, managing (as his son later reasoned from knowledge of the healing process) to "wall off the abscess and drain it into the canal of the large intestine." Charles was to have no more of the agonizing attacks.

In 1883, unrecognizable beneath a bushy beard and leading a pony laden with furs, Charles Penfield rode into the pioneer settlement of Spokane Falls. He had come six hundred miles, through the high passes of the Bitterroot Mountains and down into Washington Territory. That evening, his beard trimmed to a neat vandyke and wearing a new suit, Charles learned that Spokane Falls needed a doctor. He decided to stay and wrote to his wife to join him.

∞ SPOKANE

Six months after Charles arrived in Spokane Falls, Jean (no longer Jennie) stepped off the train with Herbert, their first-born, in her arms. The couple had been separated for almost two years, and their reunion was a joyful one. The first years together again were happy ones. Years later, Jean would write nostalgically to Wilder, "Oh! Spokane was a gorgeous place in which to live during those early days when we were all so young and sure of ourselves."

In 1883, Spokane Falls (later changed to Spokane) was a settlement of about a thousand people, mostly roadbuilders and miners, living in a scattering of rough frame houses, shacks and tents on the banks of the Spokane River. Four years before, the settlement was little more than a squatter's claim and a sawmill, but the arrival of the Northern Pacific Railway in 1881 brought the isolation to an end.

The family spent the first winter in a small house that was little more than a shack made from rough pine boards. Charles opened an office in the front room, and between consultations he would slip into the back room to toss another log on the fire to keep the house warm. Such primitive conditions were not to last, however, for that same year gold was discovered in the nearby Coeur d'Alene Mountains, and the rush began.

Between 1883 and 1888, numerous new veins were discovered. The population doubled overnight, then doubled again and again. Far away, the port of San Francisco was filled with ships left to rot while their crews scrambled to the gold fields.

It was a time of enormous energy, grand visions and riches beyond the wildest imaginings. By 1889 the population had soared to 25,000 and the Spokane Falls Board of Trade was celebrating the settlement's "Magic Transformation From A Struggling Hamlet To A Great City."

For the towns near the gold fields, it was a strange, schizophrenic period of striking contrasts. Miners who struck it rich built huge mansions a stone's throw from the rough shanties of the first settlers. They paid architects to order pink marble from Italy, delft tiles from Holland and damask wallpaper from France. They filled their mansions with gold mirrors, immense crystal chandeliers and intricately patterned silk rugs from Persia. While the miners and the militia fought and died in battles over working conditions in the mines, sold off to big Eastern companies by the prospectors, Spokane built a huge, ornate theatre which boasted the largest stage in the world. Excluding San Francisco's, the theatre was the finest west of the Mississippi, and when its builders learned that a theatre in Chicago had the world's largest stage, they instructed their New York architects to make Spokane's one foot wider and one foot deeper. The Age of Elegance had arrived.

The social ritual of making calls was performed according to strict protocol. On Thursdays, the ladies who lived in the mansions on The Hill would call on the ladies who lived in the mansions in Browne's Addition. On Wednesdays the pattern was reversed, and the visiting cards of the ladies who lived in the mansions of Browne's Addition would appear on silver trays presented by the maids in the mansions on The Hill.

Yet in the winter the unpaved streets were deep in mud, in the summer deep in dust. The sidewalks were made of wood, and during the winter the streetcars which clanged past the mansions had straw scattered on the floor to keep the passengers' feet warm. The more staid and respectable citizens—the minister, the leading bankers and lawyers and the practitioners of the more prestigious trades—co-existed peaceably with the prospectors, confidence men, gamblers and prostitutes. It was to the first group that Charles and Jean gravitated.

In this cock-eyed world the Penfield fortunes rose with those of the whole town. On Boxing Day, 1884, a daughter was born and named Ruth. Jean began teaching Sunday School, and Charles occasionally sang in the church choir. Soon the couple's relatives began to arrive. Charles' mother and father came from Bucyrus, Ohio, with his younger brothers, James and Arthur. They were followed by the Smiths, who were Charles' cousins. Thomas Jefferson, Jean's wild younger brother, arrived next. Thomas was a wonderful storyteller and a great favourite with his nieces and nephews. He became a mine promoter, built himself a big house, married, divorced, and made and lost several fortunes in the years that followed. After Thomas came the Graves, cousins of Jean's from Hudson.

Jean's father, the Hudson banker, came out on a trip west and insisted that Charles and Jean should live in the best part of town in a fine house which he would help pay for. So Charles and a friend named Walker Bean bought facing lots on the edge of town and built large, splendid places. The 1889 *Spokane Falls Illustrated* tells us that the Penfield house had a wide, diamond-shaped vestibule with finely carved wood panelling and a marble fireplace. On one side of the house was Charles' office with its own entrance. Behind were stables where he kept horses "of the very finest class." In this house, Wilder Graves Penfield was born on January 26, 1891, and here the family lived together for eight years.

∞ CHILDHOOD

Although Wilder grew to the age of eight in Spokane, he left very few real clues about what family life was like, how Spokane and the world of experiences and memories it contained affected him in the years ahead. Nor have others—father and mother, sister and brother who lived in the big house, the cousins and aunts and uncles and grandparents who came and went—left many reminiscences. In the delicate, elliptical way of the age, their reticence hints that something was amiss. Many years later, his mother would tell Wilder that the last time she and his father were happy together was on a trip into the Coeur d'Alene Mountains, the year before he was born—seven years after she stepped off the train in Spokane Falls, and nine years before she left for good.

She spoke of a large opal ring Charles had bought a few years earlier on a trip up the coast to Vancouver. The ring found its way into the possession of a woman patient who refused to return it, and there was a threatened suit of some sort. And another fragment: an angry man came to the house to talk about his wife. Jean met him at the door, and then Charles came. The two men exchanged sharp words, but Jean was ignored. Charles gave no explanation. When she asked for one, he merely remarked that it would "all come out in the wash."

These revelations awakened an early memory of Wilder's own, of "stealing along our hall once to my mother's door and listening at the keyhole to her crying and speaking to herself. It had something to do with Herbert [away at school] I thought, for she said 'bring him back,' and I sat on the floor crying too and finally went away quietly."

But if these moments cast the occasional shadow on his childhood, it was still, apparently, a generally happy and carefree one. The child's first memories, dimly recalled, are of a birthday party on the porch of the house, and a tree being planted to mark the occasion while he watched through the railings. He remembered a bird in a big green cage and himself standing staring upward and trying to imitate the deep, rich sound of its whistling. The bird was called Ruby.

Near the child, as the faces became distinct were Herbert, skinny and exuberant, and Ruth, kind and pretty with her hair in ringlets. There were maids, Norwegian girls brought over by ship and out to Spokane by the minister, recalled as shy, nervous presences, their names long forgotten.

There was his Father, with a beard, a deep baritone voice and the smell of cigar smoke, a distant but affectionate presence, whose laughter rang through the corridor from the billiard room. Most of all there was Mama, the pervasive presence. She was loving, of course, but not demonstrative; mysterious, intense, impatient sometimes, rarely laughing, but with a slow, enigmatic smile that made him want to say "Tell me! Tell me!" With her there were two others, invisible but omnipresent, God and the baby Jesus.

Across the street lived the three Bean children, delivered in sequence by Charles Penfield at the going rate of $5 a head. Margaret Bean was Wilder's first heartbreak. The children played together in the Penfields' attic, taking turns on a swing that hung from the rafters or investigating dusty, leather-bound steamer trunks. Beneath the stable was a shadowy space into which the children could crawl. They would bring spades and hoes and dig until they found bits of fluorescent wood, rare treasures long buried in the earth. And in the winter, they raced their sleds, "belly-busters," behind the Penfield house, and the younger ones vied for rides on Herbert's big bobsled.

On Saturday nights, Indians high on vanilla extract might whoop and yell and race their ponies along Riverside Drive, but on Sunday mornings the Penfields and the Beans marched to church, the children forever losing their collection nickels between the wooden boards of the sidewalks.

Margaret Bean's memories of the Penfield parents do not flatter Mrs. Penfield. To Margaret she seemed cold, remote, reserved—a "sobersides" who was "a drag" on Charles. Charles, on the other hand, she remembers as handsome and charming, a gentle and kindly doctor whose bag of mysterious bottles and powders and manner of dispensing the magic medicines almost made it worth being sick. He was gay and amusing, and always showed impeccable good taste: "when he bought a present for someone it was always the right thing." In her recollection, Charles didn't much care for church, although he liked to sing and had a fine voice. The year he arrived in Spokane Falls, he was put in charge of organizing a glee club to greet the first train to come down the tracks from the east on its way to Seattle.

During the short, blazing-hot summers, the dusty streets boiled up in clouds with every passing buggy and every breath of wind, making the town very unpleasant. By the time Wilder was two, Charles and his friend Walker Bean had begun sending their wives and children off to one of the nearby lakes for the summer months. There in the woods Charles would establish a model campsite, with tents for every purpose and a Chinese cook to take charge of the big cooking and dining tents. That done, he would return to Spokane, though he would come back several times over the summer.

Jean and Mrs. Bean ran the camp, and the children would swim and explore, pick huckleberries for "huckleberry grunt," and blackberries for pies. And at night in the tent, Wilder's mother would sing him to sleep with the familiar rhyme: "Bye, O baby bunting / Your daddy's gone a-hunting / To fetch a little rabbit skin / To wrap his baby bunting in." Wilder remembered the lullaby without irony, though ironic it was, for it was Charles' hunting trips that were the first public sign that something was wrong between him and Jean.

Charles loved to hunt—a legacy of the years he spent in the wilderness working his way west to Spokane Falls. In his consulting room in the house on Riverside Drive hung the stuffed trophies—peccary, moose, bear, mountain goat—and he would tell his children wonderful tales about each one. The arrival at the kitchen door of an

Indian guide—regarded with awe by the little Penfields who were instructed to call him "Mr. Wright"—meant that Father was tired of doctoring and was planning a hunting trip.

At first these trips were brief respites from the long hours Charles spent seeing patients in his office, making housecalls and operating at the hospital. He was a very popular doctor and, by the standards of the day, apparently a highly successful surgeon. But as the hunting trips grew longer and more frequent, his practice began to dry up. His patients grew tired of being told the doctor was away and might be back tomorrow or next month. Eventually they stopped coming. First the Penfields' coachman disappeared, then, one by one, the cook and the maids.

Family legend has it that Charles "heard the call of the wild and could not resist," and it is at this dark, wild, unfathomable side of his character that all the blame for the Penfields' eventual separation was laid. There was no suggestion that the hunting trips were a way of avoiding the more complicated issues troubling the marriage, or were connected to the female patients and their husbands. And while family legend is notoriously unreliable, it seems that something did cause Charles Penfield to change. It was as though something clicked, or unclicked, inside him at some point, releasing him from the sense of responsibility toward his family and his patients. Perhaps the process began during his trek west. Certainly, more and more with each passing year, Charles went into the mountains looking for trophies, happier to be sleeping in a bedroll on the hard ground than in his wife's bed in the big house on Riverside Drive.

Whatever the real reasons, Charles was less and less a presence in the house. When the measles came along, it was not his father with his leather case of bottles and powders in twists of paper Wilder remembered, but his mother's voice reading to him in the dead of night, shielding his eyes from the light, her arms about him rocking, and a certain hymn she crooned, making up words about Wilder to fit the tune.

As Charles turned to hunting, Jean turned to the Bible. The children closed in around her, and no doubt it grew harder and harder for Charles to return to the house. The pretence of normalcy collapsed at last in 1899, after eighteen years of marriage. Nonetheless, the breakdown was presented to the children and to the neighbours as a temporary separation until Charles could restore his practice enough to support his family. If the older children, Ruth and Herbert, had a good idea of what was going on between their parents, Wilder, the youngest, was only vaguely troubled by an awareness that all was not right and had no urge to delve into the frightening particulars. Jean had decided to take the children back to Hudson, Wisconsin, and stay with her parents, and the exciting prospect of a long train trip more than made up for the absence of his father. On the morning in late fall when they left Spokane, Charles came down to the station, bringing Wilder a compass, and waved good-bye as the train pulled out. The compass, a new parcheesi game, and baskets full of wonderful things to eat were enough for Wilder, and nothing else seemed to matter.

CHAPTER TWO ∞∞∞∞∞∞∞∞∞∞∞∞∞∞∞∞∞∞∞∞∞∞∞∞∞

Growing Up

∞∞ HUDSON

On the bright, crisp November day in 1899 when the family stepped off the train in Hudson, Wisconsin, Wilder was eight years old, a slender boy with fine, light brown hair, light blue eyes and already a distinctly stubborn jaw. He was energetic and intense and very self-conscious, as quick to anger as to laughter. "It would be a terrible responsibility to bring Wilder up," his sister, Ruth, noted in her diary in 1900, "because he is such a firefly and is so wilful—and yet he is very affectionate and easily led."

Hudson had changed considerably in the sixteen years since Wilder's mother had left. The weight of prosperity and respectability had polished many of its rough edges; it was now a town of some 4,000 citizens, with many wide streets and gracious houses.

In Hudson, as in a thousand tidy and prosperous small towns scattered across the vast American middle west, politics and morals were resoundingly conservative. By contrast with Spokane, where fortunes were made overnight and spent lavishly, hard-won earnings were escorted down to the First National Bank of Hudson where her father, Amos Jefferson, still presided, to be carefully invested. From the labours of their pioneer ancestors, a middle class was bursting into existence, a class as narrow in its outlook as it was firm and righteous in its moral vision. And yet, as the wilderness, the climate and the natives were brought to heel, pioneer virtues continued to prevail: families no longer struggled from dawn to dusk merely to survive, yet suffering and self-denial and their companion ideals were permanently enshrined.

Those were days when no mystery of nature seemed impervious to "Yankee ingenuity," with a little help from the rest of the world. Inventions like the telephone, the telegraph, radio and the horseless carriage were altering the shape and size of the world around, and what seemed inconceivable or blasphemous to one generation would be commonplace to the next.

In the narrow, exclusive world of Hudson in 1900, social success depended on being of British or German ancestry, devoutly Protestant, and—as a matter of choice, not necessity—thrifty.

Recreation in Hudson revolved around the Saint Croix River, which formed the natural border with Minnesota and on whose eastern bank the town was situated: a wide, meandering river which welcomed small boys in straw hats equipped for the day with fishing poles and picnic lunches. In summer, Hudson's more affluent citizens cruised upstream in sprucely painted motor launches to favourite picnic spots. The men wore blazers and straw boaters, the women crisp summer frocks. In winter, six- and eight-passenger iceboats flitted from bank to bank while laughter cut the cold, thin air.

This was Wilder's world for the ten years' passage through boyhood into adolescence and young manhood. Its virtues and prejudices were also his, and would remain so his whole life long. Grandson of the town's banker, Wilder was raised in a privileged circle where there was much kindness, generosity and laughter, a world where a small boy could know that important things were unchanging, and that if he read his Bible, worked hard and obeyed the golden rule, he could grow up to be anything he liked. This world was the wellspring of that certainty and confidence that distinguished him in adult life.

The two older children made the transition from Spokane to Hudson with apparent ease. Herbert was now eighteen and in college, returning home from nearby St. Paul on weekends, and spending the summers working as a teller in his grandfather's bank. He was an easy-going, good-natured young man who needed from his mother nothing more than the occasional prodding. As for Ruth, she was fifteen when they arrived in Hudson—just old enough to be absorbed by the latest dance, making new friends, and conscientiously planning for her future as "a perfect wife and mother," and aside from periodic fainting spells and headaches that passed as quickly as they struck, she too required little serious attention.

Wilder, however, had some difficulty adjusting to the new life. The legacy of his parents' separation was a mistrust of older men—a mistrust complicated by every small boy's search for models to admire and emulate. When his grandfather unwisely attempted to fill the role of his absent father, Wilder bristled.

On one occasion, not long after the Penfields arrived in Hudson, Wilder clashed with his grandfather over a thirty-five-cent train ticket. He had asked his grandfather if he could take the train to nearby River Falls on an expedition with his friends. When the banker refused him the money, claiming that he couldn't afford it, Wilder fell into a rage. Many years later he remembered his mother taking him aside afterward and carefully instructing him "not to say you don't believe Grandfather even if you think it."

For Jean Penfield, returning to the nest at the age of forty-one, the transition was even more difficult. Instead of the big, rambling house in Spokane (now empty and for sale), she and her children occupied two rooms in her parents' house on Third Street. She and her daughter, Ruth, shared a double bed in one room, with a curtain to separate them from the boys' adjoining room.

Most of her childhood friends had married and left Hudson long ago. Several times she left the children with her parents while she tried her hand at various jobs in St. Paul, but after a few months she always retreated to Hudson. "Long hours she spent playing cribbage with Grandfather," Wilder would later recall, "and I can hear her voice 15-2, 15-4 and 2 are 6 and the recurring hackneyed joke when someone won." After booming Spokane Falls, Hudson must have seemed very small to Jean. Perhaps, for the first few years, she did dream of returning, but it was never discussed, and there is no evidence that Charles wrote to say "Come back." Eventually she resigned herself to Hudson's gossip and pitying glances.

The family lived in Amos Jefferson's house for the first five years. Jean's mother had always been a small, quiet woman, and Jean ruled the family from the time she returned, working hard to keep their life together full and pleasant. Above all, Wilder consumed her attention, and she approached his moral and religious education with obsessive romanticism. In the evenings she read him stories from Dickens and poetry by Browning, which she admired not for their language but for the moral lessons they contained. And, of course, she read from the Bible. She taught a Sunday School class in which Wilder was always her best student. When a missionary came to speak of his work among the natives in Africa or the Far East to the gathered church ladies of Hudson, Wilder accompanied his mother. When she left on brief trips alone or with her parents she continued his moral instruction in her letters. "My Darling Wilder," she wrote, "Will you be my Valentine? I read a story the other day about a little boy with his first trousers—he was very proud of them as anyone could see—but more proud was he of the old lady who he helped on the street-car so carefully. The car was crowded and no one paid attention to the boy and his lady love. He stood a moment looking at the men who were seated and busily reading their papers. Finally his clear little voice was raised in protest. 'See here, you fellows, don't you know my grandma must have a seat?' After that she could have her choice of any seat in the car, for they were all offered to her. I wondered if my boy would have had the courage and the thought—I know he has the same love for his grandma."

The effect of his mother's efforts was all that she could have hoped for. Lacking the leavening presence of his more easy-going father, Wilder developed into a creature who seemed to alternate between a healthy, boyish delight in pranks and jokes, sports and games, and a serious, self-conscious, preachy moralism that mirrored his mother's. A childhood acquaintance of Wilder's later wrote to him: "One incident involving you stands out in my memory. Several of us were bicycling, probably to the swimming hole, when in our conversation I referred to my father as 'my old man.' No disrespect was intended as I loved my dad dearly. But you rebuked me gently, that I should refer to my father like that. And today, three-quarters of a century later, I thank you for your well-taken admonition."

In 1904, shortly after his thirteenth birthday, Wilder began to keep a diary, the start of a life-long habit. The big news of the first entries was that Ruth would be leaving the house to marry one of Wilder's teachers, a Mr. Inglis. "I wouldn't have been more surprised if somebody should announce that I was engaged." Mr. Inglis, Wilder noted approvingly, "is just fine going on 27" and had as a teacher acquired the nickname "Mealy." "That man is the luckiest man in the world, and if he don't toe the mark," Wilder added darkly, "I'll light on him."

Reading through the diaries it is apparent that devotion to his Mama did not preclude making her the butt of practical jokes, and rather elaborate ones at that:

"On Hallouene Wale and I had a string attached from our room around the house to the room just off of Mama's and Ruth's room. With curtains between the two, this string went in and was fastened to a pin which held a newspaper flap with a snag of marbles in it so when it was half past four we pulled the string the marbles which were in a slanting rocker with a lapboard slanting off. The marbles ran all over the hadwood floors and in under their bed and scared the life out of 'em."

The diary reveals that by spring of 1904, Wilder was planning to go back to Spokane on a camping trip the coming summer. When it was time for him to go, his mother took him aside and told him to be a "joiner," and not to be afraid that the other boys would laugh at him if, at night, he got on his knees to pray. Armed with his .22, fishing rod, haversack and, no doubt, additional wholesome advice, Wilder finally boarded the train for Spokane.

It is not difficult to imagine Jean's misgivings. The suggestion for the trip presumably came from Charles, and Grandmother Penfield no doubt added her urgings until Jean reluctantly agreed. We can only guess what she had said to Wilder beforehand on the subject of his father from the cryptic postscript to his first letter reporting the reunion, which was simply, "I'll remember—you know."

At the station in Spokane Charles met his son and they went off to the Silver Grill, "the most beautiful place I ever saw," for breakfast. "Things look awfully funny," he reported, noting the changes that had taken place in Spokane in the last five years. Charles gave Wilder a brand new hunting knife and loaned him his own 30-30 rifle, and a week later under the watchful eye of the Indian guide, Mr. Wright, Wilder, his cousin and several other boys set off for their campsite at Priest Lake, Idaho.

What they lacked in expertise as hunters, the boys made up for in enthusiasm, and it is fortunate there were no settlers living close by, for Wilder records: "Saturday at 4 a.m. we got up and got started for a mountain after goat. At 6 o'clock we went through a sort of level valley full of timber, and climbed up on a big ridge. On the end was a precipice about a block high straight up and down with a large round rock jutting out over it—we got on this to watch for game. Crack, crack, went something up the valley. We waited and pretty soon out from the bushes stepped. Well just guess. A big bear. He calmly led on down till he was below us then Rick shot and he jumped onto his back [legs] and took a hike. I was shooting with my 30-30 all the time he ran across an opposite ridge across the valley. I got in 7 shots, and other kids couldn't see him so well in the brush. I would have laughed if I hadn't been serious because at first Rick and I shot off 30-30's this size bullets [drawing of bullet shape two and one-half inches long] which make an awful roar, and Pat shot off his 38 revolver. Then he took his 22 repeater which shoots shorts and we went boom-m boom-m plink-plink-plink-plink It was funy."

One morning Wilder and two others came across some deer tracks. While one went ahead and the other two waited, "all of a sudden a doe sprang up not 50 feet ahead of us. It was a fair size doe about 5 ft. at the shoulder. For some reason Pat and I told him [the other boy] it was a faun & not to shoot. I don't know why, haven't the faintest idea what possessed us. My it seemed just to float along."

Jean, meanwhile, wrote every week, sending a Bible lesson for

Wilder to read every Sunday, which he did faithfully, usually reporting back in this manner: "I studied the lesson and it seemed to me it was all right with jesopat [Jehosophat, probably] in good company but all wrong in bad."

In August the boys returned to Spokane, where Wilder stayed with his Grandmother Penfield. There was a last visit with his father, who sent a message that Wilder should meet him at his office. Wilder waited all of one afternoon for Charles to arrive. Years later he would remember his shame when the patients who came would ask the small boy when the doctor would be in. "I blushed and could not answer," he wrote in *No Man Alone*. "Finally I watched them shake their heads and go away."

However much Wilder wanted to love and be proud of his father, the picture of his mother alone and grieving and the conviction that his father was to blame inevitably intervened, and he hardened his heart. At eight he could only sense that something serious was amiss. At thirteen, the lesson of his father's weakness had been drummed into him, and throughout his life "weak" was the adjective he would summon up to express utter contempt, to dismiss some man altogether. Always a man—the word never had any resonance for him when applied to a woman; of course she was weak, though she was expected to display those mysterious, Victorian, feminine qualities of "perception" and "intuition."

But the yearning to connect somehow with his father was strong, and it found an outlet that summer of 1904 in the mountains around Spokane. In the careful selection of a campsite, the pitching of a tent, the honing of a knife, the paddling of a canoe and the skill of marksmanship, the connection was there without effort. To this, years later, would be added Wilder's pride in his dexterity with a scalpel, thanks to his hands—strong and blunt, "the hands of a surgeon, or a carpenter," he would say—his father's hands.

∞ THE GALAHAD SCHOOL

Down Third Street from the Jefferson house was the Presbyterian church, where Wilder's mother spent much of her time. There, one evening near the end of the summer of her son's thirteenth year, Jean's dreams for his future suddenly found a focus. It was the summer of 1904, and she had gone to hear a student, home on vacation from his first year at Oxford University, talk about the Rhodes Scholarship program.

The speaker was one of the first wave of students selected from throughout the English-speaking world to receive the scholarships created by the will of Cecil Rhodes, a co-founder of the De Beers Mining Corporation and former prime minister of the Cape Colony in South Africa, from the enormous fortune he had accumulated during his life. The chosen scholars had their tuition paid and were given an allowance of £300 per annum during three years at Oxford.

The student's account of life at Oxford fired Jean Penfield's imagination; this was just the thing for Wilder. It was not just the practical aspects of the scholarship; she knew that a Rhodes Scholar would be distinguished throughout adult life. In his will Cecil Rhodes had specified that the students awarded his scholarship "should not be merely bookworms," and consideration be given to a candidate's "fondness for and success in manly outdoor sports," his "qualities of manhood, truth, courage, devotion to duty, sympathy for and protection of the weak, kindliness, unselfishness and fellowship." And of course, "moral force of character and of instincts to lead" were important qualities to look for in a candidate, "for those latter attributes will be likely in after life to guide him to esteem the performance of public duties as his highest aim."

When the talk was over, Jean hurried home to tell Wilder. Late into the cool evening they sat together on the front porch while the breezes rustled in the elm trees that lined Third Street and the new electric street lights blinked on. And Wilder listened while his mother conjured up for him a picture of the towers of Oxford and the quadrangles of the ancient colleges where young scholars studied, where faithful servants brought them breakfast and lunch, to be eaten each in his own sitting room.

Many years later he would remember, "In my fancy, I followed them to their classes, bicycling down the ancient streets and, later in the day, watched with delight as they ran across the college lawns on their way to the playing field and the river, all dressed in white."

For now, it didn't matter what he would study once he got the scholarship. He would, with his mother to guide, groom himself to be a perfect candidate. Aside from knowing that he definitely would *not* be a doctor like his father, he hadn't given the future much thought. As for his mother, she was content to let that decision be made by Wilder in consultation, presumably, with the good Lord. Anything was possible, the whole world was within his reach if he only believed it was.

"Hudson was not a small, faraway town at all," he would write. "It was the happy place. From it, roads led out to all the world. Oxford was only just over the hill. Or so it seemed on that summer evening in 1904 as we sat together, my mother and I...."

In Jean's grand design for Wilder's future, the Galahad School was the cornerstone. When he graduated from elementary school in 1905, Wilder assumed he would enter Hudson High School in the fall. But that summer his mother and three young teachers, one of them her new son-in-law, Jack Inglis, cooked up a scheme to open a small private school. With $6,000 raised by Amos Jefferson and his business associates they bought a large, two-storey stone house set on ten acres of land, two miles from Hudson and overlooking Lake St. Clair, and set about transforming it into a school.

The school would be their home for the next ten years. Jean, Ruth and Ruth's husband, Jack, moved out to the building and, along with another young teacher, Jack McQuarrie, began to prepare for the opening term. Shortly afterward, Wilder, who had spent the first part of the summer working on a farm, came out to help. The ladies of Hudson organized 'bees' to make sheets, pillow cases, tablecloths, napkins, dish towels, comforters and mattress covers. The lawns were cleaned, an outbuilding was converted into a manual training shop, bedrooms became dormitories and classrooms, and on an adjoining field a football field was marked out and rough goalposts erected. The renovations were rather crude, but in the fall, with fifteen students, The Galahad School opened its doors.

Jean's mark on the school is unmistakable. She chose the name and the motto: "My strength is as the strength of ten because my heart is pure," plucked, like the name, from Tennyson's story of King Arthur and his knights. And the analogies didn't stop there: after her father's death some years later, she built a cottage for herself and her mother on the school grounds, naming it "Sarras," after the magical city of peace where Galahad came to rest from his battles. Even her friends teased that she had established the school because she didn't want to take any chances with the education of her young champion. But it also provided a job and a home for her daughter and son-in-law, and, just as important, it was a suitable challenge for her after five restless years in Hudson. Galahad was going to be "the best little school in the north." For the four years Wilder was there, Grandfather Jefferson paid half his tuition, and the other half was part payment for Jean's work at the school. She had a small apartment there and was busy from morning to night managing the housekeeping, cooking, teaching Bible class, meeting with parents and the school's backers, and acting as "School Mother"—nursing and comforting the sick and lonely among the boys.

Wilder lived in the dormitory and, fiercely determined to be 'a regular fellow,' kept away from her most of the time. But on

Sundays they had supper together in her rooms. Afterwards she would read aloud their favourite Browning poems and would discuss the news from the world outside Hudson, Wilder's schoolwork and his daily victories and defeats.

With the vision of a Rhodes Scholarship before him, Wilder studied hard and stayed at the top of his class. Each day he practised the piano, according to the daily schedule in his diary, "from 10:40 to 11:20," between "Exercises" and "Caesar." He joined the debating society, marched with the cadets and regularly attended the meetings of "Junior Endeavour." Not a natural athlete, and neither unusually big nor especially well-coordinated, his aggressiveness and determination earned him a berth on the football team, and in his last two years at the school he was captain.

The importance of concentration was drilled into him at Galahad, and inspired by a teacher's speech on the subject, Wilder set out to teach himself to swallow food without moving his Adam's apple, and for days afterward experimented at each meal. He succeeded finally, or believed he had, and it was a lesson he never forgot.

In his second year at Galahad, he and four friends formed the exclusive Fraternal Order of Bachelors. Initiates were blindfolded and abandoned in the woods at night, forced to eat raw eggs and had cold water poured on their heads as they passed beneath a second storey window.

As well as their Sunday evenings together, Jean and Wilder made occasional forays to St. Paul on the train. They would leave after school, do some shopping, go to a restaurant for dinner and then see a play or an opera in the St. Paul Opera House. From his very first performance Wilder was hooked. The opera was *Fra Diavolo:* they had splurged and taken a box, and from where he was sitting he could see Fra Diavolo hiding in a closet. The actor could also see Wilder, for he made faces at him the whole time he was hiding. The thrill of that contact never left him. And, of course, there was the orchestra: "You could just close your eyes and the music would carry you up to the ceiling..." he wrote in his diary after a performance of *Pagliacci.*

In his diary Wilder speculated about his future. "The only two things it seems to me I would care for are the Law and ministry, and law looks more and more uninteresting. I never thought of being a minister." "The place where I can do the most good is the place I will be put in," he concluded, and a week or two later wrote, "I wouldn't be surprised if I should become a minister. I ask every night...."

Still, Wilder was in no rush to decide on his future. He had learned, from his mother and the sermons at the Presbyterian church that God had a mission for Wilder Penfield and anyone else who was willing to listen. He must remain patient and open. And while it wasn't cheating to ask for advice in his prayers, all would become clear eventually. Or, as his mother was fond of saying, "All things work together for those who love God." (Secretly she hoped he would one day be called to be a minister but, to her credit, kept silent and only let it slip years later, when he had finished medical school.)

By the time Wilder was sixteen, Jean's vision of Christian service and her sense of an intimate, mystical connection to God had become his own. It is a measure of how seriously he took religion at that age that he hesitated to accept an invitation to spend the weekend with some friends because it would mean missing Sunday School and church. His mother reassured him, suggesting that he go off by himself for an hour on Sunday "and read from your little book." He later recalled: "I don't know what book it was, but it fitted into a small pocket and had something to do with Sunday School.... I sat in the woods near a swamp and I remember a feeling of satisfaction or reassurance and a surprised feeling that it was pleasant to be quite alone. On the way back to camp I was surprised by a snake, a big one, and I killed him in terror in the belief that it was a rattler. It wasn't, but his tail continued to twitch back and forth after he was dead, and I mused over him.... How far into later life these early first impressions and discoveries go...."

The experience that day, he said, awoke in him a taste for solitude, and the urge to go off by himself from time to time "and look at life."

Wilder was maturing in other ways as well. The diary of his sixteenth year registers a subtle shift: "I am beginning to take things seriously now. Music, study and temper." The inscription on the first page, "Warning: If I catch anyone reading this I'll do my darn worst to lick him. I mean it." has been crossed out and replaced with a more mature, "Do Not Read."

That summer, he was invited to parties and boat-trips and bonfires, but Wilder's preliminary excursions into the social whirl were not without some problems: "Last night I went down to Websters to a little party and had more fun than I've had anywhere in a long time. There is an awful lot doing that I am not invited to. That's because I don't have enough money to get 'married.' And of course they don't want odd bucks butting around. I would have a hard time anyway if I had the money because Fred Anderson and William like Helen Kermott and she is the only one I would care much about..."

A photograph of Helen Kermott at sixteen is reminiscent of

Jennie Jefferson at the same age: bright blue eyes, outwardly sensible and unsentimental, but with a mysterious, self-contained aura about her. Her father and grandfather were both doctors, and her family was respectably well-off. Her father had married the daughter of a ship's captain from Southampton, New York, a flighty, spoiled, charming woman who returned frequently to Southampton to visit her family, leaving Helen, at sixteen, in charge of the house. Mrs. Kermott, it seems, had made a sacrifice in marrying a humble village doctor and coming to live with him in a small prairie town. Though we have no evidence that she ever regretted the sacrifice, she clearly did not feel it bound her to permanent exile. "Mother, if you don't have someone clean those windows soon you won't be able to even see out and then what will you do?" Helen remembered asking irritably. "Why, I'll just call for the carriage and go for a drive," was the airy response.

In the autumn of 1907 Wilder received his first address book as a present. In the back he made a note of everyone's birthday, but he left out Helen Kermott's name. He didn't want anyone to see the name of the girl he had decided he was going to marry.

In 1909 Wilder graduated from Galahad at the top of his class and as the captain of a winning football team. Each graduate was required to make a speech on a subject of his choice; Wilder's was on chivalry. In the fall he would be going away to Princeton. He and his mother had picked Princeton because in a small state like New Jersey, fewer students would be competing for the Rhodes Scholarship. Another detail about Princeton attracted Wilder privately: it didn't have a medical school, so there would be no question of his ever studying medicine.

That was a golden summer. Boyhood behind him, Wilder alone of those in his Hudson crowd was moving on to an Ivy League college. His romance with Helen Kermott blossomed. They and their friends went to dances, picnicked on a houseboat, and sang in the evening around bonfires by the river.

Perhaps a gangly, red-haired cousin of Helen Kermott's was there that summer, a lonely, unhandsome observer named Sinclair Lewis. He had visited his relatives in Hudson before, and the town in the early 1900s was surely one of those impaled forever as his Zenith, U.S.A.:

"They two-stepped on the wide porch, with its pillars of pine trunks, its bobbing Japanese lanterns, and never were there dance-frocks with wider sleeves nor hair more sensuously piled on little smiling heads, never an August evening more moon-washed and spacious and proper for respectable romance....The scene was a sentimental chromo—crisping lakes, lovers in canoes singing 'Nelly was a Lady,' all very lugubrious and happy."

At summer's end, Helen and Wilder took pictures of each other with her new camera and agreed to write. As the September evenings grew cool he walked around Galahad saying good-bye to all of the familiar places. In an empty classroom he stood by his old desk and looked out the window at "the still lake, the high dark green bank, the deadhead reflecting in the water and the fish splashing here and there," and vowed always to remember "this lake and how different it looks from day to day and hour to hour."

Finally it was time for him to leave. "School has begun," he wrote, "and the fellows are here, but I am not one of them anymore."

CHAPTER THREE ∞∞∞∞∞∞∞∞∞∞∞∞∞∞∞∞∞

Wilder Penfield, Esq.

∞∞ PRINCETON

One evening near the end of September, 1909, Wilder boarded the train in Hudson and waved good-bye to the crowd of friends and family who had come to see him off. Under his arm were volumes of Virgil and Latin Composition, which he planned to study during the day-and-a-half train ride to Princeton, so that he would be ready for the entrance exams. In the baggage car was his steamer trunk, packed the day before by his mother. Carefully laid out on top was a suit they had shopped for together in St. Paul, a splendid suit of green tweed with many pockets and flaps and buttons and vents.

That night he sat by the window staring at the full moon that hung in the east. To those who grew up in small midwestern towns like Hudson, the East in those days was civilization, polished manners, refined taste. And going east to college was to announce to all and sundry that here was one who would not spend his life behind the counter at the hardware store or working as a clerk in a real estate office or a bank, perhaps looking forward to one day taking a big trip to Chicago. Going east to Princeton was that much grander than just going east to college. After graduation, strangers would murmur "He's a Princeton man."

His second day on the train, he had just opened his books when "a big moose sat down opposite me in the same seat and began to study." The 'big moose,' whose name was Bill Chester, was also cramming for the Princeton entrance exam. By the next morning when the train pulled into Princeton Station, the two were friends.

Chester had a room in the same dormitory as Wilder, and as the latter wrote to his mother "his pocket book is about my size, though he has studied French abroad."

Wilder's first glimpse of the Princeton campus filled him with awe and delight: it was everything he and his mother had imagined, and more. Everywhere he looked were ivy-covered buildings set on spacious, carefully clipped lawns shaded by enormous elm trees. The architecture was bewildering in its variety. Some of the buildings imitated Greek temples cut from white marble, with wide steps to soaring, pillared porches and immense, ornate bronze doors. Others were massive granite Victorian Gothic, or "Oxford Gothic," with turrets and battlements and small leaded-paned windows facing into the quadrangles.

Along these paths wandered groups of demigods: aloof upperclassmen in straw hats sporting the coloured silk hatbands that identified their club; sophomores, the "enemy" whose task it was in the first few months of the school year to harass the freshmen without mercy; and the juniors, benevolent angels who were the traditional allies of the freshman class.

Along with the dormitories, dining-rooms, classrooms, the Cliosophical and Whig Societies (where students competed in "declamation and oratory"), faculty residences, administrative buildings and sports facilities, the campus included fifteen-odd Eating Clubs, the Princeton equivalent of fraternities. In 1909, they were a relatively recent development and signalled Princeton's transformation from an austere Presbyterian college to a haven of the well-to-do. Most of Wilder's fellow students came from wealthy families and had attended big eastern preparatory schools like Lawrenceville and Andover. In the words of one critic, Princeton was becoming a place "where young bloods monopolize the amenities of university life."

But there was a move underway to stem the tide, led by the President of Princeton, Woodrow Wilson. Since his appointment in 1902, Wilson had been battling with the campus aristocrats: students, faculty and governors alike. "The American College," Wilson proclaimed, "must become saturated in the same sympathies as the common people. The colleges of this country must be reconstructed from the top to the bottom...."

Wilson's attempts to uproot social privilege at Princeton echoed a growing popular outcry in the nation at large. Theodore Roosevelt's "Drive out the special interests," and "a square deal" for the common man were the catch phrases of those years. His radical notions included such—for that era—unmentionables as policies of honesty in government, regulation of big business, conservation of natural resources, and the relatively new concept of social justice. Roosevelt even invited the black educator and social philosopher Booker T. Washington to dinner at the White House, and he appointed a black man to the post of collector of the port at Charleston. But by the fall of 1909, Roosevelt had handed over the Republican party and the keys to the White House to W. H. Taft, and gone big-game hunting in Africa, and Woodrow Wilson had been handily defeated in his first major attempt to democratize Princeton University. Wilson had proposed to begin by modifying, if not eliminating altogether, the Eating Clubs. But so firmly entrenched had the clubs become—in so short a space of time—that he met with an embarrassing failure. Defeated again, in 1910, this time on the issue of the Princeton graduate school—he wanted it integrated into the campus and his opponents wanted a secluded "ivory tower" institution—Wilson would leave Princeton to become Governor of New Jersey and go on to end the Republican Party's long tenure in the White House.

So, despite the occasional ripple that troubled its placid surface, the Princeton to which Wilder came remained by and large the preserve of wealthy young eastern princes. "Yes, you bet this is a great place," Wilder wrote shortly after arriving. "Just send my piano and automobile and motorcycle and row of steins so I can be in with some of my neighbors."

However, there were at Princeton other students like Wilder, students from small towns who had gone to schools like Galahad and been raised on ideas of Christian service. And on campus there were institutions to which these students gravitated. Most important of these institutions was the Philadelphian Society, and it was there Wilder left his bags before rushing off with his new friend Chester to take the entrance exams.

The Philadelphian Society was an unaffiliated Christian undergraduate society until, in the mid-1870s, it was caught up in a campaign launched by the Young Men's Christian Association and became one of the first College Y.M.C.A.s. During the heyday of the Y.M.C.A. movement, around the turn of the century, its evangelical zeal was enormously appealing to those concerned about the deleterious moral effects of the modern age. In cities in particular, the Y.M.C.A. was seen as a way to reach the young men drawn to factory jobs and the promise of riches, many of whom were living in flophouses.

The College Y.M.C.A. was a later development, one that brought students together in prayer meetings and Bible studies, to organize Sunday Schools among the poor in the towns around the campus and to try to draw other, unconverted students into the fold.

It was through the Philadelphian Society that Wilder would make most of his friendships. The atmosphere of earnest conviction that permeated their little gatherings evoked for him the evenings with his mother. The Society's ideals, he wrote many years later, "were what I had learned to accept in the Presbyterian environment of Hudson during my childhood."

Wilder's first-year rooms, on the fifth floor of the freshman dormitory, consisted of a bedroom and a sitting-room with a fireplace. Discovering soon after he arrived that he could save $100 a year through a remission of tuition if his expenses were under $150 for the term, and mindful of his grandfather's exhortations to be frugal, he reported to his mother, "I have four electric lights and by taking out three of them my bill would be $148.50. I can use a good student's lamp as an auxiliary."

Soon after he arrived the fall term officially opened, and the first letters are full of accounts of the "horsing" that went on. The purpose of this harassment of the freshmen was to acquaint them immediately with the inferiority of their station and, simultaneously, develop in them a sense of school spirit and loyalty to their classmates. Wilder entered into it with enthusiasm: the more ferocious the battling in those first weeks, the more he liked it. He was strong and fit and reasonably agile, and eager to show he had "the stuff."

While Princeton could not compete with Harvard or Yale in numbers or in scholarship, in sports—particularly football—it competed enthusiastically with the other Ivy League colleges. At Princeton the football players were the best-known and most admired men on campus. They ate at special training tables where the food was superior and served up in huge portions. They travelled in a special Pullman car, and huge celebratory dinners were held in their honour by rich graduates at the Waldorf Astoria or the Hotel Martinique in New York. Even at practices cheering students filled the stadium, and when the team set off for an important game the whole university, faculty and students, paraded to the station to cheer them on their way.

Wilder had decided long before he came to Princeton that he would make his mark as a football player, and all through his last season as captain of the Galahad team he had dreamed of making the Princeton freshman team. When the practices began his letters reported little else. Only months later did he begin mentioning (and then rather off-handedly) what courses he was taking.

When he turned out for the first practice he found to his dismay sixty candidates, all of whom had played for big eastern prep schools and were, to his eyes, enormous. "If I am to make a good tackle," he wrote home to his mother, "I must accept that the game is a fight, a real fist fight against the man opposite you. Catch him in the face a couple of downs running and he'll let you through next time unless he is a better fighter than you." They were intimidating in other ways, as well. As he recorded in his weekly letter to his mother early in November: "At Yale the other fellows all met men they had played against and with, in Prep school, and are quite well known either personally or by reputation. They do not care for me and I feel out of place with them, at least those who made the team. A sub. doesn't amount to much after all. I noticed a difference in my value in their eyes as soon as it became apparent that Heath was outclassing me. They are the most important men in the class. With the others I feel at home. I know it is all wrong to think of what anyone else thinks about you all the time, so I am trying not to."

The green tweed suit which he and his mother had decided was the right thing for a Princeton freshman had not been a success. The raised eyebrows it provoked the first time he proudly wore it across campus had caused him to bundle it up and take it to a pawnshop in town. He replaced it with a sober, dark suit less likely to attract unwanted attention.

The sense of being excluded, an outsider, was reinforced that fall by an incident that he would remember all his life. Coming into the dining hall he overheard one of the football players mention the Galahad School, and another laugh derisively. Then one of them made a joke that Wilder could not quite hear, something about "Sir Galahad." It was obvious they meant him, and he felt "a hot flush of shame and anger" sweep over him. His determination to make the team only increased, which meant extra sessions after classes and long after the other players had left the practice field, kicking the football up and down the field by himself.

Despite setbacks on the football field, Wilder struggled on through the first term, busy every minute of each day. He joined the Debating Society and enroled in Clio Hall to study Public Speaking. The Philadelphian Society involved freshman Bible classes on Tuesday evenings and class prayer meetings on Sunday night, as well as Chapel on Sundays and several weekday mornings. "I never attended so many religious meetings etc. before I came here," he noted in his diary. "I thought it would be the other way around."

Before the fall term was over it was clear that his studies were suffering from his extra-curricular activities, especially football, and it left him in a quandary. "I am beginning to realize that there are two courses before me," he confided in a letter to his mother. "One course to make an Eating Club, the other to grind. Making an Eating Club is getting out with the fellows. I have been trying to do both so do neither well. Almost all the fellows with a very few exceptions use ponies [condensed texts]. That makes me work longer than they to get my lessons. I would do better work I'm sure if I had a room-mate. I get quite lonely and then cannot study hard. Though Bill comes up quite often."

Though anxious not to waste time thinking about home, in the evenings, alone at his desk, he would often find himself thinking of his friends and Galahad and Hudson. His letters to Helen (mysteriously nicknamed Gretchen in the last days they'd spent together at the end of the summer), are models of eloquent restraint: "Dear Gretchen," he wrote, "It is late. My studying is done but there is no time to answer your letter or thank you for the pictures. The moon is full and I feel as though I must talk to you a little while....Do you still wish on your evening star? Or is there no evening star now. I can't see west any more. There is one quite close to the moon tonight. Oh Well, it's alright if I do dream now, my studying is done. Wide."

Each Sunday afternoon he dutifully wrote to his mother, telling her the latest news and urging her to relax more. Her letters of course were full of the trials and tribulations of Galahad and the perennial servant problem, and he would reproach himself for the life of ease and luxury he felt he was leading.

Although he had met a few eastern girls at the Chesters' in New York, where he spent Thanksgiving, it wasn't until his Christmas holiday in Washington, D.C. that he had time to reflect on this new and fascinating phenomenon. An invitation had come to spend the holiday with the Price family, Washington friends of the Penfields, who moved in 'society circles.' Despite the lack of a dress suit, Wilder plunged into the Washington social whirl of formal calls, masquerades, balls, the theatre and the opera. On the train back to Princeton he wrote in his diary about an encounter at one party: "Washington girls deserve the prize for flirting. Miss King immediately got her eyes into commission. She is a good dancer....She told me she was crazy over me, that from the moment she saw me etc. Of course I could have kissed her but I didn't." The letter went on to describe a masquerade he had attended the following night. "They dance very differently in Washington from the Wisconsin way. At first I danced the way I was used to and then made a mixture of the two ways which was successful according to the girl I danced with." Miss King was there as well and apparently continued to be cordial. "Eyes like Miss King's usually get what they want, and I'm glad I made no fool of myself. It will be good to get back to the gym. I've missed it."

After Christmas Wilder started wrestling in order to build up his shoulder muscles for football. A senior named Jack Drummond, himself a wrestler, became his coach, and in February Wilder won the interclass (freshman-sophomore) wrestling match. Jack Drummond had promised to take Wilder to New York and treat him to a night on the town if he won the match, and early in April he kept his promise.

First they went to *The Skylark,* a musical comedy. The next day, Wilder wrote in his diary, "In order to show me what N.Y. was like and what really existed there, we visited a number of Cafes such as Joe Adams and a lot of others where women all painted and powdered come in and walk through. If you look at them they stop and try to engage you in conversation. There was always someone singing sometimes good voices sometimes not. Jack and a fellow by the name of Holt who was with us, always took beer and I took ginger ale till I grew tired of it and took nothing. I didn't see anyone who seemed to be enjoying himself. When we went on the street the girls often accosted us. To finish with we went to the Hay Market, a small dance hall with tables around the sides and around the balcony. They drank and danced alternately. Jack brought one up to our table. She plumped down beside me and said "hello blondy" and began kicking me. Her talk was awful and she went as far in words as it is possible to go. We left there and beat it...." Wilder concluded that he felt sorry for these girls. "They can't live long and life must be hell. I am glad I saw the degradation there and saw how easily an unsophisticated fellow could sink right down. It would be so easy. But I never want to go again for it doesn't pay to play with a thing like that."

He and Jack ended the weekend by going to a matinee performance of a play called *The City* which had considerably more appeal. It was, the diary reports, "a good problem play and right along the line of thought that was bothering me; whether or not it was better to live in a large city. The moral the play brought out was that the city either made a man or ruined him. If he was strong he conquered, if not he was pulled down. While the town allowed a man a middle course of hypocrisy."

After so many years of trying to live by his mother's ideals and win her approval, and his more recent struggles for the admiration of his classmates, it was starting to occur to Wilder that there was a third arbiter—himself. He knew he was going to be *somebody,* and knew he was destined for great things—his mother had long since convinced him of that. If he still didn't know what form all this would take, he was at least certain that the "middle course of hypocrisy" was not for him. It was not until the following year, after a summer spent helping Herbert on his newly purchased farm and "fussing" Helen Kermott, that he, rather suddenly, had to make a decision about what he was going to do with his life.

∞∞ DECISIONS

Near the end of Wilder's sophomore year at Princeton he came into his own, no longer "Sir Galahad," the lonely outsider. In the class elections in the fall, he was elected vice-president, the other offices being filled by two other members of the Philadelphian Society. His afternoons were spent practising with the football team, and his evenings preparing for the Rhodes Scholarship exam. Wilder had little expectation of getting the appointment on the first try, and he was not surprised when the board chose someone else and advised him to reapply in his senior year.

By Christmas, the anxiety of the past year had faded. He had his best friend, Bill Chester, as a roommate; he had done well in football that season and, as he scribbled in his diary early in December, "I feel at ease with everyone in the university now because there is nothing which they have that I want."

If he thought about his future, he didn't confide those thoughts to his diary. In letters home he only wrote that the idea of going into the ministry had less appeal than ever: "I went over to the Seminary....the type of men there disgusted me. Some are sound, but most struck me as uncultured, ungentlemanly weaklings. It makes me mad to think of those pups going out into the world to live Christian lives which the rest of us are supposed to model after. I don't wonder there is much sneering at the church when such men are able to thrive in it."

Although he continued to be involved in the Philadelphian Society, there too he was growing more critical. He had been teaching Sunday School to a group of Italian boys in town, and was growing weary of "the little demons." At a house party in Princeton one evening his hostess introduced him "as the one who was christianizing the Italians. Now I'm not ashamed of my work down there," he wrote to Jean, "but I was *mad* before I left their house last night."

A little later he reported that he had gone to see a student who was to lead the prayermeeting that night and found that he didn't want to do it "because he said he was all at sea....He realized simple faith would be best but could not get it. Not being any too sure of my ground myself, I could help him but little. What dope shall I hand him?" he asked his mother. "It all sours in *my* mouth too sometimes...." Although there is no record of her response, whatever she wrote back seemed to help, and the momentary doubt passed.

And then in the spring, word came from the dean advising those undecided about their concentration of courses for the next two years to make up their minds. Until now, Wilder had been satisfied with the decision to try for the Rhodes Scholarship. What he would study at Oxford if he were selected and what he would do after that were questions he was now obliged to answer.

A year earlier in a letter to his mother he had duplicated for her benefit a list of possible professions (including "millionaire") which he had drawn up. At the end he had eliminated all but medicine and the ministry, and now, a year later, the idea of being one of "those weaklings" in the seminary, concerned only with getting a comfortable parish house, seemed extremely unmanly and distasteful. Which left only medicine. Although his mixed feelings about his father extended to his father's profession, Wilder had discovered, to his own great surprise, a fascination with the mysterious world beneath a microscope. A professor of Wilder's that year was the eminent biologist and gifted teacher Edward Conklin, one of Woodrow Wilson's most illustrious recruits for Princeton. Earlier in his life Conklin, like Wilder, had considered entering the ministry, and had even been ordained as a lay preacher. And though he gave up the ministry for biology, he remained a deeply religious man, much concerned with the relation between science, ethics and religion, a subject about which he wrote several books and many magazine articles, and on which he gave dozens of speeches during his life.

At a time when Darwin's *Origin of Species* was still widely banned and "Darwinism" regularly the subject of thunderous Sunday sermons, Edward Conklin believed that scientific evidence of man's animal ancestry did not necessarily undermine either religious faith or belief in human dignity. "The real dignity of man," he observed, "consists not in his origin but in what he is and in what he may become." Conklin's point of view was stated most conclusively in his posthumously published "spiritual autobiography." Among the last words in the book are these: "No one can furnish scientific proof of the existence or nature of a divine plan in the fulfillment of which men may cooperate, but it is evident that such an ideal lends strength and courage to mortal men."

Those words are startlingly like the words with which Wilder, some sixty years after he sat in Conklin's biology class, would end his own summary of his life's work in science.

Whether or not Wilder later read Conklin's final book—and there is no reason to believe he did—Conklin had a powerful influence on Wilder's life. He was an inspiring biology teacher whose quiet descriptions of "how tiny cells within the living, growing body bud and multiply" Wilder would remember to the end of his life. In *No Man Alone,* Wilder would credit Conklin for arousing his interest in science, and for being an influence that made him reluctant, when the moment came to decide on his future, to dismiss medicine outright.

There was another reason. A few weeks earlier he and a friend had gone to New York and bluffed their way into the Presbyterian Hospital. The other student was determined to go into medicine, and he had persuaded Wilder to come along and see what it was like. Passing themselves off as interns, the two boys opened a door at random and found themselves in an operating room. In the middle of the brilliantly lit amphitheatre a surgeon, surrounded by assistants and nurses, was operating on "a gory patient who was groaning as ether was given her. Her breast had been cut away for cancer of the breast." They stayed for close to four hours, witnessing four more operations, two for removing gallstones, and a third on a small child with a chest infection severe enough to require surgery to drain the pus. During the last operation Wilder left the room for a minute or two "to get some fresh air."

Wilder described the experience rather offhandedly to his mother, and she wrote back to ask if it had affected his indecision about his future. In his next letter he grudgingly admitted that "the wonderful skill and knowledge of the surgeon appealed to me," but no, he hadn't made up his mind one way or the other. "I don't know that I want to study medicine. Don't think that because I sat through some butchering that I believe I am fitted for a doctor." His indecision did not prevent him from having some rather firm views on the subject. "In this country there are about three times too many of them now....I believe that a practitioner (who can have only a little of regular operating work) should not attempt to be a surgeon, but should let the surgeons in the hospital do it all."

With the necessity of making a decision pressing on him, Wilder found a quiet spot in the gallery of the Princeton library and at the top of a sheet of paper wrote self-consciously, "Objective: to support myself and family and somehow make the world a better place in which to live." Below, he once again made up a list of professions and began eliminating them, one by one. By the end of the afternoon medicine was the only profession left on the list. And still he hesitated, recalling a conversation with his uncle, Tom Jefferson. Tom had advised him against an indoor profession—and medicine in particular—saying that he knew the stock Wilder came from and it would come to no good if he did try medicine. This preposterous piece of advice had stuck in Wilder's mind. He remembered his father and thought that his own enjoyment of football and wrestling might confirm the truth of his uncle's warning. Would "the call of the wild" defeat his career as, he had come to believe, it had defeated his father's?

But medicine was the only thing that interested Wilder and, dismissing his fears and unhappy memories, he made up his mind to become a doctor. "This was *my life*, not my father's, not my uncle's. I would live it as I liked," he wrote sixty years later. If "the call of the wild" demanded a regular routine of vigorous exercise and escapes to the fresh air and freedom of lakes and forests, he would have to accommodate it. Besides, the fascinating world revealed by the microscope, like the skill and power of the surgeon, was a far cry from the pills, powders and uneasy associations of his father's practice.

When Wilder returned to Hudson that summer, he found that his mother had aged considerably under the strain of keeping the Galahad School open and caring for Grandfather Jefferson, who was ailing. Wilder dutifully pitched in to help with summer renovations at the school and spent much of his spare time with old friends, including Helen Kermott, back for the summer from college in Milwaukee. By the time he set off on the train for his junior year at Princeton, armed with a more recent picture of her to put on his desk, his feelings toward her were causing him to despair.

"When I look forward to being a doctor and taking 9 *more* years of preparation," he wrote on the train, "it appalls me...the girls I know now will all be old before then."

But his decision to become a doctor was unshaken, and began to manifest itself, according to Bill Chester, from the moment they settled into their new rooms in the junior dormitory. Approached by a reporter writing a story about Penfield many years later, Chester described the "intense and morbid interest" Wilder displayed in any classmate "who might get so much as a cinder in his eye." Chester remarked, "Those of us closest and most vulnerable soon learned there was only one way to avoid summary examination by the future great physician—that was to fend him off with an upturned chair, like a lion tamer."

One morning Chester walked into the washroom and found Wilder shaving somewhat gingerly with a gleaming new straight razor, of the sort justifiably known as a cut-throat razor. He had given up the safety razor, he explained, to force himself to develop a steady hand for surgery. Soon, to his roommate's horror, he was experimenting with his left hand as well.

Wilder joined the newly-organized Medical Club, but on the advice of a visiting medical-school director that students planning to go on to medical school leave biology, physiology and anatomy courses until their senior year and concentrate on getting a "cultural" education, Wilder continued with the courses required for a general degree in philosophy. These included History of Philosophy, Constitutional Government, Qualitative Analysis, French, and a course in Psychology. Required reading for the last was William James, and a little while later Wilder observed in a letter to his mother: "He [James] and I do not agree in our ideas very often. It seems largely to be a contest between his reason and my presumption....Bill and I think alot alike and we discuss the philosophy and psychology as if we were authorities." In another letter he added, "It seems to me there might be a good field for a doctor in Psychology...."

Up to this time, Wilder had managed to eke out the allowance he'd been receiving from his grandfather by an ingenious scheme of selling local tradesmen advertising on blotters, and then distributing them to each student's room. The last two years he had come back a few days early to sell the ads and make the arrangements. By this Christmas, however, he found himself short of money, and resolved not only to put out a new and bigger edition of the blotters for the following term, but to stay over the Christmas holidays as well and work in the library. He reported in a letter home that he had found a job binding constitutional records, then cutting "leads," or print, at twenty-five cents an hour. Since Grandfather Jefferson had apparently written reprimanding him for the state of his accounts, Wilder added irritably, "I have not been boozing nor gambling nor anything else, am not going to borrow a cent, have $40 to last me 'til Feb. 7, do not owe anyone a penny....Nobody has any right to worry about me because I haven't failed in making good yet."

About this time Wilder, Bill Chester and a few of their friends formed "The Dr. Johnson Society." They met in someone's room on Sunday evenings after prayer meetings "to talk and read and just sort of bicker." The original members included a clubmate of Bill's named Francis Hall, who was going into medicine, Max Chaplin, who was going to be a missionary, and Paul Myers, somewhat older than the others, "who has had interesting experiences." Other names appear and disappear, but the original five began a tradition that would survive long after their college years were over.

"Max read *The Toiling of Felix* and Keg Howard read *The Master of the Inn*," reports one letter, while another mentions that a preceptor—a senior or graduate student who led small classes known as "precepts"—had been invited to talk "politics, etc." to the group.

Princeton students had some reason to feel particularly involved in politics, for, in January of 1911, President Woodrow Wilson of Princeton University was elected Governor of New Jersey. By the time spring came to the campus, Wilson was running hard for the Democratic presidential nomination. Paul Myers was already a keen Wilson supporter, and was planning to spend the summer stumping for Wilson in his home state of Pennsylvania if he won the nomination. He did, and when the Woodrow Wilson Club of Princeton University issued its membership cards in the fall of 1912, Paul Myers was listed as president, Chester as treasurer, and the other three Johnson Club members, Penfield, Hall and Chaplin, as members of the executive committee.

In June the Dr. Johnson Club held its final meeting before summer holidays with a dinner at the Princeton Inn, and a singsong afterward. Francis Hall and Max Chaplin were to spend the summer in Europe, Paul Myers was to campaign in Pennsylvania, and Bill Chester was taking a last summer vacation. "And goodness knows what I'll be doing," Wilder finished.

Getting engaged, or sort of, to Helen Kermott seems to have been that summer's main order of business. His unusual method of courtship consisted, apparently, of telling Helen she wouldn't see much of him anymore. Returning to Princeton on the *Manhattan Limited* early in September, Wilder noted that he and Helen had spent more time together, canoeing and picnicking and going to dances, than in previous summers. One afternoon near the end he went to talk to his mother and ask her advice, and found that she had wanted to talk with him—"we were both on the same subject," he said. "She advised me and I know she was right that I must hold back since there seem to be eight more years of preparation before I can earn a living, and it is wrong to keep other men away from any girl in my own circumstances."

The next afternoon he and Helen went off for a paddle and stopped at a point of land, and Wilder announced that he would "see less of her and why, although she attracted me more than any girl I knew." That is all the information the diary provides, but in *No Man Alone*, a much later account, he gives some indication of her reaction. "She only smiled, as if in disbelief. There was no kiss. But her eyes did speak."

In the week that followed the two of them went on a canoe trip chaperoned by Bill Chester, who was visiting, and Wilder's married sister, Ruth. They paddled up the Saint Croix River to the falls. "The sky was blue each day all through. By night, at last, we slept on fragrant beds of pine boughs. The moon was full and added to its mystery, Nature seemed to have undertaken to show what she too could say to Helen without the use of words. The northern lights marched and flickered across the heavens as none of us had ever seen them before."

In his final year at Princeton, Wilder suddenly lost interest in football although he had earned his "P" at tackle, and the Princeton newspaper referred to him as "W. G. Penfield, the football player." After the final game, in which Princeton tied Yale, he wrote: "Football is one mile-post passed." Ahead was the Rhodes Scholarship competition and his success on the football team would help satisfy the "all-round" criteria for the scholarship. But he had yet to distinguish himself in his studies.

One cool, sunny day in late autumn he climbed out on the fire escape of Edwards Hall dormitory, and up to the highest platform, bringing a book he was reading. From here, between the trees, he could see the whole campus and town of Princeton spread out below. "I felt myself aloof and alone," he wrote; the sense that there was a world that lay beyond this place, beckoning to him, came as a revelation: "I fancied I was seeing the towers of the Arts and the Sciences in a dreamlike city of the intellect. There was so much to learn there and, beyond the learning, there was truth unguessed and yet to be discovered." The key to this visionary city was the Rhodes Scholarship. To get it he would have to bring his course standing up to the honours level.

By Christmas he had done it. As well, the class had elected him "Best All-Round Man," "Most Respected Man" and the student who had "Done Most for the Class Generally." However, when the Rhodes Scholarship Committee for New Jersey finally came to a decision in January —after taking the unusual and unsuccessful step of trying to have two candidates accepted—it was a student named Valentine Havens from Rutgers University who won. The committee urged Wilder to try again the following year, adding that he was certain to get the scholarship if he did.

The Rhodes Scholarship had been Wilder's goal since he was thirteen years old, and yet by the time the decision was made in favour of the other candidate, the whole procedure had stretched out for so long that he was, in a way, relieved. The ambition to be a Rhodes Scholar, romantic and appealing though it was, had been replaced by a firm determination to become a doctor. Now, he was not at all sure that studying at Oxford would be the best course, and it certainly wouldn't have been the most direct.

Then, in the midst of his indecision about what to do next, a telegram came from Herbert: "Grandfather passed away this evening. Do not think of coming." Reluctantly, since he couldn't afford the trip or the time away from his work, Wilder remained in Princeton.

The death of his grandfather would also mean that Wilder would have to finance his own way through medical school, and just before graduating *cum laude* in June, he accepted the offer of a job teaching at Galahad in the fall. No sooner had he accepted than another offer came, that he return to Princeton and coach the freshman football team. After a hasty consultation with Will McQuarrie, now headmaster at Galahad, it was decided that he would do both: coach at Princeton until the end of the football season and then return to Hudson to teach the rest of the year. Neither job had tremendous appeal, but for the moment he was simply looking forward to graduating and getting out into the world; perhaps he would reapply for the Rhodes Scholarship next year after all.

As they had planned by letter during the last few years, Jean made her first trip east to come to Wilder's graduation. They had decided that after his graduation they would go to Washington and New York, then take a boat up to Montreal and on down the St. Lawrence River to Quebec City. Despite Wilder's failure to get the Rhodes Scholarship, they found much to celebrate, and it was fitting that Jean should be there. Through his letters she had shared his experiences and met his friends and professors. When they met her they discovered she knew all about them; she hoped this one's health had improved and that one would enjoy going to law school in Chicago. The dean of the university and his wife, fond of Wilder and sorry to see him leaving, invited her to stay with them as their guest. On the night of the Senior Promenade, at a dinner given by the president, she was given a place of honour next to the German ambassador, Count von Bernstorff, there to accept an honorary degree.

Jean must have been tremendously proud of her son and would have noted the changes in him. Outwardly at least, the insecure and awkward adolescent who had set out from Hudson, Wisconsin, to conquer the east four years earlier had disappeared utterly. In his place was a handsome and confident young man, self-contained and observant, much of the defensiveness mellowed by his successes. As for his mother, Wilder wrote in his diary during her visit, she looked quite young and gay "and is enjoying what she calls our honeymoon."

After the graduation ceremony and many good-byes the two of them left for Washington, and after a day or two there, they went on to New York. From there they set off up the Hudson River, continuing across Lake George and Lake Champlain to Montreal and on down the St. Lawrence, the shores reminding them both of the Saint Croix, to Quebec City. There, in a tower room at the Château Frontenac Hotel, Jean read aloud in instalments *Le Chien d'Or,* a novel set in early Quebec. Leaving the hotel from time to time, they wandered through the streets of the city and explored the battlements of the old fort. From Quebec City they took the boat back down the river to Niagara Falls, where they parted, Jean for home and Wilder for a summer job in Nova Scotia "tutoring" two young boys.

Wilder had met the boys' father, Dr. J. M. T. Finney, that spring on a visit to Johns Hopkins Medical School. He'd gone there with the mascot of the baseball team, a dwarf named Hughie, to see if something could be done for him. It was a kind gesture, but after testing Hughie for a week the doctors at Johns Hopkins concluded that other than improving his health generally, there was no cure for Hughie's inability to grow.

A week or two after the trip, however, Wilder heard from Finney, who offered him the summer job. Actually, it was little more than babysitting, but Wilder took it readily for the opportunity to get to know the doctor. Finney was professor of surgery at Johns Hopkins and an influential figure in American medicine: an aspiring medical student could hardly make a better connection, as Wilder knew. "In the first couple of years after hospital it makes a big difference whether you have a little pull or not," he had written to his mother when the job was offered. "Besides, he is a mighty good copy for any man and I want to know him and learn from him."

The Finneys' summer place was on an island in the bay off Chester, Nova Scotia, called "Little Fish" or "Mrs. Finney's Hat." Wilder's duties for the next two months entailed giving the boys a couple of hours help each day with their schoolwork, and taking them on occasional camping trips. For this he was paid $100 per month, and could spend his considerable spare time relaxing, reading and learning to sail. Though the job was pleasant and the Finneys gracious, he chafed somewhat at the inactivity.

Then, in the middle of July, came news that his father had died in Spokane of a heart attack. Herbert and his mother went out to the funeral, and though the Finneys urged him to go with a clear conscience if he wished, he did not. Hearing of his father's death, Wilder confided to his diary, "He was always honorable enough in his way I guess, but certainly not strong or admirable. It is sort of like the taking of a skeleton out of the family closet for me. His medical library, etc. is to come to me. I have been reading Dickens'

Christmas Carol and as I write these lines I am wondering if perhaps he can still know what passes on earth, as Scrooge in his dream, and if perhaps his ghost can read what I am writing. That is foolish and yet not foolish. Certainly he still lives somehow and has a wasted life to make up for if he is ever to make good in any life. He had a fine start and had talent as a doctor and a great opportunity to do something but he let everything slip....I hope such a thing may never come to me."

Returning to Galahad near the end of summer, Wilder found his mother looking quite pale, and older. The trip to Spokane for the funeral had been hard on her, he observed bitterly, and had completely countered the good effects of their trip together in the east. Her humiliation had been made complete by the appearance, at the funeral, of the woman Charles was engaged to marry. It would be many years before Wilder could bring himself to even mention his father's name.

Wilder spent the rest of September at Galahad, noting that many of his friends had married, and only six were left, among them Helen Kermott, who seemed to be spending an inordinate amount of time with a rival. "As was true every other year at the beginning Helen ignored me somewhat. I think that if there is any understanding between her & Bill she would tell me."

The football season was about to begin and Wilder left soon after for Princeton. He lived at the Athletic Club and spent the days driving the freshman football players to their limits and the nights working late on strategy and new plays. Occasionally he took trips to New York to visit Bill Chester, and for a while "fussed" Florence Colgate, who had been a friend while he was an undergraduate. During his senior year, the Colgates had invited Wilder to spend Christmas with them, and it had been a blessed respite from worrying about the delayed decision from the Rhodes Scholarship Committee. Now, seeing him spending his time coaching football to finance medical school, Mrs. Colgate took him aside and offered to help him get started in medical school right away. "I thanked her & said no. If I had to have the money I would hate to accept it. I shouldn't accept it."

The season finished well for the freshman team owing, in no little degree, to Wilder's exhortation and determination, and he set off for Galahad, $876 richer, to teach German and English for the rest of the year.

In mid-December a telegram came from the Rhodes Committee: He had been awarded the Scholarship without even the formality of an appearance before them. The announcement was made in the newspapers and for the next three weeks telegrams poured in. One of them was from Heff Herring, an ex-Rhodes Scholar and football player teaching at Princeton. He wrote to say that the coaching committee had offered Wilder the job of head field coach for the Varsity; if Wilder took it, Herring thought he could arrange to have the Rhodes Scholarship and entrance to Merton College at Oxford deferred until after Christmas.

The offer was too much for Wilder to refuse, and so it was arranged. Impatient to begin his medical studies, he made plans to spend the summer at Harvard taking an anatomy course. He discovered to his dismay that Oxford required an entrance examination in Greek, a sight translation from Xenophon's *Anabasis*. Since Wilder had never studied Greek, he would have to make up the equivalent of a two-year course of study in a matter of months. All through the winter, aside from teaching and coaching at Galahad, he struggled along with a dictionary, a copy of the *Anabasis* in Greek, an English translation and a grammar book. In the spring he took the exam, and failed. So when he set off for Harvard he dragged along the books to study for a second attempt at the exam in the fall.

The very first day of summer school at Harvard brought a curious incident. Wilder worked long after the rest of the students had left the laboratory, and the building was completely deserted. They had begun studying the pectoral muscle that day and Wilder was so interested he hardly noticed that night had fallen. When he finally got up to stretch and looked around the room, he saw that six cadavers had been brought in during the afternoon and lay naked and horribly exposed under the bright lights. "The men did not seem so bad but two were women, one, grey haired, had, I fancied, nice refined features and it occurred to me that she was someone's mother. But worse yet—next to me stretched a woman whose skin was startlingly white. Her long hair was a bright red and her lips were parted in a grin which exposed even, white teeth and protruding tongue. The stillness was only broken by the sound of water dripping from the pipes overhead. How long did it take me to get out? I hated to turn out the lights," he wrote in his diary, "and stumbled down the hall with a prickly feeling on my spine."

Before long, however, the feeling wore off, and, so he wrote, "interest in the bodies as a piece of workmanship" took the place of the first horror. The six-week course in anatomy erased any lingering doubts of whether medicine was worth pursuing. The lecturer was brilliant, the subject gripping and Wilder spent almost every evening, often alone, working in the laboratory, then walking several miles to the dormitory to snatch a few hours sleep—before rising at four-thirty to walk back in time to spend an hour studying Greek before the class began. Still he made time to jot down a few thoughts in his diary, including a debate on the advisability of stretching the limits of one's endurance: in the textbook for his course in Psychology, Henry James spoke of tapping "lower levels of energy." If it could be done, why not *live* on the deeper levels all of the time? "Our bodies are instruments whose capacity we may not know until we try them out."

For Wilder, who saw himself as a plodder, someone who could succeed only by dint of stubborn and repeated effort, ferocious concentration would have to be a substitute for genius. In the years ahead, the result was a carefully cultivated ritual of focusing his entire attention on whatever was at hand, forcing himself to shut out anything that was not important, whether he was writing a paper, studying a book or report, or examining a patient.

From the ritual a litany emerged: "Study in a pool of light." "Keep things the same, even if a new way seems easier." "Never waste a minute." When he was fifteen, he had believed that if he concentrated hard enough he could do the impossible, learn to swallow without moving his Adam's apple. Now he was simply reapplying the same principle. The awareness, however, that he could only do all the things he wanted to do in his life by this enormous effort of will left him with an abiding envy of those brighter sorts who succeeded effortlessly, as though by some inward sleight-of-hand, while he struggled to keep up.

Back in Hudson at the end of the summer of 1914, Wilder found Helen Kermott returned from teaching in Houston, Texas, and the long, uncertain courtship came to a head. One bleak and windy Sunday with a fine rain falling, he and Helen took a walk to the bank overlooking the river, below the coulee. "She told me she wanted to ask my advice," the diarist explains. "A few days before I returned from Chester, Nova Scotia last summer she was engaged to William Webster. The night I came down to camp for a few hours, she realized that marriage to Wm was impossible. She was awake all that night. She told him the engagement could not be but he wouldn't listen to her then. All winter she would not listen to him, and when he was home this summer she avoided him. She wanted to know how much difference it would make to him."

Helen Kermott was issuing a rather obvious challenge, suggesting he stop dithering and ask her to marry him or else she'd accept one of the other offers. The provocation, as she anticipated, was more than he could stand and he broke in on her wide-eyed account and "told her I had loved her for five years, but as I considered long engagements wrong, I would not ask her to marry me. Then I changed my mind and decided to go on further but she would not let me."

The next day Wilder went to St. Paul with his mother and brought back an engagement ring, which he offered and Helen accepted. "The rest of the week we were together much."

Setting out for Princeton for the last time, he observed that the "queer, hungry feeling of doubt" that had accompanied this by now familiar train trip was gone. "Now I must work as never before for there is a much greater incentive. If I could only shorten my course!"

That autumn brought news that threatened to cancel his plans to go overseas. Midway through practice one afternoon, a student ran out of one of the nearby buildings shouting that England and Germany were at war. As the players crowded around, talking excitedly, Wilder stood there numbly, seeing his dreams of Oxford's spires and playing fields slip away from him once again. When the football season ended Wilder had given up hope of going to England, and moved to New York and a room at the Y.M.C.A., while he began his medical studies at the College of Physicians and Surgeons.

Then, six weeks later, he received a letter from a friend at Oxford saying that classes were still being held, and the departure of many of the students actually meant the instructors were giving more time to those who remained. Wilder quickly cabled Oxford to see if he would be accepted in January, and shortly after sent another to his mother in Hudson: "I'm going—where? Guess....The return cable just came, and I shall go after seeing you at Christmas."

CHAPTER FOUR

An Unusual Apprenticeship

~~~ OXFORD

It was not a propitious time to come to England. That golden and glorious autumn regiments of young men cheerfully marched off to the recruiter singing "Hullo, hullo! Who's your lady friend?" They trained on Hampstead Heath and Richmond Park while onlookers gathered to cheer or make wisecracks. Then, suddenly, they were gone overseas. Strange, foreign names now took on dreadful meaning: *Aisne, Marne, Loos, Mons.* Letters to the front were returned with KILLED scrawled across the envelope. The war that was to end by Christmas might now last a year, and the general euphoria of the first months had vanished. In January of 1915, England was settling into a deep and brooding uneasiness.

Wilder stepped off the ship in Liverpool on a cold, windy afternoon barely a week before his twenty-fourth birthday. The crossing had been rough and miserable and lonely. The orchestra had missed the boat, and the only person he had worked up his nerve to talk to turned out to be an English suffragette: "very interesting when steered away from suffrage." Each day he had written long, wistful notes to Helen.

In his stateroom, when he boarded, he had found a telegram, two letters and a Bible which Helen had sent. Though he found the Bible hard to digest at night, he wrote her, "I want to and now that you have asked me to read it with you, it will mean a lot more to me and be easy and a sort of right communication with you. Every evening," he enthused, "we will communicate by means of God's wireless. Though the communication be secondary."

Alone in Liverpool the first night, Wilder went to an evening service at a church near his hotel. The minister read a long list of boys' names and prayed for them. "They were boys of the congregation at the front," Wilder wrote, "sons, brothers, lovers; and I saw looks on many faces that told stories...uniforms in the pews, the hotel, the street showed that all the sons were not yet gone. And they prayed for the enemies' wounded as their own." The following morning he wakened to the quick, measured beat of feet on the pavement, and then the sound of voices singing about "Soldiers of the King." Looking far down the street in the paling light from the streetlamps, he saw a long line of khaki uniforms marching away to the ships.

At Oxford it was, if anything, worse. The colleges were virtually empty, as the students were among the first to answer the call to arms. "Come and die," Rupert Brooke gaily wrote from a battlefield in France to a friend, "it will be great fun." In a shabby, upper room in Albert Street, Oxford, a Committee of Military Delegates had interviewed, in August and September alone, more than 2,000 candidates and most of them received commissions. In the months that followed, intensive training courses were held in the colleges. In place of cycling undergraduates, marching cadets filled the streets.

The social brilliance of Oxford had reached a peak in the years before the war; it was the most glittering university in Europe. But by early January, 1915, when Wilder entered Oxford, memorial services in the colleges and the honour rolls on the lodge gates had become commonplace. "Emptiness, silence, reigns everywhere" at Oxford, recorded the president of Magdalen College, Sir Herbert Warren, in a letter in the waning months of 1914. "The remnant of the undergraduates, the invalids, the crippled, the neutrals, make absolutely no show at all."

There would be little enough to match Wilder's fantasy of undergraduates in white running across the green college lawns on their way to the playing fields and the river, glowing with health and good breeding. Yet if he was disappointed, his letters home do not show it.

As he rolled down the streets of Oxford in a hansom, he was amazed to find everything looking so old and "rather the worse for wear." The remaining students rode bicycles. Women, he noted with disapproval, "strode along with men's stride." Rather plain, they dressed "as though the hobble skirt hadn't been invented."

Wilder's assigned rooms at Merton College, a small bedroom and a large sitting room with a fireplace, faced Mob Quad, the oldest part of the college. Built in the thirteenth century, with thick stone walls, it was colder than anything he had ever experienced; his coal grate provided the only heat.

After unpacking, he was rubbing his hands before the coal fire when he heard a knock on the door. A man entered, introducing himself as Wilder's "scout." Although the origins of the title are lost in antiquity, the scouts performed various menial duties for the students in their rooms, and were charged with maintaining the Victorian values of an earlier Oxford. A few days later Wilder noted in a letter that the man's name was Stone: "Shall I tell you what he does? He has just laid a tablecloth over the large round table so it covers half, and has set out silver and jam and china, for one. It is almost lunch time. Now he is in the bedder—bedroom—putting it in order. Then he will come out and maybe poke up the fire and see there is water in the kettle which sits on a trivet, a little tiny iron platform that hangs on the grate. He brings breakfast here, lights the fire, and wakens me at the wrong time. That's about all he does.... The first couple of days I watched him in fear and trembling, thinking he might want to help me dress, and give me a bath."

While they may have made "no show at all" to the president of Magdalen College, those American students, many of them Rhodes Scholars, were determined to enjoy their time at Oxford. Wilder, whom another Rhodes Scholar picked out in a crowded street as an American because he was "the only well-dressed man in sight" dutifully put away his suits and stiff collars in favour of grey bags and knickers and tweed Norfolk jackets. Equipped with a list of necessities his scout presented him, Wilder went out and bought a gown (which undergraduates were required to wear when meeting with a professor), tablecloths and napkins, china and utensils, so he could entertain properly. There were few English students among the undergraduates Wilder came to know. An early attempt to become acquainted with one led to a rebuff, real or imaginary, and Wilder quickly withdrew. Those who weren't snobs, he decided, were thinking about those at the front and had no interest in making new friends—which he could understand. "Sometimes when I come into the Quad and look up at the crumbling stone, slate roof and leaded windows of the rooms whose occupants have all gone to war, it gives me a clammy sort of feeling," Wilder wrote in one of his first letters home, "as though it were a cemetery or rather, a repository of memories of those who are dead and long, long forgotten." To lonely English undergraduates unable or unwilling to enlist, the cheerful Americans and colonials must have seemed enviably carefree. But Wilder spent most of his free time at the American Club, or Rhodes House, or at afternoon and evening parties in the homes of the few American families around Oxford. When classes were over, the foreign students played rugby or rowed on the river. Around fires in one another's rooms, they reminisced about "back home" and argued about the war. In the evening, they met to sing the songs of their undergraduate college days.

Like Charles Lamb a century earlier, they came to Oxford to "play the gentleman, enact the student." Despite the accusing looks they—and every other able-bodied man—received in the streets of Oxford, they were determined to savour the opportunity. Wilder took to rugby immediately, quickly getting over his concern about making mistakes and doing "ungentlemanly stunts." "A fellow said 'Dammie' when I bumped him yesterday," he wrote to Jean, "which is the first oath I've heard since coming here. Next time I'll bump him hard and see what is joggled out of him."

Across Mob Quad from Wilder's rooms, a Harvard graduate named T. S. Eliot observed the antics of his colleagues and despaired. "O Conversation, the staff of life, shall I get any at Oxford?" he wrote mournfully to a friend, and shortly fled the unstimulating atmosphere of the university for the more cerebral company of London salons.

Wilder was too busy to notice. As he had hoped, the dearth of students meant small and intimate classes, and the opportunity for a medical student to get to know his teachers and work under them in the laboratory. The first thing he did on arriving in his rooms was unpack *The System of Medicine* by William Osler in association with John McCrae, the Montreal doctor who later wrote *In Flanders Fields*. Just looking up at the set of volumes, Wilder admitted to his mother, "makes me, mentally, worship him." Osler had come to Oxford from Johns Hopkins in Baltimore ten years earlier, and Wilder carried a carefully treasured letter of introduction to him from Dr. Finney.

Perhaps more than other young men, Wilder was on the lookout for successful, respected older men to be his models. During his time at Oxford, he came to idolize Sir William Osler. But in this he was not alone—everyone who passed through Osler's sphere worshipped him, and after his death Osler Societies sprang up throughout the English-speaking world. What evoked this remarkable response was neither the brilliance of his mind nor the wisdom of his observations; it was a much homelier and more lovable quality— what one student called simply "Osler's heart."

Sir William was a Canadian whose career had led him from the chair of medicine at McGill to becoming one of the founders of Johns Hopkins hospital and medical school. He had accepted the appointment as Regius Professor of Medicine in the midst of a very demanding life at Johns Hopkins when his wife told him, "Better to leave Baltimore on a ship than in a pine box." The position gave the recipient enormous influence and made few demands, and Osler, in 1915, was concerned primarily with gathering a medical library and writing essays and addresses. He and Lady Osler, a great-granddaughter of Paul Revere, lived in a beautiful house in Oxford surrounded by spacious lawns and gardens and known far and wide as "the Open Arms" because of the Oslers' inexhaustible hospitality.

By the time he went to see Sir William, Wilder needed his help rather badly. On his arrival at Oxford Wilder had immediately approached the head of the Physiology Department and explained that he only wanted to take the courses required in the first two years at Johns Hopkins, and to take them in the two years he planned to spend at Oxford. He had explained that he didn't care about a degree (which would take an extra year), and when the head of the department and another professor who had been called in for consultation asked why, he answered that he didn't want to waste any time. He reported the conversation gloomily in a letter to his mother; "'It cawn't be done,' they both agreed. My heart went down to see if my feet were wet.... The whole mess threw me in a fit of doubt. I wish I'd get my right hand blown off and then I'd not have to be a physician."

The only recourse was to see if the Regius Professor could intervene and smooth the way. So, with Dr. Finney's letter in hand, Wilder made his way to the "Open Arms." It is easy to imagine Osler in his favourite pose, leaning on the mantelpiece in his study, stroking his long, bushy moustache, listening thoughtfully to this earnest young Rhodes Scholar so anxious not to waste a moment. Osler, to Wilder's great relief, agreed with his plans and promised to straighten out the problems. "Osler says 'Certainly you can do it in two years here. You have 21 months, and I can fix up any courses you want at Edinburgh or some place in the summer.' He says 'You are an old man, you don't want to spend three years on this.'" "Osler says" quickly became the most common pair of words in Wilder's letters.

Sir William came to the American Club and at the students' urging spoke about his life. Wilder wrote of Osler's talk at considerable length in a letter home, ending, "He said, at the end, that his rule had been to like and sympathize with everyone. That's his creed, I think. He is the least sentimental and the most helpful man

I've ever seen—and the most lovable. You may believe that he is stimulating to me, too, and is on something of a pedestal. If I were not so dumb, I should have the nerve to hope and dream I might follow in his footsteps."

Osler, it seems, became fond of Wilder. When he went off on consultations around the countryside to one hospital or another, Osler often invited Wilder to come along. The careful way Osler listened to what the patient's attending physician had to say, his gentle, soothing manner at the bedside, the lack of pretension or self-importance that marked his diagnosis and suggestions—all this made a deep and lasting impression on Wilder. Like a thousand other fortunate medical students in the past who had come into contact with Osler, Wilder came to think of medicine as the highest and noblest calling; to be convinced that it was not enough just to heal bodies. A physician must think of his patients as suffering human beings who come to him with all of their troubles and fears.

If Osler was the perfect model of a great physician, at Oxford Wilder also found the perfect model of a great scientist, Sir Charles Sherrington. He had none of Osler's magnetic physical presence: in the physiology laboratory where he taught, Sherrington, a shy, smallish man with a little moustache and noseglasses, hurried about in a white coat with a preoccupied air, moving from table to table as the students prepared sections of tissue for the microscope. "How well I remember him peering, short-sighted, over my embarrassed shoulder," Wilder wrote many years later. "His face was smooth and almost expressionless, but I watched for the faint smile and the twinkle of humour and understanding in his eyes. 'Hmm, Penfield, you may be right,'" he would say, "'but I should have thought...' Then he would pick up the delicately pointed forceps and change the tissue of the preparation so as to set the youthful experimenter back on the right track." Sherrington, he added, "seemed quite sincere in the expectation that each student would teach him something, some time." To Wilder, the ability to encourage students and make them feel like collaborators in science rather than ignorant apprentices, was a striking departure from the more authoritarian teaching style of Princeton.

Sherrington, like Osler, was a connection for Wilder to an earlier era of scientists who wrote poems, collected old manuscripts, travelled widely, and regarded all these things as essential parts of a balanced life. Like Osler, Sherrington had left a hectic academic career elsewhere to come to Oxford, for the comparative quiet of the town, the small classes, the short terms and the beauty of the setting.

In his lectures, Sherrington had the frustrating habit of presenting both sides of each physiological problem, rather than a concise and comfortably positive statement of fact. It was in these lectures that Wilder was first introduced to the study of the brain. As Sherrington outlined the current theories of how the brain and the nervous system worked, he revealed a field of science that had barely been tapped, and in which new and startling discoveries were being made every day. As a separate specialty, neurology had emerged only in the last forty or fifty years. Neurosurgery, as a science, did not exist at all until the 1880s, when Sherrington himself was a medical student, though 2000-year-old skulls excavated in Egypt, Greece and Peru showed signs of surgical entry and evidence that the patients survived, at least for a while.

In the second half of the nineteenth century, three critical advances had breathed new life and hope into the study of the brain and nervous system. Antiseptic techniques, invented by Joseph Lister, made infection-free surgery possible; major advances in anaesthesiology removed much of the pain and terror from surgery, and then a series of brain localization experiments, in the London clinic of Hughlings Jackson and elsewhere, demonstrated that specific regions of the brain controlled motor and sensory response, and that other regions were involved with language and memory.

Great excitement followed these discoveries. In the waning years of the nineteenth century and the first years of the twentieth, it seemed that the brain would soon reveal its deepest secrets. In this atmosphere, the study of physiology led Charles Sherrington to study the reflexes related to the spinal cord, and to attempt to follow the reflexes to their source. It meant untangling and identifying the incredibly complex maze of nerves leading to and from the spinal cord and the brainstem, located at the top of the cord below the brain.

In Sherrington's basic work, he employed a "decerebrated preparation," a de-brained animal. Using painstakingly precise surgical methods, Sherrington removed the upper parts of the animal's brain, to rob it of all volition but not life. With the procedure successfully completed, the muscles controlled by the lower part of the brain and the spinal cord held the animal in a fixed, rigid position. The brainless beast could at that point be stood on its feet, motionless as a statue. That done, Sherrington could experiment with a healthy, functioning, unanaesthetized motor mechanism directed solely by the brainstem and spinal cord without the usual interference of the thoughts of the whole brain above.

It was the conclusions of these famous studies that Sherrington was teaching the students in his physiology classes at Oxford. However, it was not his reputation as a scientist that made Sherrington such an inspiring teacher, but the fact that he brought the same genius to his descriptions of the complex mechanisms that he applied in his scientific studies. Some twenty-five years after Wilder's time at Oxford, Sherrington set out in *Man on his Nature* to describe how he perceived the workings of the brain, using the metaphor of light:

"Suppose we choose the hour of deep sleep. Then only in some sparse and out of the way places are nodes flashing and trains of lightpoints running. Such places indicate local activity still in progress. At one such place we can watch the behaviour of a group of lights perhaps a myriad strong. They are pursuing a mystic and recurrent manoeuvre as if of some incantational dance. They are superintending the beating of the heart and the state of the arteries so that while we sleep the circulation of the blood is what it should be. The great knotted headpiece of the whole sleeping system lies for the most part dark, and quite especially so the roof-brain. Occasionally at places in it lighted points flash or move but soon subside. Such lighted points and moving trains of lights are mainly far in the outskirts, and wink slowly and travel slowly....

"Should we continue to watch the scheme we should observe after a time an impressive change which suddenly accrues. In the great head-end which has been mostly darkness spring up myriads of twinkling stationary lights and myriads of trains of moving lights of many different directions. It is as though activity from one of those local places which continued restless in the darkened main-mass suddenly spread far and wide and invaded all. The great topmost sheet of the mass, that where hardly a light had twinkled or moved, becomes now a sparkling field of rhythmic flashing points with trains of travelling sparks hurrying hither and thither. The brain is waking and with it the mind is returning. It is as if the Milky Way entered upon some cosmic dance. Swiftly the head-mass becomes an enchanted loom where millions of flashing shuttles weave a dissolving pattern, always a meaningful pattern though never an abiding one; a shifting harmony of sub subpatterns. Now as the waking body rouses, subpatterns of this great harmony of activity stretch down into the unlit tracks of the stalk-piece of the scheme. Strings of flashing and travelling sparks engage the lengths of it. This means that the body is up and rises to meet its waking day."

Forty years later, Wilder wrote that Sherrington had influenced his scientific thinking "more profoundly than anyone else." It was not, however, just physiological data and the spirit of scientific exploration that Sherrington imparted but a sense of wonder, and awe, at where it all might lead: "I looked through his eyes and came to realize that here in the nervous system was the great unexplored field—the undiscovered country in which the mystery of the mind of man might someday be explained."

As the novelty of Oxford began to wear off, and Wilder began to feel more at home, his uneasiness about the war grew. All of the American students were in a peculiar position which naturally worsened when it appeared America wanted to remain isolated from the war. The British press, which in the early months of the war had been obliged to rely on American and Commonwealth correspondents for war news, was virtually unanimous in its condemnation of President Wilson, and so was the general British population. At luncheons and teas, Wilder found they talked of little but the war, and on occasion, the American students were the target of some resentment. At a tea at Sherrington's in the spring of 1915, Wilder reported to his mother that a man said to him "that he was going to get the recruiting sergeant....It made me angry, as it should not have, and I asked if he meant for me. Then I told him I didn't happen to be a British subject *fortunately*. He said no more. But really, if I had a son or sons at the front, I'd speak to idle young men on the street, too. Often I see people look at me hard and rudely," he concluded, "and I know what they think."

Wilder's own thoughts on the matter were ambiguous. On one hand, he wrote, "...I hold my breath when I see England and Germany both trying to use America as a cat's paw. Trying to draw her into this trouble...." And yet for a healthy, aggressive young man, the sidelong and accusing looks were difficult to bear. More than once Wilder felt uncomfortable in civilian clothes and acutely aware of the privilege of his position at Oxford—that he studied while those who would have been his classmates fought and died on the plains of western France.

Still, emotion and guilt aside, in 1915 Wilder echoed the prevailing American sentiment that this was Europe's war, and America had no business sending her young men to die in European territorial battles. As well, Wilder came from Wisconsin, a state with a large German-speaking population, and he had grown up in Hudson with many friends of German ancestry.

In any event, the end of term finally came. Wilder, at Osler's urging, had made the necessary arrangements to study anatomy at Edinburgh in August and September, before Oxford classes began.

That left him with a couple of months free, and in the middle of June, 1915, he and two other Rhodes Scholars, one from Arkansas and another from "one of the Dakotas," set off on a tour of Europe that would take them through Italy, Switzerland and France. It was a two-month lark, and despite the warnings of a friend at the American Embassy and the reluctance of the agent at Cook's, they managed to travel through Europe without even hearing the sound of guns. Their route took them from Paris to Rome, Naples, and Florence, then back through Aix-les-Bains to Lausanne. In each city they visited the galleries and museums, and in Naples they took a side trip to the excavation at Pompeii. Only in Paris could they feel the war. Wilder wrote to his mother: "It is not the darkness, London is much darker. It is the deadness of everything. It is hard to explain. The currents of people are sluggish, and no one looks at you. Their eyes are down as though their own thoughts were sufficient company. Even the women ticket-takers and ushers seem apathetic. When you see a young man street-car conductor, you wonder if he has heart trouble or tuberculosis."

In mid-August, Wilder headed north to Edinburgh, sobered by what he had seen, and considerably more impressed with the effort the French were making in the war. In Edinburgh Wilder had his first really direct encounter with misery and poverty. "Destitution and sadness does not hide itself indoors," he wrote, "you see it sitting on the doorstep in Edinburgh." An afternoon's walk from the university out to Holyrood Palace led him through "streets of squalor and misery." Being sent off to fight, he concluded, was not the worst of calamities.

As they ran down to the tennis courts in the afternoon, the Rhodes Scholars were pursued by the cries of little boys: "Shir-r-ker—why don't you fight for your king and country?" By the middle of October he was glad enough to return to Merton and a busy fall of classes, which left him two free afternoons plus Sunday to play rugger and socialize. On Osler's advice, once again he was taking the courses that he would have little time for when he returned to medical school in America. In addition to Sherrington's Physiology lectures and lab work, he enrolled in Histology, Pharmacology, Bacteriology and Chemistry courses. For a few months, at least, concern with the outside world faded as Wilder struggled to make headway in his courses. But when the end of term came before Christmas, he had secured an invitation to return to France, along with a dozen other students.

They were invited as ambulance drivers, but Wilder decided to try and talk his way into the hospital instead. His persuasions on arrival at the military hospital at Ris Orangis were so successful that in a matter of days he was writing to Jean, "In the stress of my office duties I still have time to write you. That means a good deal, for I am a doctor now, with a nurse and a ward under my supervision. I am doing the work of a sure-enough doctor who has gone up to the front. It sort of spoils it if I say he left because he hadn't enough to do."

The soldiers were in fact, disappointingly healthy. As a sure-enough doctor, Wilder had few responsibilities beyond taking the occasional blood smear, having it stained and examining it under the microscope. It was just as well that his first patients were healthy and the nurses capable of doing the real work, since this was Wilder's first time out. Examining one of the patients he wrote, "I'm pretty sure I can feel a bullet in one man's leg, who for some reason was never X-rayed. I asked one of the Drs. about it and he said, 'well, if it is a good size you better take it out.' That sounds alright, but I never took anything but a sliver out of a finger, or piece of dust out of someone's eye. I'm going to have him X-rayed anyway, and learn how they use the X-ray."

One day while hanging about the operating room, a new doctor asked him if he could give the patient from whose leg he was removing a bullet a general anaesthetic—chloroform. Pride stopped Wilder from admitting that he had never given chloroform, and he agreed. "The orderly improvised a bottle with a safety pin in it for a dropper," he wrote to Jean. "He asked me if I'd have some vaseline. I said yes. He got it for me and I remembered that the book had said Chloroform was irritating to the mucous membrane, so I smeared it around and put it in the edges of his nostrils and lips. I asked the man if he had any false teeth, any trouble with his lungs, etc., and then started ahead feeling his pulse, and watching his eye reflexes and praying to the shade of Hippocrates." Luckily everything went well, and the patient came out just as the last stitch was being taken.

Watching the surgeons operating filled Wilder with admiration, and the urge to go into surgery himself. Here, it seemed, was an area where his dexterity and the strong, blunt hands of his father would be a great advantage. "It is nothing but skilled carpentry work with a lot of daring, knowledge of anatomy and pathology and judgement. I'm glad I've done some carpentering—the rest must be hammered out."

A couple of weeks later the winter term began at Oxford and Wilder reluctantly took his leave, with plans to return in three months during the spring break.

On Friday, March 24, 1916, Wilder boarded the S.S. *Sussex* at

Folkestone bound for France to spend the five weeks of his spring holiday at the Red Cross hospital in Ris Orangis. Just before embarking, he bumped into an acquaintance from Princeton and the two strolled about the deck chatting as the ship cast off and headed out of the harbour. On board they encountered other college acquaintances who were on their way to France as ambulance drivers.

After lunch, Wilder and his friend returned to the deck. They saw a great number of bales floating on the waves, then more wreckage and several empty rafts. A crew member informed them that two ships had been sunk there the night before. The *Sussex,* however, was an American ship and safe from attack.

But Wilder recalled that Folkestone harbour was full of ships at anchor, many more than was normal, suggesting that they had been warned of the danger. The *Sussex* steamed along close to the coast of England and then struck off across the Channel, while Wilder and his friend leaned against the rail. As they talked Wilder watched the sea gulls swimming about in the water off the bow. There was not a breath of wind, and the sun sparkled on every little ripple.

Suddenly there was an explosion and a terrific noise; the ship had been hit by a torpedo directly below where they were standing. They were thrown high in the air by the impact, and in Wilder's memory, everything seemed to go into slow motion: "By curious chance, I remained fully conscious and realized what had happened. I could see the wreckage of the broken ship turning with me, slowly as it seemed, while I rose in the air and fell again. I could hear the continuing roar of sound and I thought to myself, 'This is the end. I'm falling into the sea.' Then conviction came to me like a flash: 'This cannot be the end. My work in the world has only just begun. This cannot be the end.'"

Strange visions do, unaccountably, leap into the mind of someone suddenly facing death, as anyone who has had the experience will know. No matter how trite and clichéd they sound in retrospect, the solemn accounts of angelic choirs and heavenly trumpets that are routinely offered up by those revived from medical death at least illuminate the fate the subjects think awaits them. Looking back on his mother's absolute certainty that her boy was destined for greatness, which he had unquestioningly adopted, it is not astonishing that Wilder's subconscious flashed—instead of heavenly hosts—a reassuring message that this wasn't the end. "Call it *naïveté* or colossal egotism," he wrote of this moment in *No Man Alone.* "I *was* naïve and, surely, egotistical. Nevertheless it happened that way, and it demonstrated my deep conviction that there was work in the world for me to do."

Instead of falling into the water, Wilder landed on the wreckage of the bow on his back. Stunned, he lay there watching the debris follow him down. After a moment, realizing that the bow was slowly breaking off, he began to crawl toward the stern. His left leg "had become a flail, bending in all directions," he wrote. Somehow he made it to the stern, and a moment later the bow broke off and sank.

Most of the passengers, convinced the boat was about to go down, struggled desperately to get the lifeboats free and in the water. In a severe state of shock, and with a badly fractured left leg buckling under him, Wilder hobbled about trying to help. Those few he managed to pull out of the wreckage were unconscious, and would drown shortly anyway, he assumed. Soon he gave up and simply observed the desperate evacuation attempt. A week later he recorded the events of that day in a notebook. "Straight below me I saw the face of a man. It was white as chalk and it looked up at me through big spectacles but never said a word. I was absolutely indifferent about him. Over the edge of the deck I watched the water to see if it would rise. It was as calm and sunny as ever. The water did not rise and now people began to pass me and remark that we would probably not sink after all. One after one, the boats came back to us when they found the ship was not sinking. I moved aft and sat in a chair, where everyone in turn fell over my leg. One Swede walked on my foot and when I called him a damn fool and requested his departure he stooped down and picked up the overcoat someone had carefully wrapped about my shin. The chump never did understand why I was angry. A wind came up and waves pounded our side. Would they end up by breaking the remaining bulkheads? It grew dark and we sent up rockets which went with a great boom and showed rows of white upturned faces. The revolving light of a light house began to flash on shore. We were drifting straight toward it. All the stars came out and I identified as many as I could. The possibility of death and what it would mean to those at home came to me for the first time and it made me feel sick. A little French girl was a brick to me, wrapped me up and every now and then came back to scold me because the wind had blown someone's hat off my head. It got too cold and I asked Culbertson and Crocker to help me inside. Here was little Miss Edna Hale trying to stop the bleeding of a man's scalp. She was pressing on the wound with a big blood-soaked towel so I showed her where to press the auriculo-temporal artery below the wound and after much persuasion induced the man to allow himself to be set more upright. Great shouting and jabbering of French about 11:30 announced the arrival of a French trawler. The various people who had done so much for the wounded came in to say good-bye. I inquired and found every one of them was an American. There were scarcely any English on board except the young officer who did wonders."

For three weeks Penfield was in a hospital bed in Dover, recovering. He had been reported dead—in fact the St. Paul (Minnesota) *Pioneer Press* apparently went so far as to print his obituary—but a kindly fellow-passenger had cabled Helen and Jean that he was all right. Letters and telegrams poured in from all over, and several of the families at Oxford, including the Oslers, wrote to say that he must come and stay with them while he recovered.

To while away the time Wilder wrote several accounts of his experiences, one for some Chicago newspapers who cabled asking for a first-hand report, another for the Princeton Alumni paper, and a third—a highly dramatic third-person account which he scrawled in the back of a notebook and edited vigorously, as though to test his potential as a novelist.

The Oslers followed up their invitation with flowers—"my first"—and a comforting note from Sir William about the surgeon who was in charge of Wilder, saying that he was reputed to be a good man. After three weeks in Dover Wilder was able to get around on crutches, and he returned on the train to Oxford to spend the next few weeks at the "Open Arms," the Osler residence at Oxford.

Wilder's stay there passed all too quickly, and his admiration for the Oslers and their harmonious relationship soared. This, he thought, is how I want my married life to be. In the morning the maid arrived bearing a silver tea tray and breakfast. Lady Osler would come by to fuss over him, followed by Sir William for a chat, bearing perhaps an armful of books from his voluminous medical library for Wilder to peruse.

His close brush with death and the conviction that he had been saved for some purpose, not surprisingly, had a profound and sobering effect. During the weeks of his forced rest he had time to pause and reflect on his life. "Life has always been for me just one thing after another in fairly quick succession," he admitted in a letter to a friend, written while he was convalescing at the Oslers'. To his mother he wrote: "This morning, you will be going down to church—a true Wisconsin spring day, when a good stiff breeze has whipped up the lake and everything has budded—and you are cudgeling your brain to think just where you are going to place those other 10,000 tomato plants. I can remember those spring Sundays—11 years ago, when I used to walk back from dinner at Grandma's....My life is stretching out now. Aristotle says a man is at his height at 25. I hope not, because, as I figure it, I'm only on the first slope. But every power is here. Perhaps that is what he meant."

The idyll eventually ended, and as soon as he was able to get about with a cane, Wilder moved back into his rooms; whatever long-range effects his insight would have, for the moment it spurred him back to his books to study in earnest for the spring finals. When the results were out, he had done creditably, but the First Class had eluded him. Once more convinced that, whatever lay ahead, it was the long, hard road for someone as slow to learn as he was, he shrugged his shoulders and turned to plans for the fall. He had been accepted at Johns Hopkins medical school in Baltimore for the two years of study that would make him, finally, a real doctor. Deciding what he would do after getting his M.D. would have to wait. For now, it was enough to believe that when the time came to make up his mind, somehow or other, he would be guided.

∞∞ JOHNS HOPKINS

Wilder returned after eighteen months in England to find America preparing for war against Germany. The German U-boat campaign, of which the *Sussex* was but one casualty, had outraged the American public, and so far, Woodrow Wilson's peacemaking efforts had been unsuccessful. There was an election coming up in the fall, and Wilson knew he had to choose between being defeated at the hands of the Republicans or taking a harder stance against Germany. With great reluctance, and even as he prepared to run for a second presidential term under the slogan "He kept us out of war," Wilson set the lumbering machinery of government in motion. That summer, while Wilder basked in a hero's welcome in Hudson and spent much time with Helen Kermott, giant preparedness parades were held in the big eastern cities. Though the south and the mid-west (Wisconsin in particular) were still lukewarm to the war frenzy, Wilder had made up his mind that war was long overdue— the attack on the *Sussex* had removed any lingering doubts.

Tolerance was never his long suit, as the following account of a pacifist meeting he attended reveals:

"At the...meeting the other night John Dorsey said—'Well there's no one I've seen in this crowd that I'm afraid of.' And there was no one who could be suspected of violence. There were many nice looking women. But only a sprinkling of men and they were a second rate puny looking lot. I don't know that I blame the women very much for being there after all. Although I disagree with their aims.

"A socialist talked as we were leaving and after a disgusting preliminary said—If war came he was one who would not fight. John & I shouted out that we would fight and there came from several men's voices in the audience—'Here's another that will' 'Here's another that will.' Then John fell to cursing the man in a loud voice and with all too full a vocabulary so I had to hush him up. They were true pacifists and no one even reproached us, but a mild little usher suggested we take a seat and seemed quite contented when we ignored him...."

Although Wilder was willing to fight, his weeks at the Red Cross Hospital in Ris Orangis had given him a taste of practical medical work, and he hoped somehow to do his bit looking after the wounded rather than actually carrying a gun. And though he felt America's entry into the war was long overdue, he regarded the prospect of war with dread, knowing that his medical training would be delayed still more. At Oxford he had in eighteen months satisfied the course requirements for the first two years of medical school. Now he had two more years ahead at Johns Hopkins in Baltimore before earning his M.D. And after that, no doubt, a year or two of internship. At twenty-five, he was restless to be done with the preliminaries, frustrated at finding himself so much further from completing his studies than most of his Princeton classmates. He was also growing anxious to resolve the uncertainty in his relationship with Helen. She was waiting patiently enough, but he wanted to marry, have children, be a real and respected doctor, live in a big house and enter a state of grace—in short, to be Sir William Osler, without delay.

When September came, Wilder said good-bye to his mother and to Helen, who was going off to college in Milwaukee, and set off for Baltimore. Johns Hopkins was to be a sharp contrast to the rather relaxed pace of studies at wartime Oxford. When the first few weeks had passed, he wrote to his mother that he wished the other students wouldn't seem so bright and mature. "There seems to be no 'dud,' no one who will cheer me by knowing less or learning more slowly than I."

Considered then the best medical school in the United States, Johns Hopkins trained doctors through a rigorous combination of lectures and lab work, and on-the-spot apprenticeship. A legacy of Osler, who had helped establish the program of medical studies, the Johns Hopkins teaching method involved the students' following the doctor or surgeon around the wards and departments of the hospital from bed to bed, in effect learning about diagnosis by diagnosing patients. As the students advanced in this innovative program, they would assist in the treatment. It was effective training, but Wilder found the pace gruelling at first, and his slow progress discouraging. "At night from my window," Wilder wrote home, "I can see way across Baltimore these letters in electric lights: POWER. And I often think it stands for the thing I am seeking every day in my books and lectures, and yet I always seem further away from it."

Wilder's letters home throughout the fall of 1916 continued to reflect the changes that followed his brush with death on board the *Sussex*. One of the changes was a growing curiosity about himself and the influences that had shaped him. Prompted by an essay he was writing for a course in psychiatry taught by the famous Adolf Meyer, he wrote to his mother summing up her influence on him. "Certainly it has been the biggest factor in my life. Way back I can remember your telling me to be an 'out and outer' before I left for Spokane. I'd never heard the expression. But you said, 'the boys will not laugh at you, but will respect you.' It was that that decided me to say my prayers on my knees up at Priest Lake, even if the other boys did see me. A talk from you started me to thinking about Oxford. Your ideal of Christian Service gradually, and to an imperfect degree, became mine. Your sane view of the Bible and religion helped me through a year of doubt at Princeton as well as a letter or two written by you at that time, and it *was* a critical time. It has always been your wise suggestions at the right moment that were the most important determining factor in each doubtful formative crisis...."

But as Wilder grew older his relationship with Jean began to change. Although he still asked for her advice, it was more and more out of habit. And his mother, for her part, was turning to him more and more as an advisor, and even as a confessor. Wilder wrote to Helen about it after Jean came back to Baltimore with him for a visit:

"I was set to write you last night but Mother needed a good long talk so after I had worked some we talked several hours. You said when she was planning to come that there would be need of sympathy and time and I thought of it last night. She has come to a time of change. My father was not the man who could lead her. She was the stronger and the result was the usual one. He was smothered, gave up trying to live up to her standards, turned to others and finally let go. Mother had to become then both father and mother to us. She could not be the quiet, resigned type then, she must be a doer. And now has come the time when her children have grown up & become emancipated. The school which she really created and dominated has grown up, or Jack & Will have, and now her work there is at an end. And now she has the different woman's role to play. She may let the struggling slip and learn what the peace a faith such as hers should bring. Its a bit hard and often, I think, a claw of bitter memory comes out of the later years in Spokane to make her still writhe a little from the pain of an old wound. Think of going to your best friend and hearing in her delirium the evidence of your husband's infidelity...."

As Wilder's and his mother's roles slowly reversed, Helen's became more and more the voice Wilder heeded. After returning to Baltimore for the winter term, having spent much time with Helen over Christmas in 1916, the couple's correspondence reflected a new intimacy and a deep yearning for the magic world they created when together, that even the presence of Wilder's mother could not, for once, dispel. He was all too aware that as his relationship with Helen developed he was leaving his mother behind for the first time, and that realization brought pangs of guilt. "It seems queer I could get the homesick feeling with mother here," he wrote. "But that is what it was & is."

That winter and spring, a flood of letters poured between Wilder and Helen. They resolved to write each other in French to practise, and he mooned as effectively in that language as he did in English.

They had long since decided to wait until Wilder had finished his medical training and could support them, and he had already laid plans to return to France during the holidays the next summer. Then, in April of 1917, two events changed the outlook drastically. On April 6, America declared war on Germany, and the trip to France seemed an even more perilous prospect than before. A few days later a letter came from Wilder's older brother, Herbert, who knew of their impatience to get married. If he wished, Herbert wrote, Wilder could borrow against his share of Grandfather Jefferson's estate—enough for the two of them to live while he completed his studies and internship.

That was all Wilder needed. On April 20 he sent off a special delivery letter to Helen at Milwaukee Downer College, where she was studying: "Dear Helen. Will you marry me? No 'sometime' or 'after years.' Will you marry me in June and sail with me June 9th for Paris? It rests only with you...." There was a certain element of risk in crossing the Atlantic now that America was in the war, but "to go down together would be better than for one to go alone it seems to me."

Helen agreed. A date was set for early June and Helen went to the dean of the college to ask for permission to shorten her course so she could go with Wilder to France. The dean listened to her pleas and agreed with a sigh and a bit of practical advice: "Don't forget to bring your rubbers, my dear."

The wedding was held at the Kermotts' in Hudson on a rainy evening early in June. The house and the wide porches overlooking the river were filled with white flowers: lilacs, spirea, honeysuckle, lily of the valley and white roses shining through green leaves and candlelight. Many of their old friends came with husbands and wives and babies, many of the young men in freshly-issued uniforms, slapping each other on the back and talking eagerly about the war. After the service the old crowd gathered on the porch to sing together for the last time, and to say good-bye.

Three days later, on July 9, 1917, the newlyweds boarded the *Espagne*, bound for Bordeaux and thence to Paris, where the American Red Cross Hospital had set up new quarters in an old mansion on Rue Piccini. Helen would work at the hospital too, as an auxiliary nurse—rolling bandages and working in the hospital surgical supplies room.

And what of the marriage in those first few months? Although in retrospect the marriage has an air of inevitability—preceded as it was by five years of serious flirtation and a three-year engagement neither Wilder nor Helen were prepared for the sudden intimacy of married life. During their engagement they had been together only a few weeks. They had both changed and grown in three years, with only the gossamer thread of letters to keep pace. Through these *billets doux* proclaiming eternal love, high ideals, and reverence for the sacred (and safely removed) married state, they had loaded the courtship with a burden that marriage was hard pressed to match. "After eight days on shipboard my patience was wearing thin. Perhaps hers was...." Wilder wrote sixty-odd years later. This was not to be a calm and gentle marriage: they were both stubborn, headstrong and touchy, and the difficulties of those first few weeks were a warning of the tempestuous interludes that punctuated their life together from beginning to end. Wilder was forewarned by the disaster of his parents' marriage—a weak and philandering father and a moralistic, driving mother. Helen was the child of a flighty, irresponsible mother and a father who had settled for second best in his career in order to marry young. Aware, perhaps, of how much of each of their parents was in them, Wilder and Helen embarked on marriage determined to impose strict discipline on these wayward genes.

∞ PARIS

Two days out of Bordeaux, the *Espagne* sailed into the war zone—a fact that became suddenly and alarmingly clear to the newlyweds.

"Saturday afternoon I was reading to Helen on deck," Wilder wrote his mother. "She watched something for some little time—a minute or two—and finally called my attention to it. It was a round black object like a pole at the distance of, perhaps, a quarter of a mile, and just even with us. Instead of rising or falling it was horribly steady. It reached about three feet up out of the water and its steadiness made me turn cold. She thought it was moving. I could not be sure. We were broadside to the thing. I tried to believe it a buoy. In two or three minutes our stern gun, a 75 millimetre, went boom! and a pillar of spray rose just beyond. People were dashing downstairs for their preservers. I saw another shot fired and then our bow-gun, a 98 millimetre, got into action and the water rose like a geyser very close to the periscope.—I went below for the preservers. The booming continued. People ran back and forth but smiled and called out to one another. We were going very fast and in a crooked course. On deck the passengers, in their preservers, were gathering nearer their appointed boat places. We went to our place. Some women were crawling into complete rubber suits—waterproof from feet to neck where the head emerged. The feet were weighted and padding full of air over the shoulders. They presented very grotesque figures. No passengers saw any torpedo.

"That night a very great many, especially ambulance drivers of whom there were over 200 on board, slept in their deck chairs. But we went below, only arranging our clothes as a fireman might. Helen's big, heavy coat was very useful. She was as cool as could be."

They arrived safely on June 18, tired and strained from the crossing, and caught the train to Paris. For Helen this unusual honeymoon was her first trip outside of the United States, and she was, at first, nonplussed. "Arrived in Paris we could get no vehicle for some time till I left Helen a minute to get a taxi from a nearby throughfare," Wilder wrote. "I found her saying 'non, non' to the most disreputable old ruffian who was trying to carry her bags to the subway or carriage or something. She said he was the third she had repelled...."

The war had changed France dramatically since Wilder was last there, a year before. Of the hotel in the Latin Quarter where they stayed at first (for ninety cents a day), he remarked, "I'd been there before and knew it to be quiet and nice. Now—it was dark of course but the carpet was worn. The old landlord had been succeeded by his daughter whom we found puzzling over accounts with a soldier. They announced that there was no warm water and never would be. They have ceased to pretend to keep up and there is a feeling of we're up against it, let's make no pretense."

The large American colony in Paris included a number of Princeton friends and others Wilder had met in 1916 in Ris Orangis. An American couple, the Christies, acted as surrogate parents to the young Americans who flooded in during the early years of the war to volunteer as ambulance drivers, hospital orderlies and Red Cross workers. Mr. Christie was associated with an American life insurance company, and he and his wife held frequent parties and dinners for the volunteers, took them in when they needed a place to stay temporarily, consoled them, used their influence to disentangle the intimidating web of French bureaucracy when necessary, and were known to their young friends as Ma and Pa Christie.

"Mr. Christie says there is a class here who get along perfectly well, the rich are not growing any poorer but the soldiers' families fare not so well," Wilder explained to Jean soon after their arrival in Paris, in a letter describing how he and Helen had found, through Mrs. Christie's efforts, a nice room that would be their first home. "As I write now, Helen is straightening her stuff. I'd no idea a girl could use so many little things, all of them indispensable, apparently. Our room is big, running water and lots of mirrors. Through the two big French windows come the clump-clump of horses' feet or whirr of a machine in a nearby street, or there comes a buzzing from an aeroplane and, far up above we can see the airman rising to start like a big fly buzzing over the trenches 50 miles away."

"We are quickly growing accustomed to things," he wrote a few weeks after arriving in Paris. "Aeroplanes overhead, war bread, mourning, foreign tongues—and even each other." At the Red Cross Hospital, Wilder worked in a ward under the supervision of a doctor, changing dressings in the morning and assisting in the operating room in the afternoon. Helen was in charge of the linen department, and each morning after breakfast in their room they set off arm in arm for the fifteen-minute walk through the fashionable sixteenth *Arrondissement* to the hospital.

Early in July the first American troops landed in France and Paris celebrated. The war had devastated both sides; the Germans, rumour maintained, were starving, and the French were faring little better. America's entry was expected to bring the conflict to a quick and victorious end for the Allies. All of the Americans in the hospital were given the day off and Wilder and Helen eagerly made their way to the cemetery where the troops were to decorate LaFayette's

Tomb, a gesture to acknowledge America's historical debt to France.

"...at the gate of exit we found a great mob surging. I asked one of the gendarmes if Pershing was coming that way and he said no, they were getting placed for his exit. There were more women than men. They appeared to be working women and girls. Almost all had bouquets of flowers. As we watched they came running from somewhere and lined the street for several blocks. Flag vendors passed back and forth till everyone wore the stars and stripes. How they chattered and laughed and crowded! Over the street corner was suspended a banner which said 'Welcome to the American soldiers—Long Live America.' By making a detour we reached the other side of the cemetery just in time to hear the roll of a drum coming up the street.

"Fortunately, being of a taller race, we could see over the heads of the crowd. First came some French poilus in faded blue, then a mounted French guard which wears the same uniform as in the days of Napoleon. Big helmets and plumes of horse tail. Then came the khaki. Even as I write a chill runs down my back. Then I could hardly contain myself. First Pershing, looking strong and fine, on horseback followed by his staff. They bowed and smiled at the shouts of applause which preceded them down the street.

"On returning to our rooms Madame Combes asked us with some anxiety 'Are they going to bring their own food?' There's the rub."

Every day Wilder and Helen eagerly read through the American papers for news of what was going on at home. In the frenzy as America geared up for war, anyone who spoke of peace was at least "a slacker," probably a socialist. Wisconsin, a state that had vigorously opposed America's entry into the war, rushed to declare its patriotism the moment war was declared. It was the first state to pass legislation endorsing the declaration and the first to fill its quota of recruits. Even Hudson had its brief moment of glory on the front page of the European edition of the New York *Herald*. One morning early in September, as Wilder and Helen were eating breakfast, they spied the following story:

"Much amusement has been caused in America by the attempts of the People's Council of America to hold a peace convention. After Milwaukee had refused to permit the meeting, as likely to cause rioting, a small trainload of pacifists had been touring the Middle West seeking to hire a hall.

"After Minneapolis had refused to harbor them, Hudson, Wisconsin, whither they emigrated from Minneapolis, forcibly ejected them. When Mr. Louis P. Löchner, the organizer of Mr. Ford's peace mission to neutrals, arrived in Hudson with the Peace Council leaders, they were met by a determined band of citizens who forced them to listen to a number of speeches opposing peace, and then bundled them back to the train and commanded them to betake themselves elsewhere. No violence was offered to the pacifists, though cries were raised in the crowd in favor of pillorying them.

"At the same time that Wisconsin was dealing summarily with the German peace talkers," the article went on, "a large audience in New York was vociferously cheering Mr. Roosevelt, who declared that men of the type of Senators Stone and La Follette [of Wisconsin] should be sent back to Germany, where they properly belonged."

On reading this bit of news Wilder wrote to his mother, "I thought that if Jack [commissioned as Captain in the U.S. Army] was there, perhaps he would be speaking, and I'm sure Herbert was there and speaking his mind, and Helen wondered if her father was there...."

The news that Will McQuarrie, the principal of Galahad, received a captain's commission arrived shortly in a letter from home, and Wilder learned, too, that a draft notice had arrived in the mail for him. "Two captain brothers and I a conscript! Why in the name of Heaven don't you or Herbert write me about that draft?" he wrote to his mother. "I shall not go around pleading exemption. If they would rather have me as a combatant private, I suppose I'll have to go. But there is no glamour about the thing for me, and I feel that I am doing my duty anyway."

Wilder's duty at the hospital was becoming more and more interesting; in the last month he had begun doing minor operations himself, removing pieces of shell and shrapnel. In addition, he reported, "I am now doing carpentry work on an apparatus to elevate a whole man." The man was suffering from a broken hip and an infected wound, which made moving him about to change dressings and bedding extremely painful.

The apparatus Wilder built was a success, and Dr. Blake, the head of the hospital, praised his ingenuity. Soon after, Wilder ended his weekly letter home, "Address me at the hospital, and you might put the Dr. on as Blake wants me to act as such, and I go by that title." And a few days later: "Well, what do you think I am now? Clothed in khaki, a Red Cross uniform only, but bearing three stripes of a captain. We are never addressed as Captain, but doctors take that rank in Red Cross. I bought the uniform of one of the doctors here, as he was getting a U.S. uniform. He sold it to me for $10,.... I went all over Paris buying the belt, cap, khaki shirts, ties, collars and socks. Now it seems better. One is not so conspicuous in uniform. I'd like to go downtown and see if anyone will salute me."

Despite these small vanities, Wilder welcomed the arrival of a new doctor to take charge of the ward. "I want to work under a good man. I don't give a whoop about being in charge of anything. I want to learn." However, now that a real doctor had taken over, Wilder was no longer called Doctor Penfield, and far from having charge of an entire floor of the hospital as before, he suddenly found himself back in the shoes of a lowly medical student. The new arrival, Wilder wrote, "at times takes great pleasure in emphasizing the *Mr.* instead of Dr. He was very nasty, but is better now. Oh well, I'll get along but I wish I had my degree—or never heard the title of Doctor."

With winter came other frustrations. No heating was permitted before November 1, despite the bitter cold and damp, and a fire in the grate was "the rarest, most expensive, beautiful and soul-satisfying thing in Paris!" The war news was discouraging. Although by the end of 1917 some 200,000 American soldiers were in France, their arrival had not magically turned the tide, as the optimists had predicted. In October, the Italian army suffered a defeat at the hands of the Austrians, and the Allies were obliged to hurry troops from the Western Front to help the Italians push the enemy back.

And Helen, who they thought had been suffering from fatigue, turned out to be pregnant, a matter of great joy, of course, and some concern. "This is going to be a hard winter in Paris," Wilder wrote. "Sugar can only be gotten on ration cards now, and not always then. Coal many cannot get at all, and there is now a rule that hot water for washing and baths, which is only allowed twice a week, shall only be a certain temperature. Wood is rare. There is no coal in the *departments* outside of Paris. There are bread cards now, though the quality of the war bread is not so bad as during the summer.

"Meatless days have been given up but sweetless days (2) still exist and no milk, or anything containing it may be sold after 9 A.M. There will be much suffering as prices are going up. Yet the French seem absolutely resolute, although they talk and find fault with their government. Germany seems to have started for Petrograd on the sea route. It makes the war outlook very gloomy. Years perhaps."

Although Wilder had planned to work through the winter and defer returning to Johns Hopkins for his degree, the older doctors advised him to go back home and finish his training. Paraphrasing the advice in a letter, Wilder reported, "Any young man who has remained at home can be pardoned for joining the army on graduation and before he has an internship, because he doesn't know. But you have had a chance to see how many men of experience we have here, and can see the need at home. You ought to take your internship after graduating.

"Dr. Taylor came in and agreed with him [the older doctor], but added 'It's easier to join the army.' Another Dr. interposed 'After the war will come the greatest competition and upset the country ever saw. All these doctors now drawing $2,000-$4,000 will be dumped onto the country to earn a living. Only those well equipped will weather the storm. Right now every hospital is begging for interns. They have to have them. There is much greater need for me to be back home than there is here.'"

Finally, with some reluctance, Wilder cabled Johns Hopkins to see if they would accept him late, and when an affirmative reply came he and Helen booked passage on the S.S. *Rocambeau* leaving Bordeaux for New York at the end of November, 1917. They left Paris by train early on a bitterly cold Sunday morning. Even as the train sped through the gently rolling countryside between Paris and Bordeaux, where the leaves of the oak trees had turned to copper, the soldiers and other passengers "began to look strange and foreign to us, just because we were going home and already looked through the eyes of the man across the sea," wrote Wilder.

∞ THE HIGH ROAD

Despite a passenger list that included no less than seven American generals and the redoubtable Winston Churchill, then minister of munitions, the S.S. *Rocambeau* safely made harbour in New York on the morning of November 26. Wilder and Helen collected their luggage, stopped long enough to celebrate their return with a meal of "Ham sandwiches with white, white bread, *real coffee*, and fresh cream, cakes and syrup" at the lunch counter in Pennsylvania Station before heading for Baltimore.

During the next two years their lives followed the traditional path of married medical students and interns of modest means: for Wilder the routine meant long hours, exhausting work and fierce competition; for Helen it meant loneliness, cramped apartments, boredom and, soon, a baby as sole companion for much of the time. Hovering nearby always was insecurity about the future: would Wilder do well enough to be admitted as an intern? Where? What should he choose as his specialty? Who would be his next teacher and inspiration? Although Osler and Sherrington were the guiding lights in his firmament, Wilder was always on the lookout for men of stature to apprentice himself to, men who could teach him what he needed to know. But all this took time—would the money hold out?

Against all these odds, the couple survived and even flourished. Helen took the threadbare existence in her stride, knowing it would pass. "The week we spent apartment hunting was disagreeable work but I was as happy as I have ever been," Wilder reported in his weekly letter. "Helen and I are coming to understand each other better all the time, and it means more to me every day. I'm glad Helen is just the girl she is. She is so capable that she is always a help, not a drag, and she is not going to slow down my work the way many wives do. I am awfully proud to have Mrs. Finney and my old friends here know Helen. Oh, well, I'm glad we are hitting the trail together."

Helen wrote regularly to Jean as well: "Yesterday I mended some kind of a diagram about 9 ft. by 3 ft. And last night I sat up in bed and listened to a lecture on the subject. I was surprised at how interesting it could be made. And I love to hear him present a case. He gets so interested, talks so clearly, states the thing so logically."

At Johns Hopkins, medical students were permitted to select their own course of work for the final trimester before exams. Wilder had done well in his physiology classes, and his professor Dr. William Howell offered to pay him $100 to perform demonstrations for first-year students. Wilder agreed and, since Howell was chairman of the U.S. senate committee investigating the best ways of treating shell-shock, asked if he could undertake some research for the committee. The most promising investigations at the time were in replacing blood by other substances in order to raise blood pressure. Howell complied and assigned Wilder his first research project: injecting gum arabic into the veins of dogs and studying their reactions. He also suggested Wilder try injecting "anything you think of," Wilder reported to his mother with excitement. "I shall have a chance for some latitude. Now that is what I've been hoping for; to be given a real problem and the assurance that if the work be completed it will help the cause for which I am not yet fighting, and it makes my late internship all right, too, you see. I probably can't get any startling results, but it is the sort of thing I am most interested in."

At the end of May Wilder took his final exam, and a week later Wilder Jr. was born. Sitting in the waiting-room Wilder scribbled a note to his mother. "Waiting! And as at all such times my thoughts turn to you, for I know you understand and think in the same range with me. She is a wonderful woman, mother....I was rather dazed, you remember, at the wedding? The same feeling has returned to me now. I can't realize what's happening in the outside world. And again it seems as though I were playing football and had been hit on the head enough to daze and only leave me the consciousness that I must go on playing. That was an old feeling in football, but now there is *nothing to do.*"

Two weeks later he had recovered sufficiently to joke: "We brought Helen home on Thursday, and the boy tagged along as though he were permanent."

A doctor at long last, Wilder forged ahead through the summer with his research, occasionally exasperated, but more often feeling that he was making real headway. "I've rigged up some apparatus to follow the pressure in the veins as well as in the arteries," he reported to his mother. Although the results weren't definite, they were encouraging nonetheless. "Of the five dogs done last week, one died on the table [and] the others wag their tails in their cages when I approach. Each lost from 75-85% of his blood, and none has an infection."

In September, 1918, Wilder, Helen and the baby went to Boston, where Wilder had been accepted for a year's internship at Peter Bent Brigham Hospital. Shortly after arriving, Wilder finished writing up his report on the blood-pressure experiments and, feeling some foreboding, sent it to Dr. Howell. "Now that it is finished it seems so inadequate, so incomplete and it does not agree with Dr. Bayless in England nor Dr. Cannon," Wilder's letter home warned. "I do not think Dr. Howell will do anything with it."

But he was in for a surprise. Not only did Dr. Howell approve the thoroughness of Wilder's experiments and conclusions, he arranged to have the report published in the *American Journal of Physiology.* Wilder sent copies to Dr. Finney, Sir William Osler and others: "I feel proud even though my first born is ugly and rather misshapen," he confessed. Osler responded with characteristic warm encouragement: "Dear Penfield, That is a very nice paper—congratulations. When you are an old man—no hurry—you will look on it with much pleasure. It is always nice to start with something good. That primary constriction in the vessels is interesting...." By the time Osler received the reprint of the report Germany had surrendered. In the lull that followed the victory celebrations, Wilder realized he must decide what to do at the end of his surgical internship in Boston. Late in November, he wrote to his mother to explain the plans that were slowly evolving in his mind. "With peace comes the freedom to make plans for one's own future. Helen and I shall go on for several years, at least three, working in hospitals. It should be longer but will depend on how long we can keep the wolf from the door.

"The old choice comes up, for immediate practice and income or to aim farther toward real excellence and a greater stake. Helen is all for playing for the bigger sphere—and so am I. So we shall postpone practice for as long as maybe, and eventually work in a big place in association with a big hospital if we are lucky.

"Helen told me this morning about Dr. [Helen's father—known simply as "Dr."] and Dr. Sippi. They went abroad to study together, to Vienna. Both on the same footing. Dr. Kermott was quicker with the language and did more and faster laboratory work. On returning to America he was impatient for a practice and income at once, and went to a small town where one goes fast.

"Sippi returned to Chicago, got into association with the University, and hadn't a cent, nor, hardly, a patient, for years and years while Dr. flourished.

"At present, from other sources, I know Sippi has perhaps the largest gastroenterology practice in the country, is a Professor at Chicago and his name is a household word among doctors when they speak of medical treatment of gastric ulcers—The Sippi Treatment. I may never be a Sippi, but I'd like to try it. It isn't the money, (I'd guess his income at $100,000 a year, perhaps) but its the big sphere of influence and the doing something that appeals to me. Success—whatever that is."

Although the decision to specialize rather than go into general practice was now made, Wilder had yet to decide on a specialty. He was in a peculiar position. On the one hand he loved doing research, and found it a field where his dogged, meticulous habits and his ingenuity, developed during years of trying to keep up in a highly competitive field of study, served him extremely well. On the other hand he wanted to be a surgeon. He was still a very physical young man. He liked using his hands, and he was fascinated by the power surgeons held: the power to heal, to enter into battle with disease armed with a surgeon's knife. Dr. Finney, one of his heroes, was a surgeon of international fame. And the practical consideration of the disparity between the incomes of researchers and surgeons weighed in the balance.

Wilder needed peace and quiet when he had an important decision to make, and few were as important as this one. So in March he and Helen left Wilder Jr. with a friend and spent two weeks in a little cottage at the seashore in Rhode Island. "Here we are, having a glorious time," Wilder reported. "We arrived yesterday in a pouring rain—it had rained for three days. Today it has developed into a nor-easter, blowing a perfect gale, with rain that stings your face.

But I borrowed a saw and axe and we scoured the sea coast for logs, and now we have a dandy fire in the grate. I saw wood, eat, read, sleep—with a good pard.—Pretty nice."

During their retreat, Wilder and Helen talked at length about the various possibilities for the future and, by the time they returned, had agreed that Wilder should aim for brain surgery. To some degree, according to Wilder's own memory of it, the decision was provoked by his observation of Dr. Cushing in brain surgery. Wilder had spent many hours in the last six months assisting Cushing during brain operations and making rounds to tend to his patients. At the end of the day Wilder would come home and fill notebook after notebook with his observations of Cushing's innovative techniques and making notes to himself on how he thought they could be improved. He had been much impressed by Cushing, despite the surgeon's abrupt manner—as well he might be. Cushing was considered the best brain surgeon in the world, and thanks to him brain surgery was slowly gaining acceptance as a specialty. As Wilder would write in *No Man Alone,* "Cushing had proven, or rather was in the process of proving, to the world that although brain surgery had become the most dramatic and dangerous of specialties, it could be carried out with a reasonably low death rate. In a sense, he had succeeded in making the specialty respectable in the eyes of the public and, at the same time, had given it dramatic lustre.

"But Cushing's patients were largely sufferers from brain tumor or from painful neuralgia. These conditions interested me little at that time. On the other hand, the memory of the 'undiscovered country' I had glimpsed through Sherrington's student lectures did intrigue me greatly. It was something I could not forget. Cushing was showing the world *how* to be a brain surgeon. Perhaps, I thought, if I could return to Oxford for graduate study and learn what was known about the neurophysiology of animals, I might gain a broader view of man, find more instructive approaches to human neurosurgery. I wanted to know all that was known about the human brain, neuropathology, neuroanatomy, neurocytology. Then, I argued, I would learn clinical neurology and finally go on to the operative technique of neurosurgery."

Such an approach to surgery of the brain was unheard of in 1918. Brain surgeons usually came to their specialty through general surgery, not from laboratory study and clinical neurology. Clinical neurologists were inclined to regard neurosurgeons with suspicion; their field was studying patients with disorders, diagnosing the causes and recommending treatment—usually drugs or something less dangerous than radical surgery. Surgeons, for their part, pointed out the limitations of other treatments, and in the case of disorders such as tumours, which often killed the patients anyway, argued that neurosurgery was better than nothing.

In such an atmosphere of mutual mistrust, what Wilder was suggesting was almost heretical. A neurosurgeon who could confidently do his own basic research and lab tests, and diagnose his own patients, would be neither fish nor fowl. He would have to prove himself both to neurologists and neurosurgeons and, in a sense, his success would be a rebuke to both.

This was Wilder's first challenge to conventional wisdom in his chosen field, but it would not be his last. And like many of the other challenges he would issue, this one had the rare mark of inspiration. By the success of his example in the years ahead he would pave the way for generations of scientifically trained neurosurgeons to come.

Money was the only stumbling block to a return to Oxford to work with Sherrington. Although in theory Wilder had one year left of his Rhodes Scholarship, the rules were that Rhodes Scholars had to be single. Nonetheless, Wilder wrote to the Rhodes Trust and a few weeks later learned that in his case the trustees had made a special ruling "in view of the war and my part in it." When he reported the exciting news to his mother, her enthusiastic support for this adventure prompted Wilder to ask her if she wouldn't like to make the trip with them, and to his surprise she said Yes.

Wilder wrote Sherrington to ask if he'd be welcome, and early in September a brief telegram came saying simply, "Laboratory delighted accommodate you stop." And so, on October 1, 1919, Wilder, Helen, Jean, Wilder Jr. and Ruthmary, born ten weeks earlier, set sail from Boston aboard the S.S. *Winifredian,* "a ship that was slow and steady and cheap."

Little coaxing was needed to convince Jean to join them on this trip. She had spent the last few years tending Ruth, who had been frequently and mysteriously unwell. But with Ruth's husband, Jack Inglis, back from the war, Jean was finally free to pursue her own interests. She brought a portable typewriter, determined to write "movie scenarios." Though none of these efforts seem to have survived, she did keep a voluminous scrapbook of the year she spent in Oxford with her son and daughter-in-law. Snapshots of Jean on board ship show her on deck in a heavy coat, staring at the lens with a determined and unyielding look. She had never lost the air of being one of the intellectual and spiritual leaders of a small town, a woman who felt she'd been destined for better things, prepared to suffer silently—but not too silently. "Our fellow shipmates were mostly

Irish and English people of little education," she wrote. "About the only ones with whom we became acquainted were the ones at our table—called by ourselves the *Elite*, by some of the others the *Intellectuals*."

"During twelve days of rest and relaxation at sea" Wilder wrote many years later, "my purpose in life took clearer shape. Life had changed for me. I had someone with whom to share the planning now. Indeed, my wife had brought me certainty and an unexpected kind of security. Even if my professional career did not work out as planned, there could never be a better life than this!"

Oxford, Wilder discovered, was a different place now that the war was over. For one thing, Sir William Osler, "the man who had been my first friend there," was ill. "When I called at 13 Norham Gardens, sounds were strangely hushed," he recalled. "Some weeks before, while driving across England to see a patient in consultation—it was during the great railway strike—he had caught cold and come down with pneumonia. Complications had followed. He was in bed at home now, dying."

The Penfields found lodgings in town, and Wilder paid a visit to Professor Sherrington. "I told him my all-embracing plan. He nodded when I said I hoped to master all of the basic approaches to the nervous system! He might well have laughed aloud, but he only smiled. Then he added quietly, 'You could perhaps begin by helping me to study a problem that puzzles me in regard to the reflex action of a cat's hind leg.'"

The idea of being a partner in Sherrington's research was thrilling, but after a few experiments, Sherrington was elected president of the Royal Society of London, and suddenly had no time to continue his research at Oxford. For partnership Wilder turned instead to Sherrington's two assistants, joining Cuthbert Bazett in an experimental study of decerebrate rigidity, and Harry M. Carleton in research studies of the microscopical structure of the nervous system.

Perhaps the most important thing Wilder learned at Oxford in that year of graduate study was how to carry out research, although needless to say he did not "cover the whole field of neurophysiology."

By summer, 1920, Jean had decided to go home. She and Helen had got along remarkably well during Wilder's frequent absences, but her constant enthusiasms had been exhausting, and both Wilder and Helen welcomed the peace and quiet that followed. By now, most of Wilder's and Helen's relatives had made their way west to California. Jean, Ruth and her family, Herbert and his, had all become permanent Californians; there were no Jeffersons and Penfields left in Hudson, Wisconsin. A few years later, Helen's parents joined the exodus, so that no roots on either side were left in the midwest.

By the time of his mother's departure, Wilder was spending more and more time in London. When the Rhodes Scholarship ran out, Sherrington applied for a Beit Memorial Fellowship on Wilder's behalf. The fellowship was granted, and Wilder decided to continue his graduate studies in the city where he could use the medical libraries as a resource while he spent the next year learning the art of neurological diagnosis.

In 1920, the National Hospital at Queen Square in London boasted some of the best neurologists in the world—a new generation that had replaced the pioneers, Jean-Martin Charcot, Sir David Ferrier, Hughlings Jackson and others, who had established the specialty of clinical neurology. The leader of the new generation, Gordon Holmes, was an amiable and unpretentious Irishman who became Wilder's friend and mentor; Holmes and his wife Rosalie would introduce the Penfields to their favourite form of relaxation, three- and four-day rowing expeditions on the Thames.

Though Holmes and the other London neurologists subsisted on their private practice, on certain days of the week they would see patients without fee in the Queen Square public wards, and conduct teaching clinics there.

A sign would appear on the bulletin board at the hospital: "Dr. Holmes [or another] will examine patients at 2 o'clock," and graduate students from around the world would come to learn the art of neurological diagnosis. "These graduate students," Wilder wrote in *No Man Alone*," were well aware that the key to diagnosis was knowledge of the complicated functional pathways of the brain and spinal cord. Diagnosis would make it possible to label, and then, at least, to comfort and guide these patients—even if no physician anywhere had, as yet, learned to cure the ailment."

Gordon Holmes' teaching clinic, Wilder continued, "showed me what neurological teaching could be, at its best." He went on to describe one of Holmes' clinics in detail as an example:

"On the tick of two, the door burst open and Gordon Holmes entered. He stood for a moment while he inspected his audience, tall and erect with black eyes and dark curly hair. When the resident physician wheeled the patient into the room, Holmes sat down abruptly in the single seat reserved for him in the front row.

"The patient, in a dressing gown, sat upright before him. Thus, Holmes faced her squarely, as everyone else did, while the light from the high windows over his shoulder fell upon her.

"She was an appealing young Cockney woman. As she entered, she looked up, frightened to see the audience. But Holmes spoke, and she looked back at him, and continued to keep her eyes on him throughout the interview as if she had forgotten the others. She needed help and this man gave the impression that he would give her help if there was help to give.

"We realized that Gordon Holmes was seeing this young woman for the first time. There was no time to lose since another patient must be seen before the end of the period. When Holmes examined, there was always a sense of urgency. There must be no mistakes, no misunderstanding. A life could hang in the balance.

"He questioned and we heard the patient make a simple statement of her complaints. It was simple, perhaps in spite of herself, guided as she was by this compelling interrogator.

"'Notice the smile,' Holmes remarked in a clearly audible undertone. 'Notice, too, that the angle of the mouth moves less actively on the left than on the right when she laughs. You remember that she told me she has lost consciousness on several occasions. She told me too that each time she did so, it was preceded by difficulty in finding her words. She was aphasic.'

"Then to the woman, he said, 'Are you left-handed?'

"'Yes,' she replied.

"Holmes drew the dressing gown aside and asked her to lean back against the chair. He broke a thin wooden spatula and used the tapering end as a wand to stroke the abdomen.

"'When I stroke the skin,' he said to us, 'here on the right side of the abdomen, the umbilicus moves to the right quite briskly. Not so on the left. There is only a flicker there in the upper quadrant. In the left lower quadrant, the abdominal reflex is absent.'

"He scratched the soles of her feet with the spatula; glanced back at us, then turned and stroked them, once more, with great attention.

"'I think Babinski's sign is positive on the left,' he said. 'The great toe makes a small abnormal movement upward there, but not on the right.'

"He talked to the woman then with brief kindness, and asked the clinical clerk to prescribe phenobarbital to protect her from more of the attacks. As she left the room he turned to us.

"'So much to live for, with a husband and two little children! The attacks are epileptic. The cause is a lesion in the cerebral cortex of the right cerebral hemisphere. Like most left-handed people, the speech area is in the cortex of the right instead of in the left hemisphere.'

"He made a drawing on the board to show what he believed to be the limits of the speech area and the pathway of the motor tracts. Even slight interference with these tracts by any sort of lesion would cause the reflex abnormality he had demonstrated by scratching the abdomen and the sole of the foot on the left, and the underaction of the smile on the left. Then he drew the location of the lesion where it was causing the epileptic attacks.

'What is the lesion?' he asked. 'It can be an abnormality of a blood vessel or it could be a scar. But I'm afraid this is a tumor. It is located too near to the speech and the motor area for me to call in the surgeons safely.' Although he did not say it in so many words, it was clear he felt he must protect the patient from the blundering of a surgeon.

"I would never be content, I thought, to be such a neurological surgeon. I must learn what was known about two subjects: pathological lesions, and neuroanatomy. Finally, someday, I would study two other things: the mystery of epilepsy, and how the human brain does what it does."

Attending the clinics at Queen Square and visiting various research laboratories around London occupied much of the spring of 1920. But in order to qualify for his research degree (B.Sc.) from Oxford, Wilder had to keep an official place of residence there, so he would bicycle out from London at the end of each week, some fifty-miles uphill and down. Helen would frequently bicycle out twenty miles or so to meet him on the London road, and they would stop at a roadside inn and have tea together. Wilder had devised saddles and stirrups for the bicycles so that Wilder Jr. and Ruthmary could be taken along, howling with delight as they raced down the hills.

In mid-December Wilder received his B.Sc. from Oxford, and a few days later the family moved to London. They had found a small but comfortable flat forty minutes from Queen Square where Wilder was conducting most of his research, and were lucky enough to get a maid to wash the dishes and clean the flat: a living-room, nursery, bedroom and shared kitchen and bath.

These were happy times for Wilder and Helen from all the evidence of letters and memories. During this period they developed friendships among the young London doctors and their wives, like Gordon and Rosalie Holmes, that would prove to be lasting.

Still they were anxious to return home to America. Wilder was eager to practise the knowledge he was acquiring with such painstaking effort. "It is such a little thing that turns the scale in brain operations, and I see things done even by [Percy] Sargent [chief surgeon at Queen Square], who is a splendid surgeon, which I, personally, think are the causes of an occasional death. That sounds egotistical no doubt. At any rate, in the next 30 years I believe there will be great strides in our knowledge of the nervous system and our treatment of it and I want to take part in both changes."

He and Helen were not quite clear where they would settle, finally, but Wilder had been tentatively offered a post at the Ford Hospital in Detroit by Dr. McClure, the medical director. Naturally, the job was contingent on a personal interview with the hospital administrator.

A few weeks later Wilder wrote that plans to return to America were set: "We have reserved passage on the *Olympic*, the largest British steamer, for May 25, crossing in seven days. We have a two-berth cabin with a couch for Wilder, and in that way pay three full fares at the minimum rate of 33£ 15-0, second class. I hope that McClure will not write and say he thinks I had better wait any longer," he added, "as I want to come home. It is partly a longing to be *home* and to be with warm-hearted Americans again."

CHAPTER FIVE ∞∞∞∞∞∞∞∞∞∞∞∞∞∞∞∞∞∞∞∞∞∞∞∞∞

A Young Surgeon to Watch

∞∞ NEW YORK

On June 1, 1921, Wilder and Helen stood together at the railing as the S.S. *Olympia* steamed into New York harbour. They were flat broke, and Wilder had only vague prospects of a job. Still, they were home.

Passing quickly through Customs, the Penfields loaded all their worldly possessions, including two enormous crates of books, into a cab and set off for Pennsylvania Station. Helen was to take the children to Wisconsin to await the outcome of Wilder's interview in Detroit. As the driver navigated through the busy Manhattan traffic, the two of them stared out of the windows in amazement at the way people bumped into each other without apology, the clothes the women wore, the obvious affluence, the easy familiarity and friendliness. Strangest of all, and most disturbing, was the nasal quality of American speech. Suddenly they felt like foreigners.

In the confusion of installing Helen and the babies into one lower berth and getting all the baggage stowed away, Wilder forgot to give her the tickets. After the train pulled out, he discovered them in his overcoat and spent several frantic minutes dashing about the station trying to find someone to set things right. Eventually a ticket-taker made the necessary calls, and after waiting to hear that new tickets had been brought on board at Philadelphia, Wilder stopped cursing himself and started for Boston. The annual meeting of the American Medical Association was being held there, so Wilder had decided earlier to delay his trip to Detroit long enough to renew his American contacts.

On arriving in Boston good news and bad news awaited him. The bad news consisted of discouraging reports about the Ford Hospital: "Ford driven" according to the scuttlebutt, and no animal experimentation permitted because Henry was prejudiced against it. The good news began with a letter from Cuthbert Bazett, now at the University of Pennsylvania, offering Wilder $3,500 a year to teach Physiology. Heartwarming though it was to feel wanted somewhere, Wilder didn't want to teach, and the pay was too little for a family of four. Nonetheless, the invitation would make it possible to explore the Detroit offer with more self-confidence.

While in Boston, Wilder stopped in at Peter Bent Brigham Hospital to visit with Dr. Quinby, the urologist-in-chief, for whom Wilder had done a bit of research during his internship there, three years earlier.

"When Quinby saw me entering his office," Wilder later wrote, "he called, 'Wilder! I thought you would come. We didn't know how to reach you.' The greeting thrilled me. It was good for the lonely, unwanted feeling that had been mine since I landed in New York. 'Allen Whipple,' Quinby continued, 'came here from New York to inquire about you. Great opportunity there—wonderful man, Whipple—just what you want, I'll let him know you've come back.'" Before Wilder even had time to reflect on this unexpected bit of news, a cable arrived from Whipple himself asking Wilder to stop in and talk before heading for Detroit.

Whipple's interest in Wilder developed from a curious stroke of fate. The year before, in Paris, Wilder had met a young doctor named Harry Murray who was attending medical conferences there. Murray was now working as an intern with Whipple, and happened to mention Wilder Penfield and his unusual approach to brain surgery through the basic sciences and clinical neurology. Whipple was intrigued.

The Presbyterian Hospital, of which Allen Whipple was the newly appointed surgical chief and professor of surgery, was in the midst of great upheavals. In the spring of 1921, it had become the primary teaching hospital connected to The College of Physicians and Surgeons (P & S), Columbia University's medical school. Instead of the traditional part-time plan, whereby members of the attending staff of the hospital earned their livings in private practice, the medical and surgical services would become full time, endowed by the Rockefeller Foundation and the General Education Board. And the plans were extended to include a new medical centre that would be built at 168th Street and Broadway on the site of the American League baseball park. The centre would have all modern facilities necessary for medical treatment, research and teaching.

On July 1, all the doctors previously on the attending staff were to resign. Walter Palmer, the young, newly elected physician-in-chief and professor of medicine, was coming from Johns Hopkins and bringing with him a brilliant group of assistants. And Allen Whipple, a young and then relatively unknown product of P & S, was elected to assume command of the surgical service, with only two attending surgeons and two associates. Wilder was being considered for a post as an associate.

When the meeting in Boston was over, Wilder went to New York to see Whipple. Before the interview was through he had been offered the job—"just what I would have conjured up if I had been the possessor of Aladdin's wonderful lamp," he wrote in a letter to his mother two days later, hardly able to control his excitement. "Well here I am in New York, and our star of fate has paused above this hot, thundering city," he began, then went on to describe Whipple's proposal. "I make rounds every morning in some ward, have one special operative morning, (he knows that I will need instruction at first) and operate, some, on other mornings. Have one morning when patients are referred to me!! in the outpatient; give one clinic a week!!! and do *all the neurological surgery*. Best of all the research facilities are great and someone else will prepare my sections, thank goodness. That is for nine months in the year. One month will be for travel to other clinics (possibly on a fund!). One month for vacation and one month for concentration on any research." Whipple explained that the job was being offered to Penfield because of his training in physiology, and that P. & S. was prepared to help him complete his surgical training.

However, the job possibility in Detroit was still pending, and Wilder felt obliged to keep his promise and at least listen to what they had to offer. Fortunately they made it easy for him to refuse. "I saw the Henry Ford Hospital and never have I been more thankful than when I was able to refuse to go there. As far as equipment is concerned the place is the last word, and financially it was a little better, as they offered $5,000 [Whipple had offered $4,500]. We could, probably, live less expensively here too.

"But Liebold the superintendent, Mr. Ford's secretary, is hopeless. I told him I wanted to continue research. McClure urged on him the necessity of providing facilities for research. He was ridiculous. He said, well we have a good laboratory and if there is any problem that needs solving, we will just turn it over to specialists there and we will get these things solved. He talked on about medicine as any conceited ignoramus might. I would get practically no operating, and would do anything the hospital might require from fussing around fussy patients up."

From Detroit Wilder wired Helen at Devil's Lake, Wisconsin, where she and the children were having a holiday with her parents. Detroit was impossible. Would she settle for New York? Or would she prefer Philadelphia, where the offer from Bazett was still open? Her reply was "Timbuktu if you like."

Wilder and Helen were ready to put down some roots. They had been living out of suitcases in rented rooms since they were married in 1917, four years earlier. Wilder Jr. was now three, Ruthmary nearly two, and they would soon have to start thinking about schools.

Writing to his mother in mid-August, Wilder mused, "I wonder if we shall always be here. If all goes well—about 10 years, I should say. Then—who knows? I want 10 good years of undisturbed work professionally, and we want to grow in *somewhere* socially. But this seems a barren and rocky wilderness as far as friends are concerned."

The wilderness was the New York suburb of Yonkers, forty minutes from the hospital by train, where he and Helen had eventually found an apartment they could afford. For $90 a month they rented a small, fourth-floor walk-up with a splendid view of the Hudson River, which was its only redeeming feature. "Along here it looks exactly like the Saint Croix," Wilder wrote to Herbert. "The Palisades are a little higher than the Minnesota shore and the river a little wider, but it is hard to realize it and we get the same kind of sunsets across the river."

His lack of surgical experience made Wilder feel at a disadvantage, which he tried to make up for by working longer and harder. He was gone each day from seven in the morning to seven at night, and home was a badly needed refuge from the long, exhausting hours at the hospital. "I told Whipple, the Chief, I would never bluff a thing I couldn't do," he wrote Herbert on his third day at the hospital. "It is mighty uncomfortable at first, though, to admit the men below me, who of course are often my senior in years, know more about a thing than I do."

Wilder was considered to be the hospital's neurosurgeon from the beginning, but for the first two years he was required to take his turn at general surgery along with the two seniors and the other junior on the surgical staff. From time to time he was also required to make rounds in the surgical ward with the interns and other junior staff members, some of whom had more actual surgical experience. "But only one, an assistant resident, showed the contempt he apparently felt for me, the young attending surgeon who had been set over him. From time to time, I detected a pitying smile—or found myself embarrassed by an unnecessarily awkward question," Wilder recalled in *No Man Alone*.

How to respond? The contempt—real or imagined—was not the sort of thing Wilder's touchy pride would permit him to ignore. "At last, I could take it no longer," he went on. "There are limits to the control of anger. At least there are to mine. After making rounds in the surgical ward one day, I led him to a place where there were no observers. We faced each other alone. 'I need your help to make our service run as it should,' I said. 'From now on you're going to play this game and play it fair. You know very well what I mean.' I had meant to keep cool. But a wave of anger blew off the lid. 'If you don't I'm going to knock your (blank blank) block off and I'd be delighted to do it right now.' It was not an idle threat. I had boxed, and I was strong and fast. He stood for a moment in silence. Then he declared himself to be a loyal member of the team."

Always a fighter, Wilder saw a challenge left unanswered as a sign of cowardice. There is an exhilaration in his accounts of incidents such as this that is rare elsewhere in his diaries and letters, the same exhilaration he felt on the football field in the crunching tackles that were his specialty. By disposition he was not a calm, calculating quarterback; he was a born tackle, a player who had made his mark on the college team for his man-to-man assaults. This account was written over fifty years later, by a man then in his eighties, still smouldering at the contempt. And still (as his description goes on) trying to justify his threat—which must have astounded the assistant resident—of a thumping. "From that moment onward, he put on the garb of admiring respect and we worked together as friends do. I wondered, as years passed and he became a successful surgeon, what thinking went on in the back of his mind. There are, I know, many kinds of respect and differing forms of friendship. Medicine in a large hospital is, after all, something like football. Teamwork and loyalty are essential to success. I am not now excusing myself or suggesting that violence or the threat of violence is always the best approach to harmony. But it did work this time."

However, Wilder's loyalty and dedication to teamwork soon impressed his colleagues. He was prepared to suffer criticism delivered in the spirit of teamwork by someone whom he admired. Just before Christmas, Allen Whipple sent a tactful and appreciative note to his young surgeon. The note thanked Penfield for his "constant and unquestioning support and loyalty since we began the cruise in the Good Ship." Whipple's note continued: "Your standing just as much guff as we could give you and ready to take more. Your steady and constructive improvement in general surgery, your understanding of neurological problems have been a joy to me and the rest of us, but best of all is your interest in and training for original work, and I expect great things of you."

∞∞ FREDERICO

The first patient admitted to Wilder's care was a little Italian boy, Frederico, who was suffering from a brain tumour. The only hope of saving this boy's eyesight, and his life, was an operation to remove the tumour. Rather nervous at the prospect of such an operation, Wilder asked for a consultation from the Department of Neurology. To his surprise, the professor of neurology himself, Frederick Tilney, came to see the boy. He came unannounced and left a note on the patient's chart: "No Operation." Wilder thought the statement arrogant and infuriatingly categorical. Tilney's attitude was precisely what Wilder had encountered at Queen Square Hospital in London: the neurologist knows best and the neurosurgeon must accept his decision as final.

Wilder examined the boy again and called Tilney on the telephone. The pressure from the tumour was growing and would blind the boy in a matter of days or weeks. If they could only locate the tumour exactly, they might risk an operation before it was too late.

It was late at night when Wilder called; Tilney was abrupt and rude. No, he had no time to re-examine the patient with Wilder. The boy would die anyway; an operation would be pointless. Wilder's angry reaction was characteristic: "Frederico was my patient. I would welcome advice. I would not accept dictation." As for Dr. Whipple's reaction to the dispute, he "looked grave when I told him what had happened. He agreed in principle. Next day he talked to Tilney at a meeting of the medical faculty and came to see me afterward. The whole issue of the disposition of the neurological department, he said, 'is to be decided in a few days when the dean of medicine, William Darrach, returns from Europe. Unless there is a real chance to cure the boy or to save his life, please don't push the issue too quickly.'"

Frederico was Wilder's first neurosurgical patient, and this incident the first inkling of trouble ahead with Tilney. By Wilder's account, Tilney wanted to gain control of all neurological and neurosurgical cases in any of the university hospitals. In addition, he wanted all the neurosurgical operations to be carried out under his eyes in the New York Neurological Institute by the Institute's own neurosurgeons. Whipple, for his part, was determined to strengthen the surgical service at the Presbyterian Hospital—it was that plan that had caused him to hire Wilder in the first place. At the end of the week Whipple told Wilder to go ahead with an operation on the boy if he thought it best.

Wilder didn't really know *what* to think. Tilney was probably right: it was hopeless. But Wilder was not quite ready to give up, not with his first patient, not with a little boy when there was the faintest chance of saving his life. If only he could locate the tumour exactly, then he would know whether an operation would kill Frederico. Or worse, leave him crippled, mute, helpless.

While Wilder was studying in Europe, reports of a new procedure called ventriculography had been published by a brain sugeon named Walter Dandy at Johns Hopkins. Dandy claimed the procedure could show the position of a brain tumour with greater accuracy than any existing method. Unfortunately both Harvey Cushing in Boston and Charles Elsberg at the New York Neurological Institute regarded the operation as dangerous and unnecessary. Dandy, for his part, not only showed contempt for the opinion of these two reigning monarchs in the field, but had refused to join the newly formed Society of Neurological Surgeons.

Undeterred by the possible repercussions, Wilder wangled an invitation to Baltimore to watch Dandy perform a ventriculogram, to see for himself. The technique that Dandy was perfecting required the surgeon to insert a long, hollow needle through a hole in the skull, deep into the ventricular cavity of the brain, to draw off the ventricular fluid and inject air. The exchange of air for fluid did not appear to distress the patient and on X-rays the air produced a shadow clearly revealing the exact shape and position of the ventricular cavities and the position of a tumour, if there was one.

It was an amazing revelation. Not only could Wilder use it to locate brain tumours in patients who were brought to him, but the clear picture it gave of the brain would help in all sorts of other studies of the organ. No longer would a neurosurgeon have to accept the dictates of neurologists. With ventriculography, and other techniques that would surely follow, the surgeon could be his own neurologist.

Returning to New York in some excitement, he performed a

ventriculogram on young Frederico. The procedure worked perfectly, but it revealed that Tilney's diagnosis had been correct. The tumour was too deep to risk removing it.

Wilder sent for the boy's parents and explained to them: he dared not operate and, what's more, it seemed as though the tumour was malignant. The parents were recent immigrants, but the boy's uncle spoke English. "I'm afraid your boy is going to die," Wilder told them. Then, unwilling to remove all hope, he added "I may be wrong. Doctors *are* wrong sometimes, you know."

Many years later he wrote that it became an important matter of principle with him never to remove all hope: "Men and women in a darkened room will look at the light, however tiny. Stubbornly, they may even live by it and rejoice in it—provided the door is not quite shut."

Two or three weeks later came a call from the uncle. Frederico had seemed fine at first; then he had got worse, and the day before he had suddenly died. It was morning when the call came, and the funeral was scheduled for that afternoon.

Here, from *No Man Alone,* is Wilder's own account of his reaction: "I felt I must know the answers that only an autopsy would give me, but the boy was at home, and the funeral to take place in a few hours. So many questions. Could I perhaps have saved this lad of ten? I remembered how he had looked at me with his appealing dark eyes when I realized that vision in them was a light about to fail. Some pictures one never forgets.

"In the autopsy room at Oxford, Sir William Osler had taught me how to remove the brain. At the same time, he had made me realize that a postmortem examination is admirable, a splendid thing in which the physician takes pride. It brings always the hope that this patient did not die in vain. Fortunately, too, I had carried out autopsies later, from time to time, for the pathologist Godwin Greenfield, in London.

"I made a quick decision and asked my intern to come with me....

"We took the subway downtown and emerged in the poorest Italian district. As we climbed the stairs of a gloomy tenement, I explained to him that there might be danger here, due to misunderstanding. I gave him the empty satchel, which was empty except for the instruments—and we agreed that, if we should succeed he was to vanish with with the precious specimen in the satchel, leaving me to talk with the parents.

"The front room was crowded with people. They were obviously dressed in their best. The mother, in black, was weeping. I tried to explain. There was a shocked silence in the room and then a hubbub.

All the talk was in Italian. Some were shouting, 'No, no.' At last the uncle took me out into the hall. 'I know you done your best,' he said. 'Now you wanna save—maybe another Italian boy? Maybe this might come to Frederico's little brother? Yes? All right, I guard the door. You sure you make him look the same when you're finished? Sure? Okay.'

"I remember my feeling of reassurance in the presence of this ally. He was intelligent, gentle, intuitive, he had understood everything. That feeling was reinforced when I realized what a big fellow he was, a northern Italian who towered above all the others.

"In the back room, the child lay on a table, beautiful in death. He was dressed in white silk! Doctors are like other people. Nothing could have been more distasteful to the intern and to me. But this had to be done. We worked feverishly, with sidelong glances at the flimsy double doors that separated us from the front room.

"The uproar that interrupted the quiet talk from time to time in that front room might have been used for the sound effects in some operatic mob scene. But, at last, the job was done, the boy dressed as before. All was the same that met the outward view. I opened the door and entered the front room, while my stalwart intern slipped away down the stairs with the satchel.

"I told them the boy could not have been saved. But perhaps we would learn enough to save other Italian boys, someday. The uncle helped me out of the front room and I, too, slipped away and down the stairs, with a sense of vast relief, to the welcome anonymity of the New York subway."

The autopsy confirmed the diagnosis, and proved that the ventriculogram had clearly shown the exact location of the tumour. Despite the disapproval of the other clinicians, Wilder decided he would continue to use Dandy's new technique.

Despite the satisfaction of learning a new diagnostic technique, the death of his first patient left Wilder feeling depressed and useless. He had no better luck with the next two patients. At midnight one night Wilder was called down to the hospital to perform his first major brain operation. A man was brought into the hospital unconscious and about to breathe his last. It appeared that he had an abscess deep in his brain, and so Wilder operated. He worked over the patient until six A.M., and then was forced to stop before even reaching the abscess when the patient's condition suddenly worsened. Then, for a couple days, the patient's condition improved inexplicably. Just as suddenly it reversed and Wilder took the man back to the operating room. This time the abscess was located right away; it was "like a great lemon filled with pus." Wilder did what he could, but a few hours later the patient died.

Hardly had Wilder adjusted to this defeat when a woman was admitted, also in a coma. In a letter to his mother he described the event: "We figured out the location of trouble and I turned down my first 'bone-flap.' That means making a trap door in the skull that may be closed when you are through. This time it turned out to be the malignant kind of tumor that cannot be removed completely. So I took a piece out for microscopic study and quit. Last night she died." At the end of the letter he added, "Brain surgery is a terrible profession. If I did not feel it will become very different in my lifetime, I should hate it."

Wilder's despair echoed that of many neurosurgeons of the time, as so often their patients subsequently died—some as a result of their efforts and some despite them. Only Harvey Cushing, in his surgical clinic in Boston, was demonstrating a respectably low mortality rate. But he operated primarily on tumours and extremely cautiously at that, and he was often forced to leave behind a portion of a tumour that would grow and kill the patient months or years later.

It was partly because of the hopelessness of brain surgery that Wilder turned with such fierce delight to laboratory investigation and experimentation; there only the lives of rats, hamsters, dogs and monkeys were at stake. There were other reasons. The thrill of scientific exploration was one; every day new discoveries were being made. And Wilder was determined to prove that he was still a neurologist even as he learned the craft of neurosurgery. More important was his determination to prove that a surgeon could be both a scientist and an "operator"—and the best of both. His own laboratory conclusions reinforced his knowledge of the brain whenever he operated, and the invaluable understanding that came from operating helped direct his laboratory explorations.

With all this in mind, in April of 1922 Wilder confided in a letter to his mother, the best solution would be "a Neurological Institute including surgery. It is along that line that the real future of neurology lies."

∞∞ SPAIN

Wilder's investigations in the laboratory stemmed from a seemingly banal question, posed to him one afternoon in the fall of 1921, just months after beginning work at the Presbyterian Hospital: "What is the cause of epilepsy?"

The speaker was Bill Clarke, professor of surgical pathology at the College of Physicians and Surgeons—not a man given to asking silly questions. Penfield, by virtue of his studies in pathology in London and at Oxford, had been assigned as one of his first academic duties to instruct in a course given by Clarke. On this fall afternoon, Wilder had come across Central Park to the medical school to discuss his forthcoming teaching responsibilities, unaware that Bill Clarke's startling questions had instructed and directed most of the other surgeons on the staff of the Presbyterian Hospital. The search for an answer to Clarke's query about epilepsy would have far-reaching effects not only on Wilder's life but, through him, on the treatment of epilepsy and the understanding of the brain as a whole.

Epilepsy, "the falling sickness" of ancient times, had been noted as a disorder for thousands of years, but until the last hundred or so it had been regarded with superstitious awe as symptomatic of possession by evil spirits. It was a particularly distressing disorder. Suddenly and mysteriously, its victims collapsed, went rigid, rolled their eyeballs, frothed at the mouth, soiled themselves—and when the fit was over few had any memory of the episode.

Ironically, wars are occasionally great boons to science. A study of soldiers with head wounds received during World War I had revealed that at least thirty per cent of those with "penetrating injuries" to the head subsequently had epileptic attacks. The obvious conclusion was that there existed a connection between head wounds, scarring of brain tissue and epileptic fits.

Penfield had learned the best methods of staining and preparing microscopical sections of the nervous system during his years of study abroad. Was he interested in studying how the brain heals from injuries? He was. Clarke suggested that a series of experimental wounds in laboratory animals, examined after different intervals of time, would be a good place to begin. Clarke's technicians would do the work if Wilder would carry out the operations and teach them the techniques. The students could study the sections. And in the process Wilder might learn something that would serve him well as a surgeon.

For the next two years, Wilder devoted much spare time to this research, but in the fall of 1923 he was forced to admit that he had come to a dead end. The techniques he was using would only show the cells in ghostly outline, and he could learn nothing from them. In desperation he tried another staining technique, one he had experimented with at Oxford. The technique, which involved impregnating the cells with a solution of gold and silver, had been pioneered in Spain by a scientist named Ramón y Cajal. Wilder had brought a

Spanish dictionary along to the library at Oxford, where he copied out some of the methods Cajal described. Although the results had not always been successful, on occasion the cells were brilliantly outlined as a result of the technique.

So, in the fall of 1923, Wilder, once again armed with a Spanish dictionary, made his way to the New York Academy of Medicine. There he found pictures that seemed to represent the cells he could not stain and a method for staining them, described in Spanish. Returning to the Presbyterian, he began to teach an orderly from the public ward to use the Spanish procedure "With the very first sections, the outlook changed. It was the Oxford experience all over again. Very exciting, but also very confusing. What I saw was difficult to interpret. Occasionally cells stood out, clear and complete, as I had never seen them before," Wilder wrote.

Cajal's research had earned him the Nobel Prize eighteen years earlier, and since then he had gathered about him in Madrid a school of Spanish cytologists. Unfortunately, the reports of their work had been published only in Spanish journals. But in the drawings published by one of them, Pio del Rio-Hortega, the cells, which were no more than ghostly outlines in Wilder's standard preparations, stood out sharp and clear. Wilder's attempt to duplicate the technique had been more successful than the results he had achieved in two years with the standard method, but it was still a far cry from the brilliant pictures del Rio-Hortega was publishing.

Wilder went to see Alan Whipple. If he was ever going to understand what went on in those brain cells, he would have to go to Spain and learn the silver and gold impregnation technique from the masters. Could Whipple give him six months off and help him raise the money to take Helen and the children to Madrid?

If Wilder was sure he ought to go, Whipple could get along without him for six months, but as to the money...Whipple at first just shook his head. There wasn't enough left in the budget. Then he recalled an operation he had performed free of charge on the daughter of Mrs. Percy Rockefeller, just after the full-time plan was inaugurated. She had seemed grateful; perhaps she would be willing to help.

The end of March found the Penfields halfway across the Atlantic. Whipple had succeeded, and Mrs. Rockefeller, and others, had provided the funds for the trip. Wilder had dashed off a letter to Pio del Rio-Hortega, and without waiting for an answer, enrolled in Spanish lessons at the Berlitz School. Twice a week Helen took the subway ten miles downtown to take each lesson with Wilder, and they invited a young Puerto Rican who worked at the hospital to dine with them six days a week so they could practise their Spanish.

It was only now, in the middle of the ocean, that Hortega's reply reached them. Forwarded by wireless from New York, one word only: *Venga* (Come). As Wilder would later write, "I looked up the word *venir,* to come. *Venga* was the imperative form usually applied to a child or a dog. *Bien venido* was recommended to signify 'Come and be welcome.'"

There, aboard ship in the middle of the ocean, Wilder sat down and wrote to his mother: "The changes in the brain itself I did not understand and have only begun to study. I can get no farther until I learn something about neuroglia cells in Madrid—and here we are in mid-Ocean.—and where are we going as far as the future is concerned?...

"I've done nothing but prepare and still I am preparing. I do not see the way toward hydrocephalus or epilepsy or any worthwhile problems and so I go on trying to learn, hoping the method will become apparent. But there is not the slightest guarantee that any clue lies in the direction I am taking. I am at the height of my power and still reaching out for new weapons...using none.

"Anyway, our bridges are burned," he concluded, "Our blue flower is truth. Only by finding it shall I succeed."

No doubt boredom with New York, however temporary, and lust for adventure played a part in the decision to go off to Spain for six months. So much of Wilder's internal life, it seems, was experienced in terms of adventures, challenges, mysteries and revelations. In this Helen was his match, and it was at times like these that she was most content. Each night on board ship they studied their Spanish lessons, then danced a little and went to bed to read *Rosinante to the Road Again* by John Dos Passos. The story delighted them, but it was the title that seemed deliciously appropriate. Rosinante was the horse that carried Don Quixote from La Mancha out into the world to set its wrongs right. A horse, Cervantes wrote, "so lean, lank, meager, drooping, sharp-backed and raw-boned as to excite much curiosity and mirth."

They landed at Vigo, and after leaving the children in their hotel with Alice, the maid, Wilder and Helen set out to explore. Down through the old part of the city they wandered, along narrow cobbled streets, past tiny, crowded houses. Dusk was falling. Women and children sang "in their queer tremolo," the boys played in the streets. And through the gaps in the houses they could see the bay and the sun setting against grey crags. Spain!

From the window of the hotel the next morning Wilder stared

out, "at the strangest scene I ever saw.... Streams of women, some barefoot, some with slippers, almost all dressed in black, were carrying on their heads all that the market contained: vegetables in huge baskets, fish, everything. Sometimes they stopped to talk, baskets two or three feet high balanced on their heads, gesticulating and laughing. Men loafed about, many in tatters or else dressed up in splendid military uniforms, with a dagger in the belt at one side and a revolver on the other.

"Soldiers are everywhere. They must mean a heavy burden on the peasants. Someone must pay for their salaries and finery. Perhaps," he mused, "the women."

Several days later they moved on to Madrid by train, and found lodgings in a *pension*. Here, they discovered that the name of Ramón y Cajal was known to everyone. But though the master was virtually a national hero, Hortega was unknown. "On further inquiry," Wilder recalled, "I discovered that Hortega had a laboratory of his own in the *Residencia des Estudiantes* (a university students' residence) situated in the outskirts of the city.

"On the first morning after our arrival, I walked out along the Avenida Castellana, marveling at the beauty of Madrid in early spring. The laboratory was housed in a single, L-shaped room. I knocked. When no one answered, I pushed the door open and saw a series of tables, one after another, placed beside each window in the outer wall. At each table, a man was sitting, with a microscope and small glass dishes and bottles before him. I advanced hesitantly. Not knowing what to say, I said nothing. Turning the corner of the room, I discovered more men at tables. At last, someone rose, a little man who had been sitting at a larger desk placed at the far end. There were no technicians, no secretaries, no doors into other rooms.

"Those seated at the tables had looked up as I entered," Wilder continued, "while the hum of conversation ebbed away and silence fell. Here was a test for my Berlitzian command of the Spanish language! But I made the plunge. The man at the desk smiled politely and came to meet me. This was Pio del Rio-Hortega—a slender man in his mid-thirties, with high forehead, black hair and a small moustache. He had the strong, handsome features of a Castilian noble and the quiet dignity of a gentleman. He seated me at the only vacant table. It was next to his desk. I was heartened to realize that I was expected at any rate."

This was, for Wilder, an important meeting. As a student in Sherrington's laboratory at Oxford, he had first heard of Cajal the master and Hortega the brilliant disciple. It had seemed a romantic story: the young doctor Cajal returning from his military service in Cuba, who used his army pay to buy a good German microscope and a few books and dictionaries. Working alone, he learned all there was to know about cell structure in the 1880s. One day Cajal happened to try the silver staining method of an Italian, Camillo Golgi, which impregnated nerve cells with a silver salt. Suddenly he could see the cells as individuals, clear and distinct.

With his own modifications of Golgi's technique he could see what no one else had ever seen, the details of nerve cells and their connections. From this followed a theory, "the neuron theory of cellular independence," which eventually earned him a Nobel Prize and brought to his laboratory disciples such as Pio del Rio-Hortega. But still they laboured alone in Madrid, cut off from the rest of the scientific world by geography, language and, increasingly as the years passed, resentment at being ignored.

This labour in darkness, without recognition, seemed inspiring and romantic to Wilder. At Oxford, he and his lab partner had taken to calling each other Ramón (after Cajal) and Pio (after Hortega). Wilder was Ramón.

That first morning, Hortega gave Wilder his first lesson in the Spanish technique. First, tissue from the brain of a rabbit, frozen hard, was cut into thin slices resembling small, blank squares of white paper. One by one, these "sections" were passed through a solution of silver, and then through a complicated washing and drying process. That done, a drop of balsam was used to hold the section in place between two thin glass covers.

The brain slice was now ready to be examined under the microscope. If the method had been properly carried out, the cells that had absorbed the silver would stand out clearly while the rest of the section would remain invisible.

Wilder learned quickly, and before long realized that with care and patience and a few modifications of his own he could apply the same techniques to almost any of the cell structures in the brain. It was common knowledge that scar tissue forming on the surface of the brain as a result of a blow or a wound could be the cause of an epileptic fit. The question was, How? With this technique Wilder could examine the scar tissue he removed from his patients during surgery and perhaps find an answer to Bill Clarke's question.

After four and a half months, Wilder and Helen fled Madrid and the terrible heat of August. They visited Lyons briefly so that Wilder could watch René Leriche and talk with him. Leriche was pioneering operations on the sympathetic nerves, operations to relieve pain and improve circulation. From there they travelled to

Paris, where Helen walked the children in the *Tuileries* and Wilder wrote a summary of Leriche's work, hoping to have it published in New York when he returned.

Though the adventure was over, they would soon strike out again. Meanwhile, and for the rest of their lives, Spain and Spanish art, music and literature would conjure up this romantic and golden interlude.

∞∞ THE MONTREAL OFFER

The Penfields were to stay in New York for four more years. They were, Helen wrote, "more boring if more satisfying times," a time for consolidation in various areas of their life. Wilder was thirty-three, Helen thirty-two when they returned from Spain. They wanted to have a few more children, and to stay in one place long enough to make some real friends. Wilder had to continue the slow, careful process of establishing his reputation as a surgeon and scientific investigator: there were meetings to attend, papers to write, associations to join. Now that he was back from his foreign jaunt, everyone wanted to take advantage of his newly acquired techniques. He was expected to study and report on all the neurological specimens coming into the surgical-pathology laboratory, all the autopsies that came into the medical-pathology laboratory. The professor of medicine wanted Penfield to see the consultations on the Medical Service and in the Medical Outdoor (out-patient) Department, in addition to all the neurosurgery on the wards and in the Outdoor. As well, Wilder wanted to continue his part-time work as a neurologist in the Vanderbilt Clinic, across Central Park. But most of all he wanted a proper laboratory of his own to continue his study of the cells of the brain and nervous system.

The first order of business on returning to the hospital, however, was smoothing the feathers that Dockrill, his cantankerous lab technician, had ruffled in his absence. When Wilder hurried to the lab he found Dockrill sporting a black eye and learned that he and the chief technician in the pathology lab had been in a fistfight the day before.

Edward Dockrill was a clever young Cockney adventurer who had jumped ship in New York after sailing around the world as a cabin boy for some years. Soon after Penfield joined the staff at Presbyterian, word spread throughout the hospital that he was looking for a technician to work in his small room in pathology. At the time, Dockrill was working as an orderly on the public wards. He immediately applied for the job, claiming he had worked at Queen Square in London as a technician. "He needed medical treatment badly," Wilder reminisced cryptically. Since he provided no details we can assume the problem was something unsavoury. Not only did Dockrill need glasses to correct his vision which caused a decided squint, Wilder quickly learned that he was no trained technician.

Still, Dockrill wanted the job badly and, despite the doubts of the chief of pathology, Wilder took him on. The metaphor of Dockrill's former occupation pleased him: "I had my first assistant, a cabin boy. My ship was under way!"

Dockrill had shown himself an eager and quick-witted student, as well as ambitious. In Wilder's absence, he had placed a new and rather ostentatious sign over the door of their little room. It read: NEUROPATHOLOGY. Dockrill had been busy, and not just at defending his boss's territory. What little Wilder knew of the Spanish methods before he left, he had taught to Dockrill, and while he was away Dockrill had worked hard to perfect the technique as best he could. The slides were excellent. Wilder complimented him on the work and told him Whipple had agreed to give them a larger room for their work, and a bigger budget.

When Dockrill seemed reassured, Wilder turned to leave and saw a young man he didn't recognize coming down the stairs. The chief of pathology had warned that a National Research Council Fellow interested in neuropathology had drifted into the lab in Wilder's absence and had been given permission to look over the specimens of the nervous system until Wilder returned.

The first things Wilder noticed about Bill Cone were his build and unusual looks: a picture-book Sancho Panza to Wilder's Don Quixote. Cone had big shoulders, a big head and short legs. He was dark and heavy featured and customarily wore a slightly sad expression. He and Wilder stood in the hall talking for a while, taking each other's measure. Cone, Wilder learned, had acquired an interest in neuropathology by working in the lab of a psychiatric hospital during his summer holidays from medical school at the University of Iowa. When he graduated in 1922, he had been awarded a National Research Council Fellowship to continue his clinical work in neuropathology. He had come to New York to train in neurology under Tilney, the Columbia professor of neurology whose imperious instructions not to operate on Frederico had so offended Wilder.

Tilney, however, was too busy with his private practice and with organizing the New York Neurological Institute to teach Cone, and besides, there was as yet no laboratory at the Institute. So Cone had come to the Presbyterian Hospital.

Wilder and Bill Cone entered the lab and plunged immediately into an argument about neuroglia cells, while Dockrill beamed genially. They would argue so, with a microscope between them, off and on for the next thirty-five years. These arguments occasionally took on a ferocious tone, which intimidated students and perplexed colleagues. Whatever their dissimilarities, both men were ardent and ruthless debaters, with strong tempers.

What did they think of each other at that first meeting? Cone of this intense, prematurely balding character who talked like a scientist and was a surgeon, with his dignified and slightly chippy manner that could instantly disappear in a dazzling warm smile? Penfield of this short, burly researcher six years his junior, quick to argue, equally intense? It didn't matter. They both knew and cared about the same things, and they needed each other. Wilder needed an assistant to work in the lab and in the hospital, and Cone was looking for a teacher in neurology, a laboratory to work in, and, to some extent, a direction in his life.

Cone began as an apprentice and learned astonishingly fast. "Soon," Wilder remembered in *No Man Alone*, "he seemed to double my potential. He became my alter ego throughout the hospital. He acquired the art of neurosurgery and patient care as if by instinct. He learned from Whipple and the other masters of general surgery in the hospital as I had done, leaping over the intern and residency sequence, reading widely, and approaching his specialty with the basic understanding of pathology and anatomy that he had already mastered."

Cone was a superb colleague, and would be satisfied for many years to be Wilder's alter ego, despite flattering offers which regularly came to him. They became friends before long, and to the Penfield children, he was soon Uncle Bill. His wife, tall, attractive, blonde and witty, became Aunt Avis. The Cones had no children of their own, and so they lavished much attention on the little Penfields; there, too, Bill Cone was willing to stand in for Wilder.

"So much to do and so little time:" the words ring through Wilder's diaries and letters expressing the fear of imminent failure, carefully hidden from all save his mother and himself. Concentration, he knew, was the key for someone like him; that and a competent secretary at work and a competent wife at home. The latter he had already in Helen, the former he soon acquired as the small room in the pathology ward expanded into bigger quarters and became "The

Laboratory of Neurocytology." He worked twelve or fifteen hours each day. Often he was called back during the night to perform an emergency operation.

Wilder knew, from observing the lives of his colleagues, the price that doctors' families often pay. Early on he decided that his family would be different, that he would be both surgeon and father, a part of his family's life, and not just an occasional, tired visitor.

After a year in the apartment on Valentine Lane, Wilder and Helen had moved a step further away from the city and into the country, to Riverdale. The commuter train journey was not much longer for Wilder, and Riverdale felt more like a small town than a suburb of a big city. They had found a house for rent on the grounds of the Riverdale Country School: the house was one of four just built to accommodate staff families as the school grew, and the rent was $1800 a year. Wilder managed to get that down to $1500 by offering to act as advisory football coach one or two afternoons a week, and running a two-week football conditioning session in September.

Life in their new home was carefully organized to make the most of the time Wilder was home. Breakfast was at seven sharp. The shiny new penny in front of each child's place, their allowance, was removed if they weren't there to sit down with Daddy. After all, if they did not breakfast together, they might not see him at all, since he sometimes stayed late at the hospital. In the evening after Helen had read to the children, they might be allowed to wait up in bed for him, knowing when he was coming by the barking of the dog, Tuck Two.

Sometimes he would bring them in their bathrobes to the living room: Ruthmary on his shoulders, Wilder (too tall for that sort of thing) behind, and they would sing.

Ruthmary: "I remember the French songs best, acting out *'Savez-vous planter les choux,'* marching up to bed on the final *'Maman, les petits bateaux qui vont sur l'eau, ont-ils des jambes?'"*

And another memory from Riverdale: "Daddy had realized on his way home that the Barnum and Bailey circus was leaving the next day, and that he had promised to take us. So after dinner we were wakened and dressed and off we went. At a side show...I remember Daddy questioning the giant about headaches, while I slipped his ring over my hand as a bracelet. Yes, the headaches were terrible. But he looked fine to me!"

One evening in the middle of a dinner party given by friends with whom the Penfields were staying for the weekend, a thunderstorm began. They had brought the two children, who were asleep upstairs. Remembering that Ruthmary had suddenly begun to fear storms, Wilder excused himself and left the table. He woke Ruthmary up and brought her outside, where she sat on his lap on the wet grass under a big black umbrella and they sang together. She was never afraid of storms again.

Despite his efforts to maintain the balance in his life, Wilder would occasionally reach the limits of his concentration and lapse into a walking daze: forgetting where he parked the car, pocketing a letter and dropping the house keys in a post box instead, getting on a train and going in the wrong direction for half an hour before realizing his mistake. It was up to Helen, with the help of Alan Whipple, to make him take time off now and again to recover. These were wonderful stolen moments. The truants would leave the children behind and disappear for a weekend to a hotel downtown or a cabin by the sea. They would indulge in the rare luxuries of sleeping late, taking long walks and discussing the future far into the night.

On his desk at home there was always a paper or two waiting to be written, conclusions to be drawn which often eluded him until he slowly and carefully wrote them out in long hand and could see them on the page before him. In this Cone was, unfortunately, no help. Lacking the patience for writing and the ambition for the recognition it brought, he left Wilder to draw attention to their joint investigations.

Wilder enjoyed writing. It helped him to crystallize his thoughts, and he relished the challenge of writing clearly and well. Most of the time he was working on strictly scientific papers: "Acute Swelling of Oligodendroglia", or "Microglia and the Process of Phagocytosis in Gliomas." But in 1926 he got a chance to try something different, a biographical sketch of Ramón y Cajal. Although the piece was written for a scientific journal, this was an exercise in a different sort of writing, and it thrilled him: "It has called forth more letters of congratulations than anything I have ever written," he reported proudly to his mother.

The next few years passed quickly, during which there were changes at home and at the hospital. Despite two or three miscarriages the Penfields were determined to have more children, and on February 7, 1926, a "rather long" baby girl with bright red hair was born and christened Priscilla. In January Wilder had operated and removed a piece of brain the size of an orange from a boy who had degenerated into "a sort of vegetable with almost constant convulsions." A month later the boy walked into the hospital free from attacks and much improved, and Wilder showed him off proudly at the weekly surgical conference.

In the early spring of 1926 Wilder was invited to a conference of the American Neurological Association to talk about brain wounds, and in May he was asked to write a chapter on neuropathology for Nelson's *Loose Leaf Surgery*. In June came a long-awaited invitation to be a member of the Society of Neurological Surgeons, a select group with a membership restricted to twenty-five.

Despite the increasing burden of his work, which kept Wilder, and often Helen (who did his typing and helped him draw diagrams) working late into the evenings, the couple kept two nights a week free to go to the theatre, dine with friends, or walk about downtown. Some friends attempted to interest them in bridge, but after a few evenings they gave it up. "What a waste of perfectly good cerebration," Wilder wrote. He was difficult to play with anyway, since he hated being the dummy and would always bid, no matter what cards he held in his hand.

During this period, Wilder was growing more and more conscious of his age: "I called Wilder Jr. from the ice today," he wrote his mother one Sunday afternoon in February, 1927. "Some other boys called, 'Hey, Wilder, your father wants you.' In a flash I heard an echo from 30 years ago, and it said 'Hey, Wilder, your mother wants you.' We look older, but inside that same boy lurks and sometimes he is surprised to find that he no longer exists." The letter continues, "Little Johnny Rabbit died today, a baby on whom I had operated three times and hoped to beat the hydrocephalus at the fourth operation on Tuesday. Some day I will beat it—or will I?"

One morning in early June, 1927, Wilder arrived at the hospital to find a letter waiting for him. It was from a Dr. Archibald, Professor of Surgery at McGill University in Montreal, and surgical chief at the Royal Victoria Hospital. The hospital was looking for a neurosurgeon. Archibald himself had been doing some brain surgery, along with his own specialty, chest surgery, and had been sending the most serious neurosurgical cases to Harvey Cushing in Boston. Montreal was big enough to support a full-time neurosurgeon, he wrote, and in fact whoever came would have a virtually unobstructed field: the only other neurosurgeon in Canada was just starting up in Toronto.

That night Wilder talked the offer over with Helen. While neither one of them particularly wanted to move from New York, and didn't relish, as he confessed to his mother a few days later, "the cold winters of that North land," he was starting to feel as though he had reached a dead end in New York.

The long-awaited transfer of the neurological and neurosurgical work in the city into the new medical centre now nearing completion, was scheduled for the spring of 1928. With the move, Wilder had come to believe, would go much of the freedom he had enjoyed in the last six years: freedom to choose his work and to study and treat patients as he liked. The Neurological Institute, under the direction of Wilder's adversary, Professor Tilney, would restrict his efforts once the move had taken place. So far no one had approached Wilder to describe his place in the new scheme, although an offer of some kind would, no doubt, come. But his freewheeling days were about to end.

A second problem, as serious as the first, was that the older neurosurgeons in the city seemed to get all the patients—or at least all the wealthy patients. What patients were left for their juniors, like Wilder, were the hospital charity cases. "I have waited in line long enough," Wilder wrote in his weekly letter to his mother, the subject on this occasion being Archibald's preliminary offer. "Practice has not been good this year." He went on to say that he had sent a wire back to Archibald, emphasizing that he was "very interested if they wanted pathological, experimental and operative sides of neurosurgery developed, and if I wouldn't starve in the process of transplantation."

Archibald came down to New York a few days later to see Wilder operate and talk with him. After the operation the pair went to lunch and talked until past seven in the evening. Archibald agreed that the money to guarantee Wilder a certain minimum for a few years might be found, but was more hesitant about Penfield's ambitious plans to build up a complete modern neurosurgical clinic. Nevertheless, before returning to Montreal, Archibald promised to scout around and see what could be done.

Two weeks later Wilder left for London to attend the first British-American Neurological Conference: eight Americans had been invited to present papers, and Wilder was one of them.

Visiting London again after seven years was almost like a homecoming. Skirts were higher, just as in New York, but otherwise the city seemed unchanged, and a tandem bicycle, he observed, could still cross Trafalgar Square without attracting stares and hoots of laughter. Gordon Holmes, Percy Sargent, Godwin Greenfield and others who had been friends or teachers were all there, delighted to see Wilder again, and flattering about the progress he was obviously making. The student had returned a neurological investigator in his own right. He had time for tea with the Sherringtons and a brief chat with Lady Osler on the platform at Victoria Station. She was off to Belgium to dedicate a cross commemorating fallen British soldiers and to visit her son Revere's grave. News of the Montreal offer had reached her through the grapevine: had he decided whether to go?

As the train whistle blew she recalled the cable she had sent to Sir William when he sought her advice about moving to Oxford so many years ago: "Don't procrastinate, decide at once." This bit of advice spurred Wilder to write a long letter to Archibald. Reporting to his mother afterward, he outlined the letter's content as follows:

> Canada needs a neuro-surgical clinic and Montreal is a suitable place to develop one. There would be needed,
> 1. A neuro-surgical interne
> 2. A research fellow
> 3. Segregation of neuro-surgical beds
> 4. Special examining room in hospital
> 5. Association with both Royal Victoria and Montreal General Hospitals.
>
> It is only possible to develop one operative team in one hospital but to have sufficient operative material it would be necessary to draw from both hospitals.

In the intervening months, Helen gave birth to a fourth child, a boy duly named Amos Jefferson Penfield, and the happy event seemed to inaugurate a period of good fortune. First, a damage suit that had been pending since 1916 (for knee injuries sustained while on board the S.S. *Sussex*) was decided in Wilder's favour; the court awarded him $15,000, which to the Penfields seemed a huge amount of money. Shortly afterward, two wealthy couples were involved in a car accident right in front of Presbyterian Hospital. One was dead on arrival; Wilder operated on the head injuries of the three others, and their gratitude had the effect of dramatically improving his private practice, hitherto *not* financially rewarding.

With the change in their fortunes, and the unbroken silence from Montreal, Wilder and Helen began to make plans to stay in New York. Then came a telegram from Archibald: all arrangements had been made. Could Penfield come to Montreal for a meeting? He took the train to Montreal the same day.

Though Archibald had spared Wilder the details of the intricate diplomacy surrounding the proposal to bring a full-time neurosurgeon to Montreal, it was clear that the main purpose of the invitation was to see if Penfield could pass muster before the autocrats of the Montreal medical world.

When it came time much later in his life to write about the events that led him to Montreal, Wilder was able to present at least a superficial account of what was going on beneath the surface in 1928. Though he cared about those aspects of hospital politics that affected him and his plans directly, he had no taste for intrigue himself, and thought political behaviour unseemly and distasteful in others—though he was aware of the enormous power others wielded, and even had a certain uneasy respect for it. Fortunately, Wilder's personal political arsenal contained large measures of dogged determination and self-esteem: if the hospital board would give him what he wanted, fine, he would come to Montreal. If not, he would decline courteously and dismiss them and their empire altogether.

Montreal was a city jealously proud of its medicine. Rich Montreal businessmen fought ruthlessly for appointments on hospital boards as a sign of their status, then fought equally ruthlessly to retain control. The news that a young neurosurgeon was coming for an interview passed quickly through Montreal's high society: What was he like? Where was he from? Would he fit in?

After a rather hasty tour of the hospital and a lecture to medical students on locating tumors in the brain (which Penfield had agreed to give), he was taken to a luncheon in his honour at the exclusive Mount Royal Club. There were twenty-five guests, and Sir Arthur Currie, Chancellor of McGill, presided. Various heads of departments from the Royal Victoria Hospital and the Montreal General Hospital were there as well. Among the guests were several who had agreed to back Archibald's plan to bring Penfield to Montreal, notably Dr. Lewis Reford. Dr. Reford was a powerful ally. He was married to the daughter of Montreal millionaire Duncan McIntyre, and connected by marriage as well to A. A. Hodgson, a rich and influential Montreal businessman. The Reford Hodgson families had agreed to contribute anonymously to the support of the proposed laboratory of neuropathology, which Wilder had insisted on as a condition of his acceptance. To his mother Wilder reported that Archibald "made a speech about my past history and the desire of every one that now Montreal should become the Mecca to displace Boston, etc. Very embarrassing." There were other speeches, including one from the head of Neurology at the Montreal General to say that if Penfield came members of his department would co-operate as much as they could.

That night Wilder caught the train back to New York, and for a week waited for the formal offer that had yet to come from Montreal. Finally he wired Dean Martin at McGill to ask if it was safe to burn his bridges. Martin wired back, "Burn your bridges." A long letter arrived the same day saying that the guarantee to make up the financial shortfall in the first three years of his practice would be made shortly. He would be appointed Professor of Neurological Surgery at McGill, and his title at the Royal Vic would be Surgeon-in-Charge of Neurosurgery.

Bill Cone, despite a flattering offer from Alan Whipple to stay on in New York, decided to go with Wilder to Montreal, where he would be chief of the clinic and a partner in Wilder's surgical practice.

Wilder had told Archibald that he would come to Montreal in March, and the family would follow when school was out in June. But in the week that followed, he and Helen decided to postpone the move for six months and travel to Germany. The decision was in part the result of a sudden reluctance to plunge from one life into the other, but the primary reason concerned an eighteen-year-old patient of Wilder's named William Hamilton.

Three years earlier Hamilton had been struck on the forehead by a falling brick, and some months later had begun to have epileptic fits. The boy was referred to Wilder, and he decided the time had come to put into practice what he had learned in seven years of studying brain scars. He knew from his experiments that in the part of the brain damaged by the falling brick there occurred sudden electrical discharges at the time of an epileptic attack. These discharges blocked the action of the delicate mechanisms that must be active to maintain consciousness; in effect, the epileptogenic explosions caused a short-circuit in the boy's brain. Although Wilder could not yet answer the question, "What causes the electrical discharge to happen so suddenly and mysteriously?", he had learned how to remove the scar from which the discharge often originated without leaving a second scar on the brain.

Three weeks before going to Montreal, Wilder had operated on William Hamilton. Had the boy been older or the attacks less severe, Wilder might have proceeded more cautiously once the brain was exposed on the operating table. However, it was a mark of Wilder's approach to surgery that he was willing to take risks that more conservative surgeons shunned. As the operation progressed, Wilder realized he would have to remove more than half of the patient's right frontal lobe. It was one of the first, if not *the* first lobectomy, or removal of a large portion of the brain.

In any case, when Wilder returned from Montreal, the patient was up and about and begging to be allowed to go home. He appeared well, and the psychological tests revealed no loss of "mentality," as far as could be seen. Gratifying though this was to the surgeon, another question immediately followed: If each part of the brain has a separate and important function, how could the removal of such a large section not affect the patient?

Wilder couldn't say whether or not William was cured. Perhaps another scar would form after all, and cause another series of attacks worse than the first. If so, the radical removal of such a large section of the brain was unjustified. Before he could perform other such operations with any confidence, he knew he would have to answer that question for himself.

While Wilder was waiting for a formal offer from Montreal a doctor returning from a visit to clinics around Europe stopped him in the hall to tell him about the work being done by a German neurosurgeon, Otfrid Foerster. Presumably news of Penfield's operation on an epileptic had made the rounds. Foerster was operating with apparent success on epileptics, many of whom were suffering from head wounds received in the war. If Foerster had operated on a series of patients who had epilepsy, then he must have the follow-up studies that would tell Wilder what he needed to know. When Penfield notified Montreal that he would be delayed for six months while he went to Germany to watch Foerster in action, the immediate response was $1,500 to help with expenses and Archibald's blessings.

And so, on March 21, 1928, the very day that Wilder's colleagues moved from the Presbyterian Hospital to the new medical centre uptown, the Penfields set sail for Germany.

As on their trip to Spain, Wilder and Helen left without having received a formal invitation, but a welcoming cable from Foerster was waiting when their ship docked in Hamburg. With all their luggage for the move to Montreal and the four children, Wilder and Helen took the train to Breslau, where Foerster had his clinic. For the next six months, while the children learned German from their playmates in the little village of Obernigk, where the family had found rooms in a *pension,* Wilder reviewed Foerster's techniques and results:

"There were 12 cases in Foerster's series. The patients had survived, and they could now be reported, from one to five years after operation. The results were excellent from the patients' point of view. It was clear that Foerster was carrying out the right operation. My experimental studies showed why it was right. Together we could see the ways of improvement now. There were details in his procedure that I would adopt. Some I would change....

"In the weeks that followed, I worked out the story of healing and scarring in the human brain, a wonderful sequel to my animal series. I wondered what Bill Clarke would say if he could stoop above me and look over my shoulder...."

In mid-September, Helen, Wilder and the children sailed from Hamburg to Montreal. Cone planned to be in Montreal by the time Wilder's ship arrived, and two research fellows, one from London and one from California, were preparing to join him and Wilder in the laboratory they would open. The Montreal adventure was about to begin.

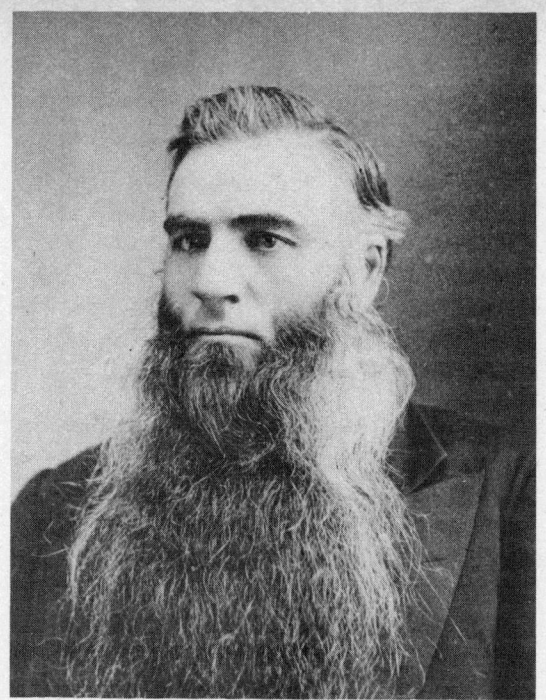

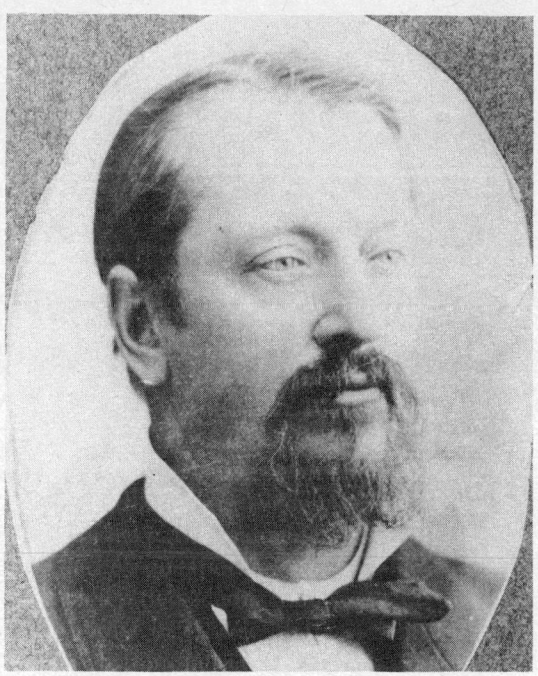

Dr. Ephraim Penfield (*top*) and Amos Jefferson, grandfathers of Wilder Penfield.

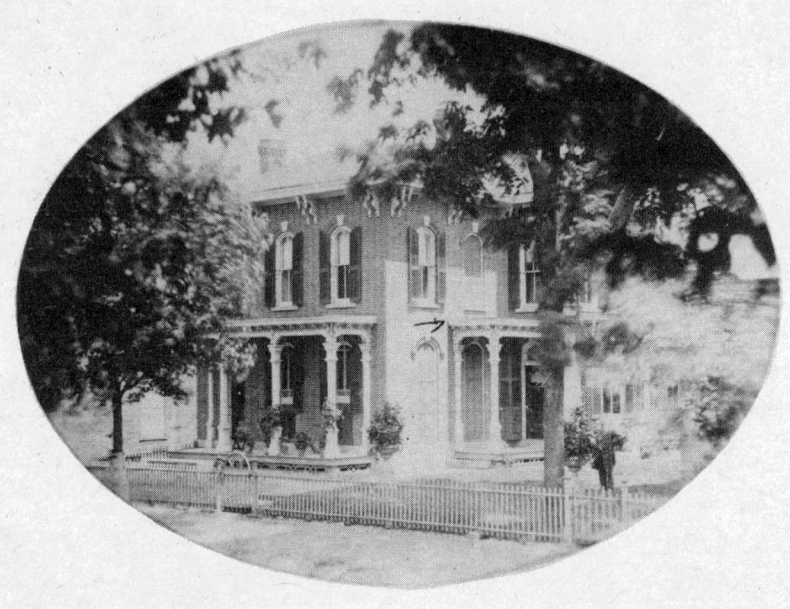
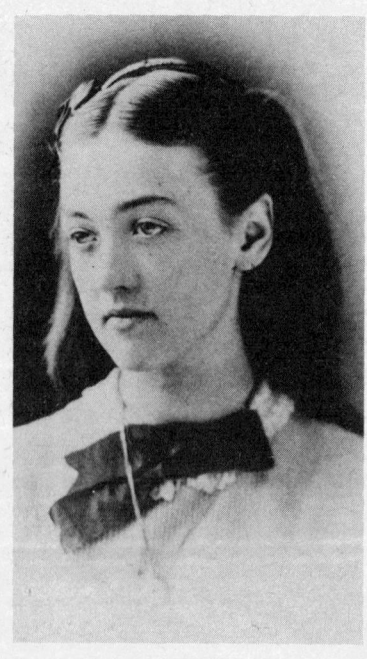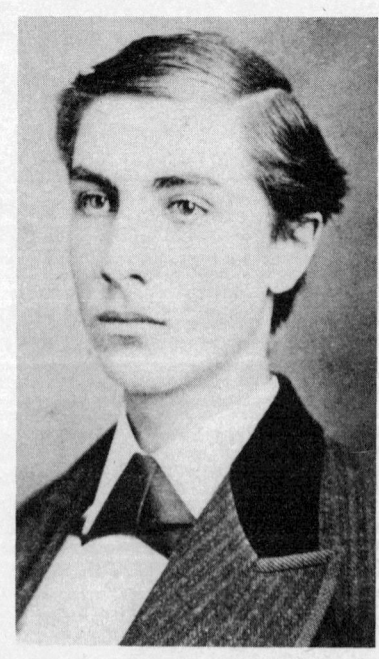

TOP OPPOSITE: The Penfield family home in Bucyrus, Ohio, where Wilder's father Charles was born. (Arrow points to Dr. Ephraim Penfield's private office entrance. The doctor is standing on the lawn.) BOTTOM OPPOSITE: Charles Samuel Penfield, age 17 (1875) and Jennie Marie Jefferson, age 15 (1874). BELOW: Charles Penfield circa 1885 and Jennie Jefferson, age 19 or 20, when she was engaged to marry Charles.

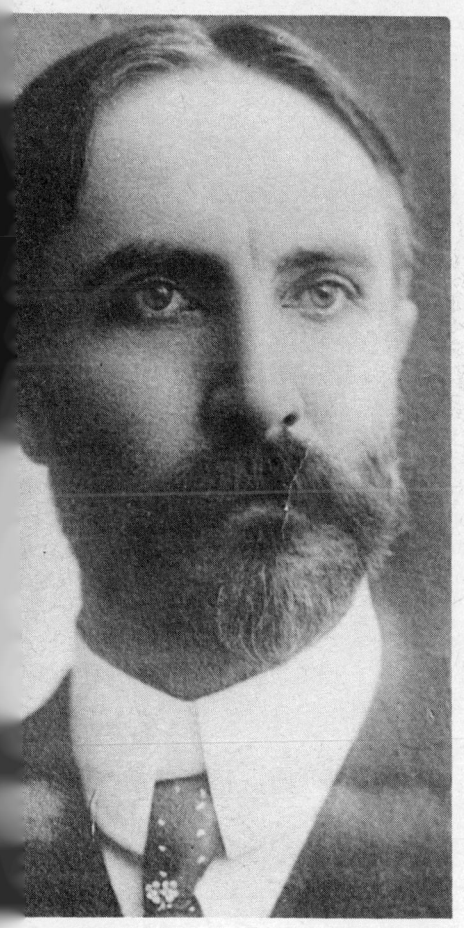
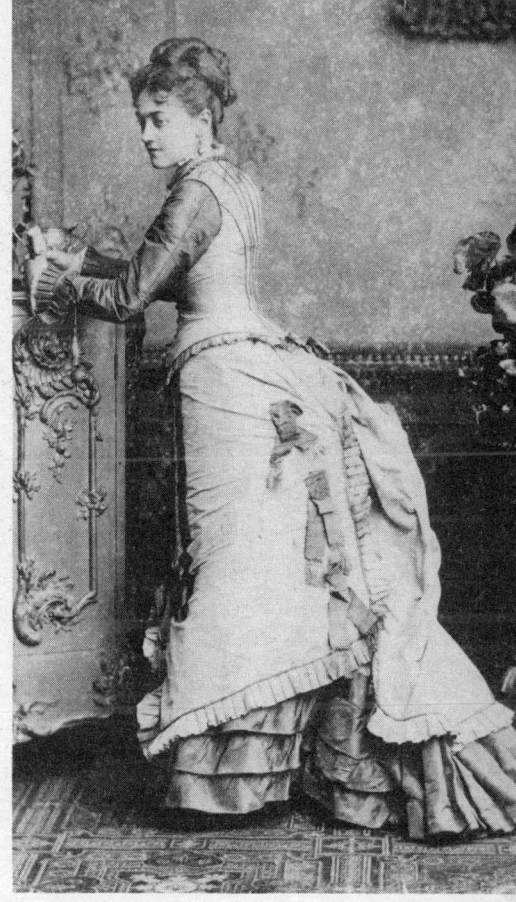

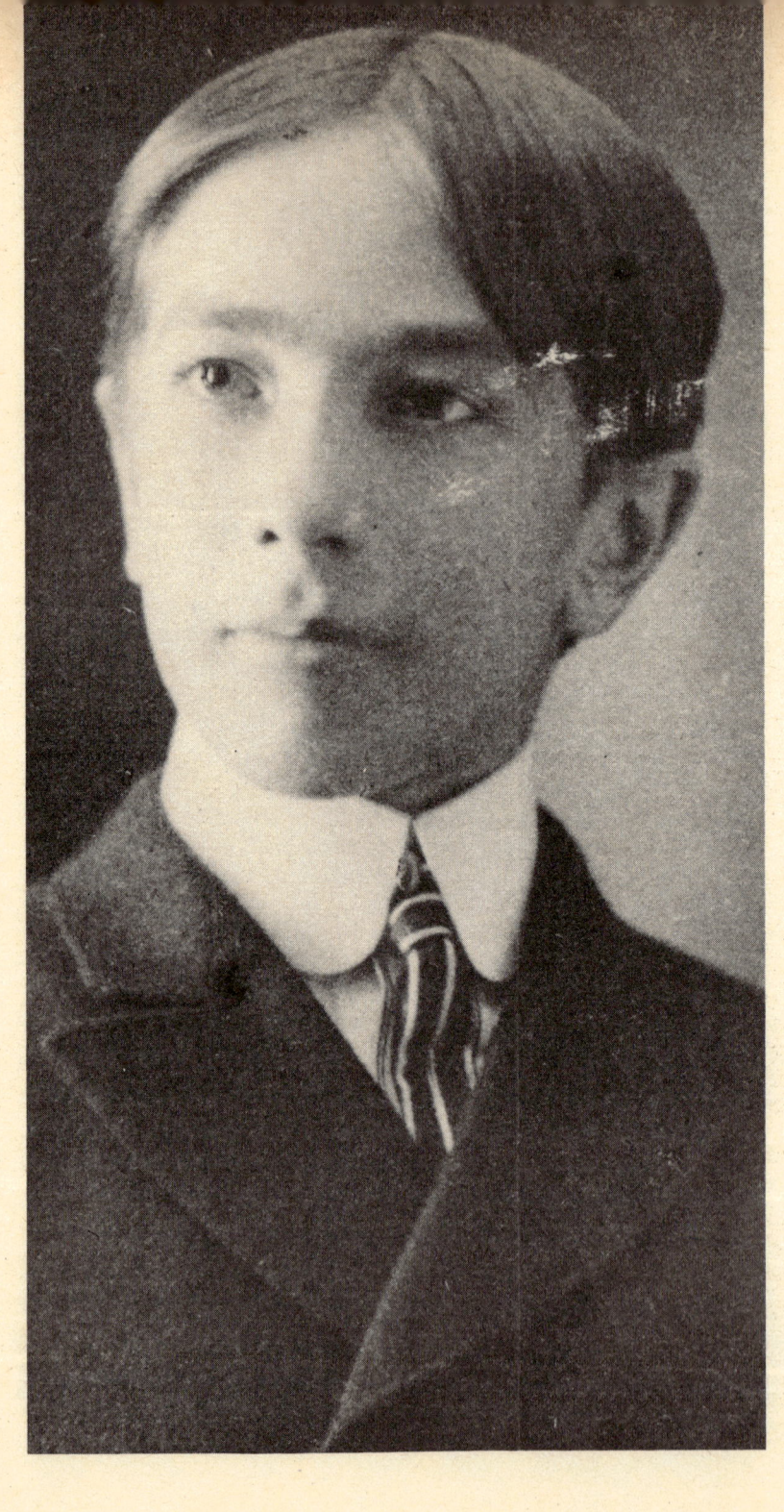

OPPOSITE: Wilder, age 13 (1904). BELOW LEFT: Amos Jefferson's house on Third St. in Hudson where Wilder grew up. BELOW RIGHT: Wilder as captain of the Galahad School football team, age 17 (1908). BOTTOM: The Penfield clan at Galahad School circa 1907. *Rear left to right,* Grandmother Penfield, Jean, Wilder, Aunt Addie. *Front,* Herbert Penfield (with son George), Herbert's wife Mary, Jack Inglis (with daughter Elizabeth), Ruth Penfield Inglis.

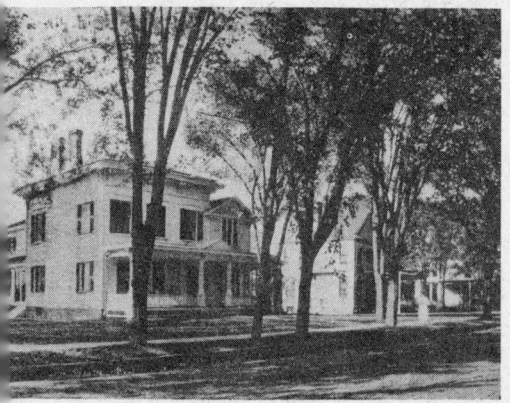
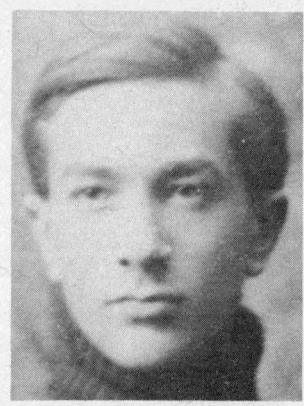
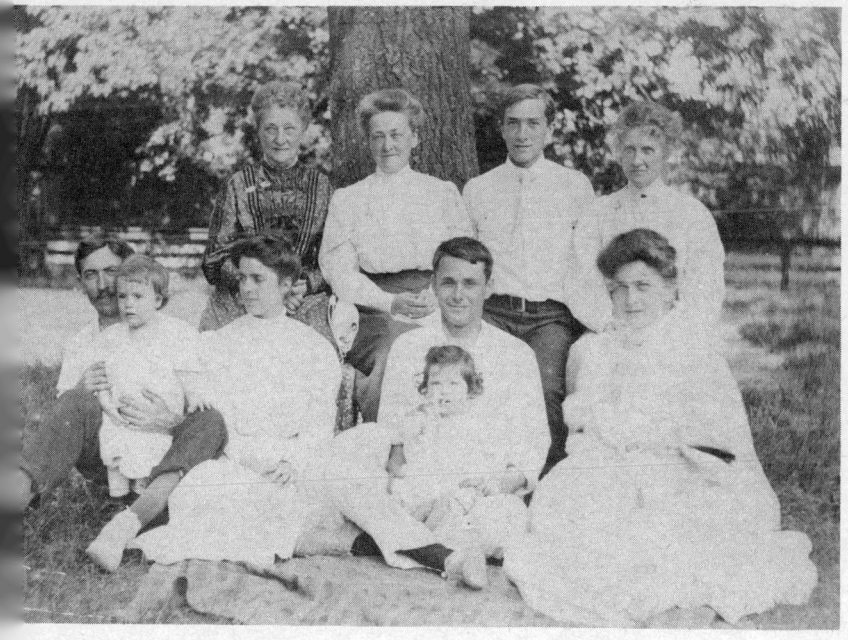

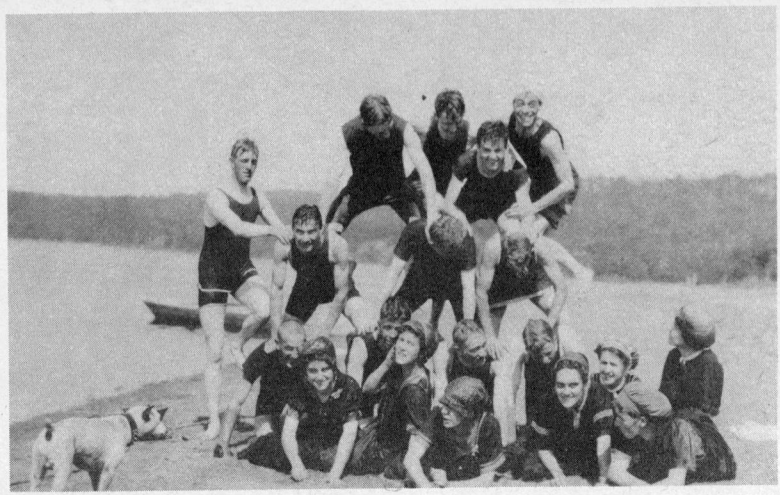

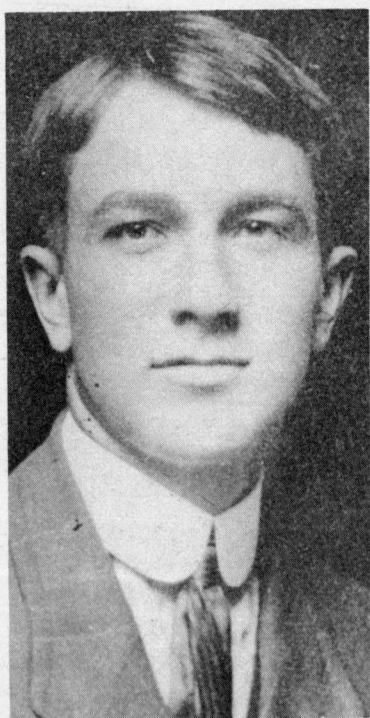 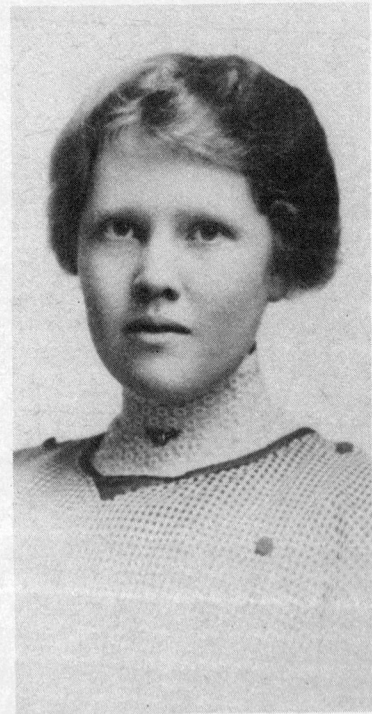

TOP: The Hudson gang circa 1910. (Wilder is centre of first row of kneelers.)
ABOVE: Wilder as Princeton undergraduate, age 19 (1910) and Helen Kermott, Wilder's future wife, age 20 (1912).

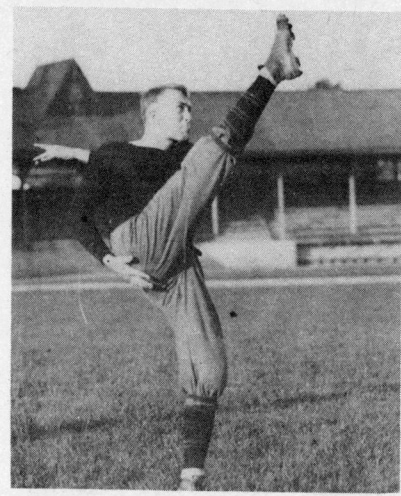

Wilder kicking a football during Princeton stadium practice (1912).

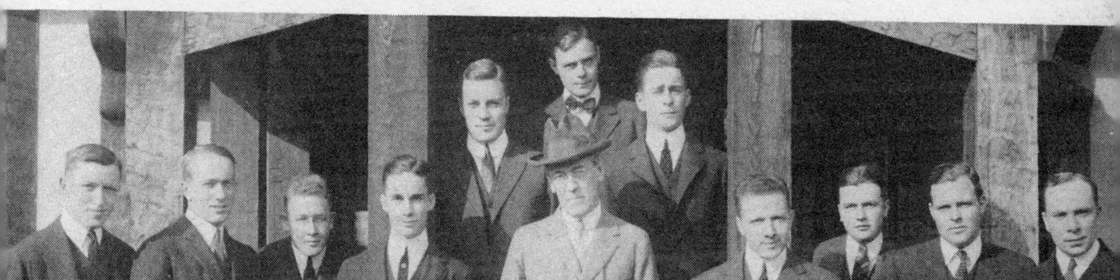

The Woodrow Wilson Club of Princeton University (1912). *From left:* Max Chaplin, Wilder, Francis Hall (sitting). Bill Chester is behind and to the left of Woodrow Wilson. On Wilson's left is Paul Myers. (All were members of the Dr. Johnson Society.)

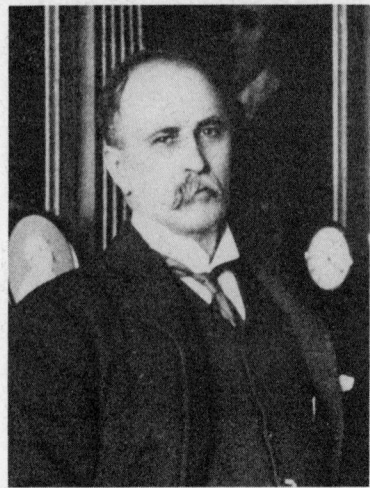 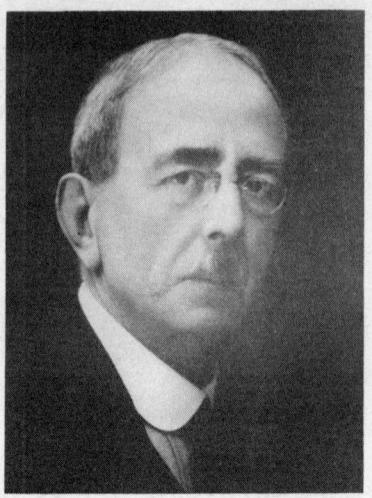

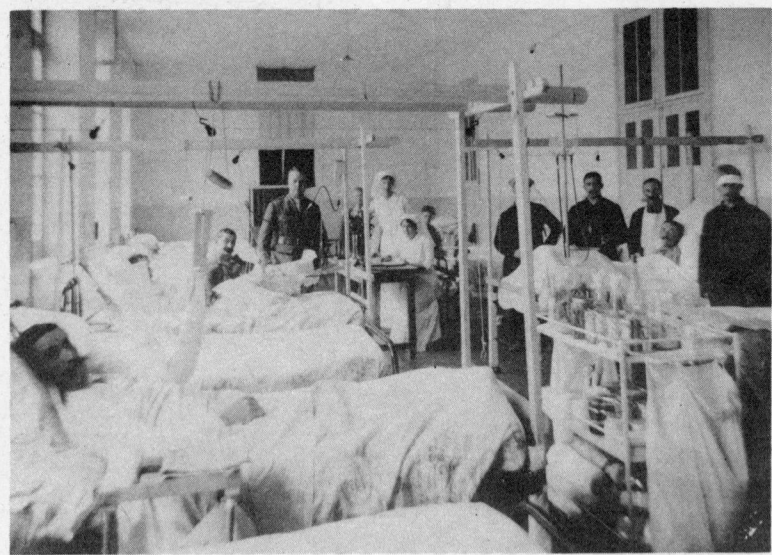

TOP LEFT: Sir William Osler.   TOP RIGHT: Sir Charles Sherrington.
ABOVE: A Ward in the military hospital at Ris Orangis, France (1916).
TOP OPPOSITE: The S. S. *Sussex* after bow was blown off by a German torpedo.
BOTTOM OPPOSITE: Wilder and Helen as newlyweds in Paris in 1917.

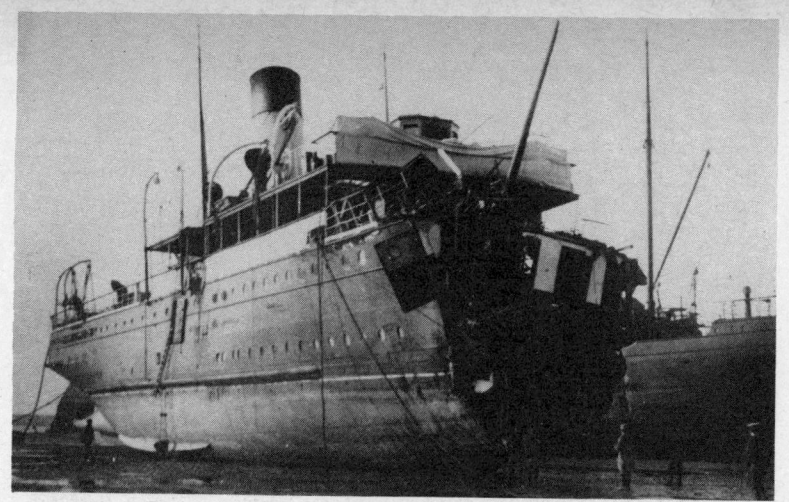

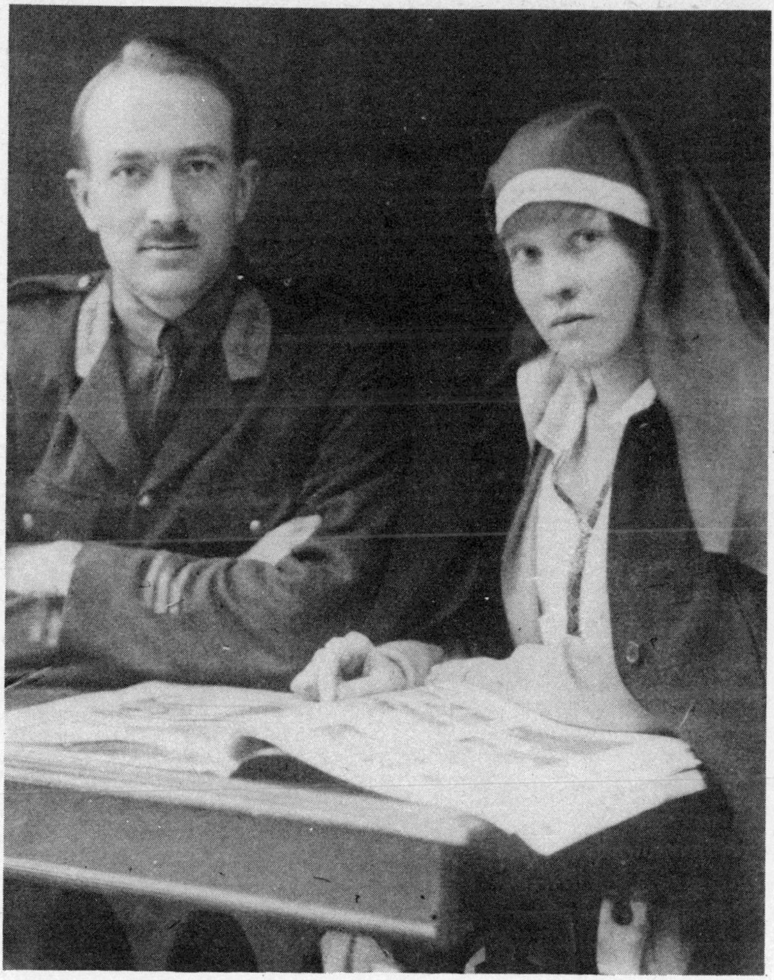

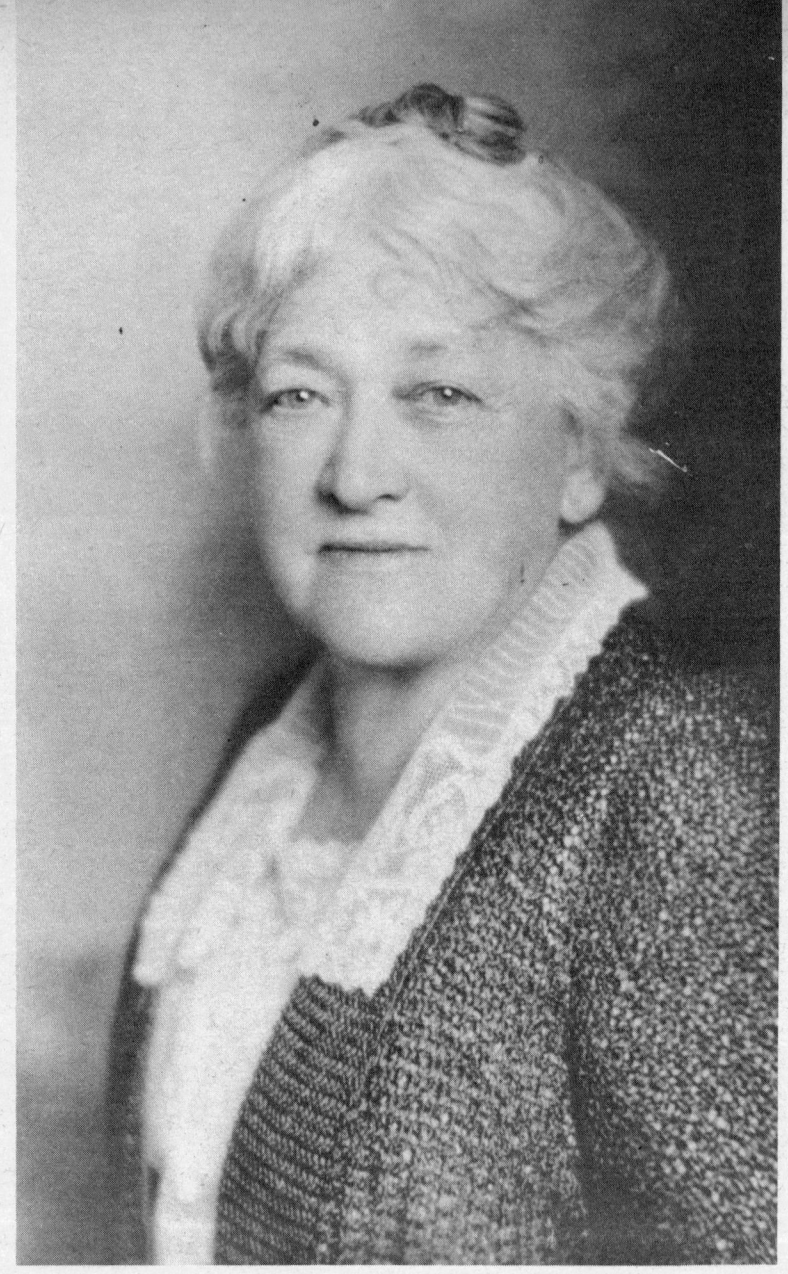

Jean Jefferson Penfield in middle age.

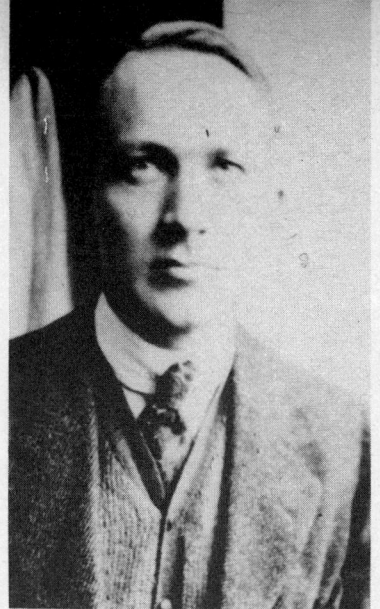 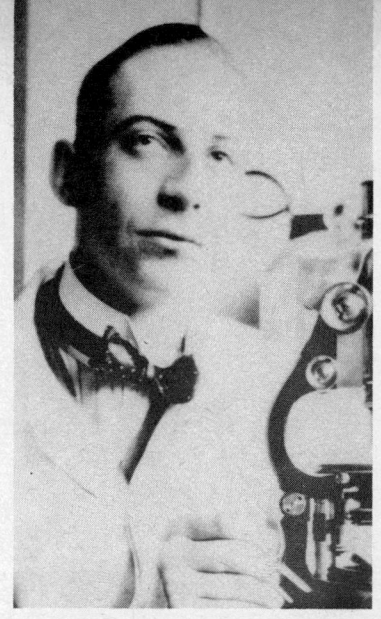

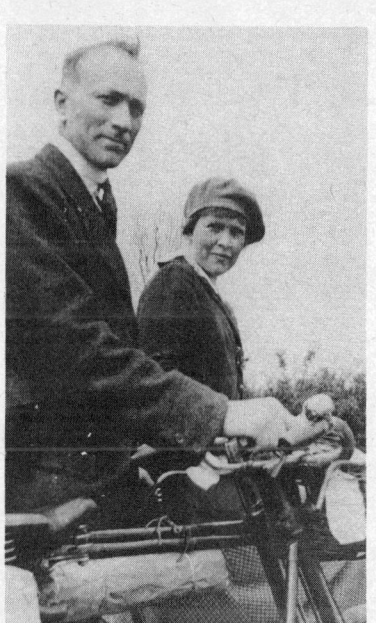 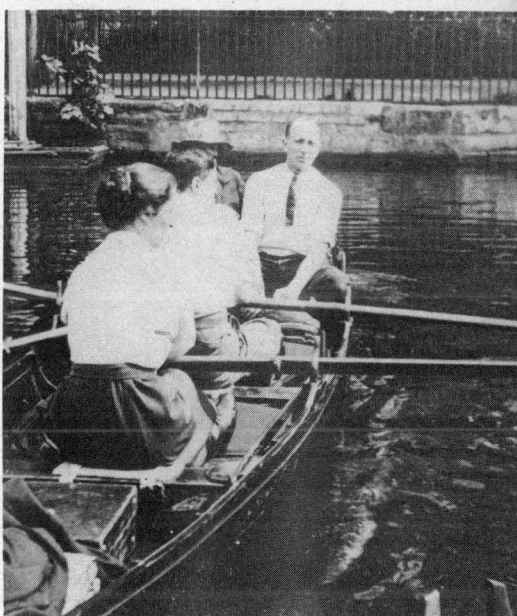

TOP: Wilder (left) and his lab-mate **Harry** Carleton at Oxford in 1920. Wilder's nickname was Ramón (y Cajal); his partner was Pio (del Rio-Hortega). ABOVE: Wilder and Helen cycling near Oxford and skulling down the Thames with Dr. and Mrs. Gordon Holmes.

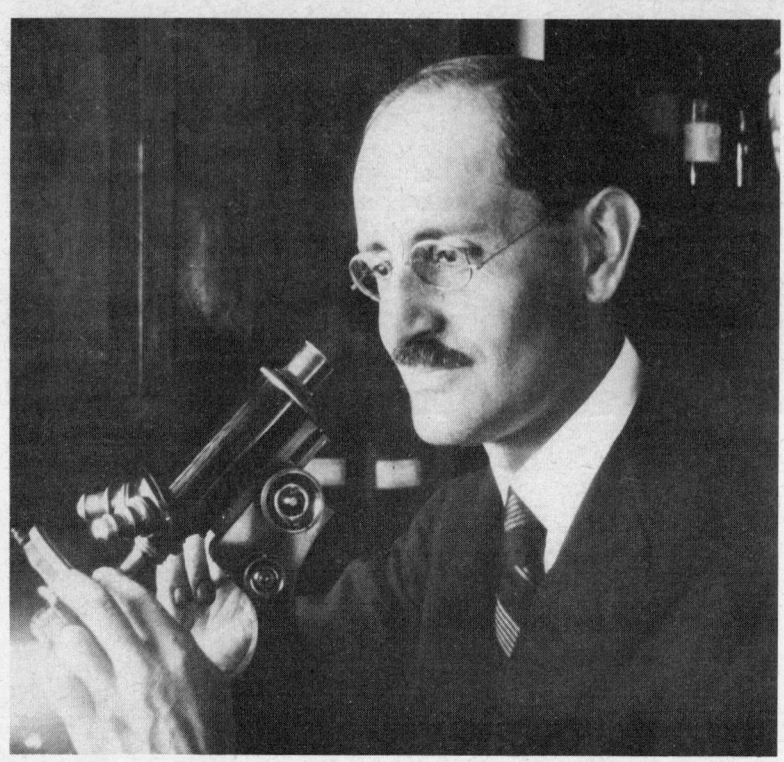

ABOVE: Pio del Rio-Hortega, Madrid, 1924, photographed by Wilder in Hortega's laboratory. RIGHT: Dr. William V. Cone circa 1928. TOP OPPOSITE: Helen and three children in 1927 (Priscilla, age 1, Wilder Jr., 9, Ruthmary, 8.) BOTTOM LEFT OPPOSITE: The Penfield family in 1935. *Left to right,* Ruthmary, Priscilla, Wilder Jr., Jeff, Helen, Wilder. BOTTOM RIGHT OPPOSITE: Wilder with his mother Jean during his last visit to see her in California in 1935.

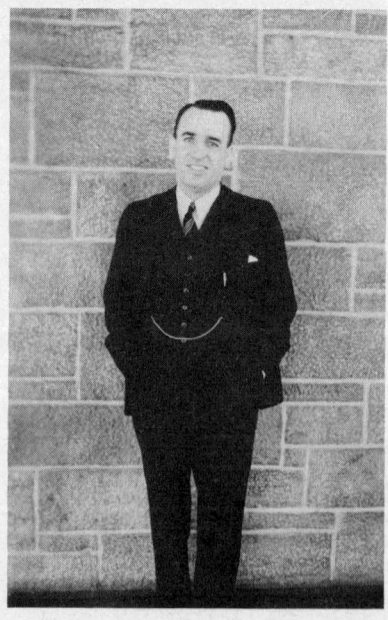

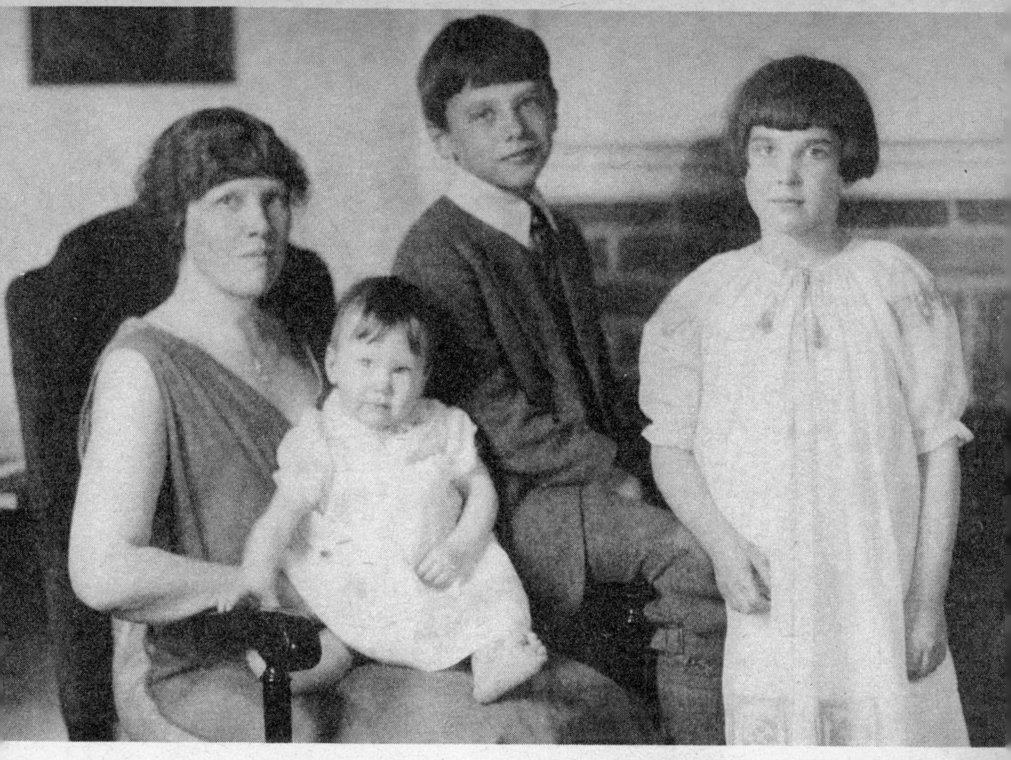

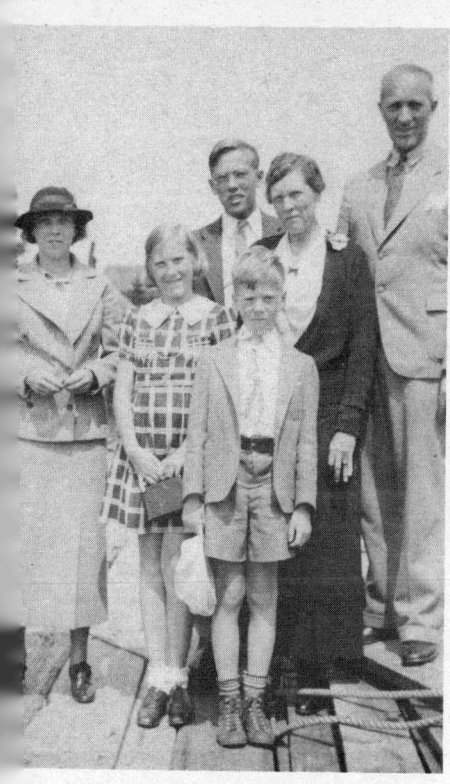
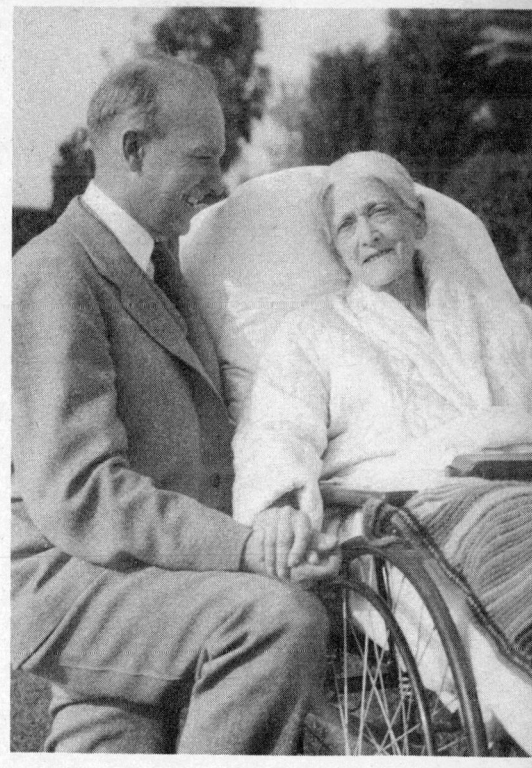

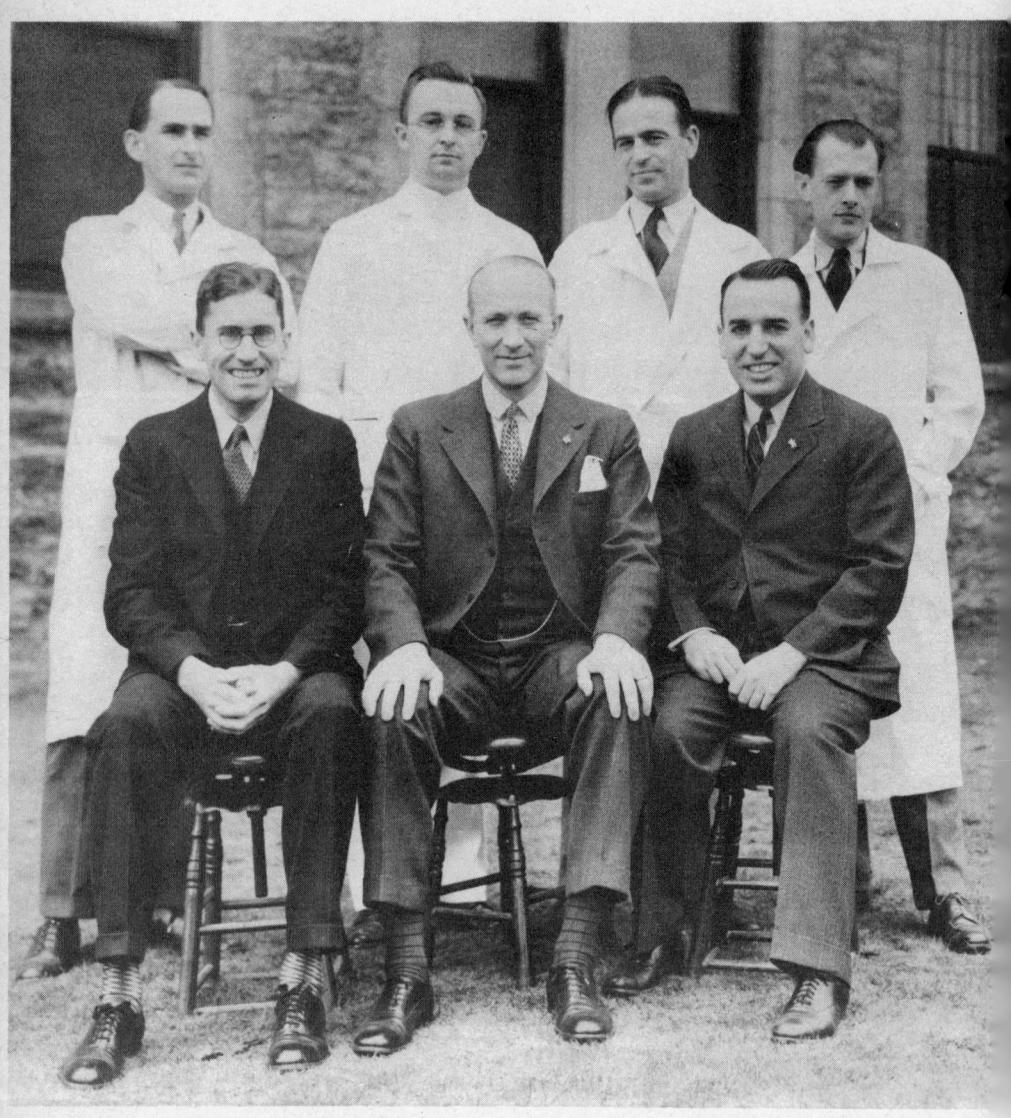

ABOVE: The "Old Guard," 1934, the first group of young neurosurgeons trained by Penfield and Cone in Montreal before the opening of the M.N.I. *Seated left to right,* Arthur Elvidge, Wilder, Bill Cone. *Standing left to right,* Arne Torkildsen, Lyle Gage, Joseph Evans, Jerzy Chorobski. TOP OPPOSITE: The Montreal Neurological Institute under construction and soon after opening. BOTTOM OPPOSITE: The bridge over University Street connecting the M.N.I. to the Royal Victoria Hospital.

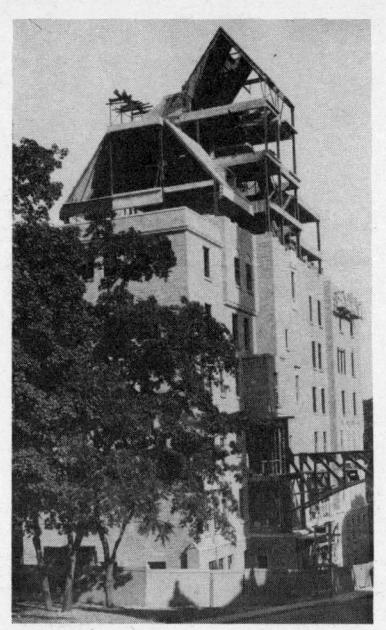 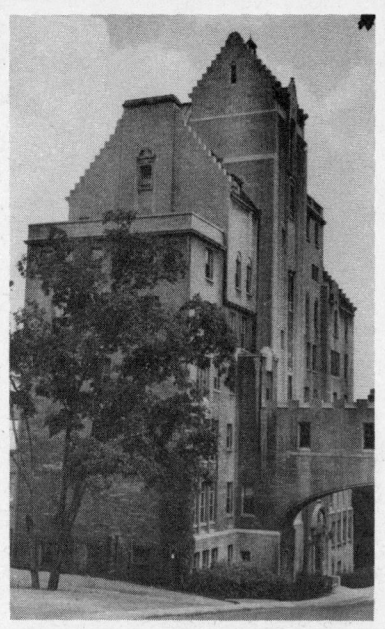

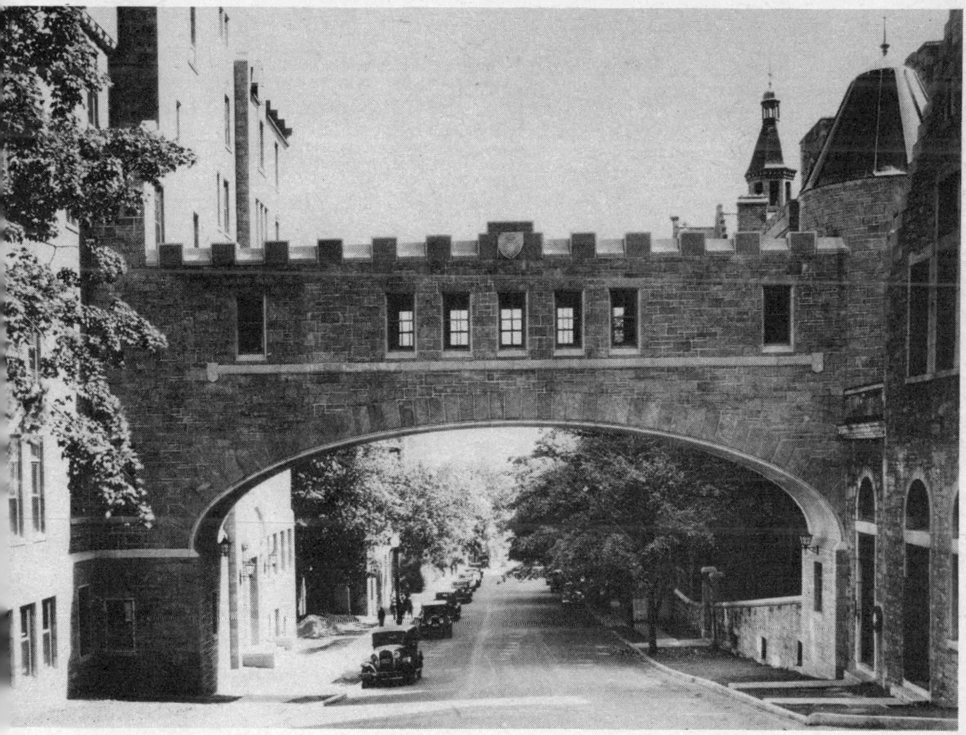

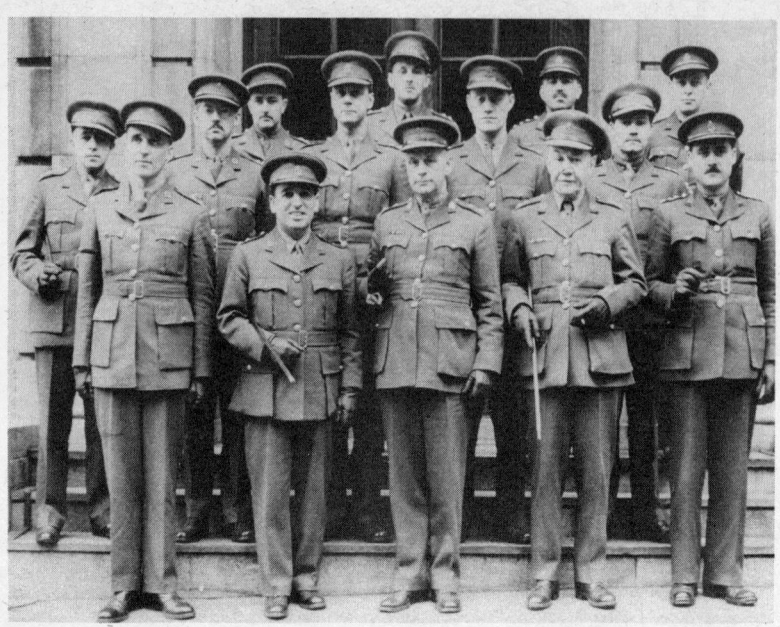

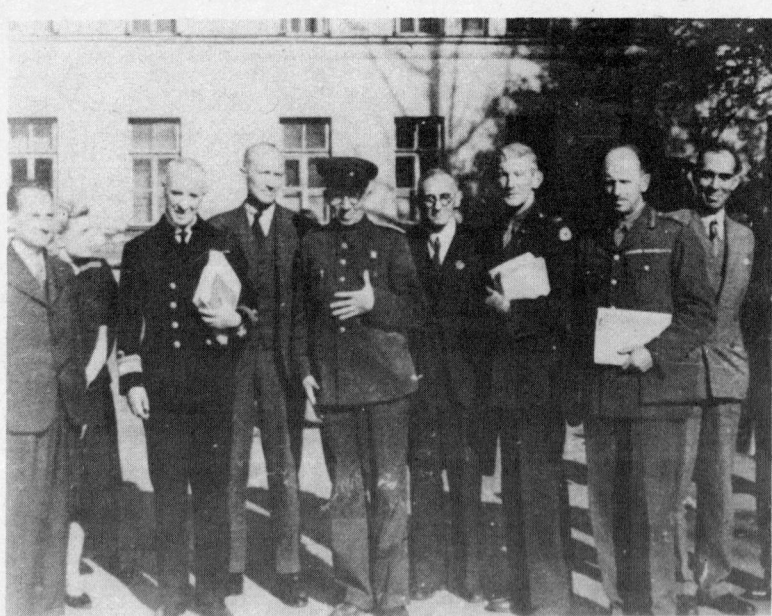

TOP: The Number 1 Neurological Hospital team at Basinstoke, England, in 1940. In front row are Bill Cone (*second from left*) and Colin Russel (*second from right*).   ABOVE: "The Russian Mission," July 1943. Wilder (*fourth from left*) poses with his Soviet hosts and other delegates.

PART TWO

*And time yet for a hundred indecisions,
And for a hundred visions and revisions...*
T. S. ELIOT

CHAPTER SIX

His Own Master

MONTREAL

As the tugboats gently nudged the S.S. *Montnairn* into her berth at Quebec City in the early morning of September 26, 1928, Wilder stood on the upper deck, oblivious to the bustle and excitement of the other passengers, looking up at the turrets and towers of the Château Frontenac Hotel, high above on the cliff. He was looking for the windows of the tower room where he and his mother had spent several memorable days during their trip to celebrate his graduation from Princeton, fifteen years earlier. Quebec and the grand hotel that dominated the city would always remind him of her and that first trip, but on this occasion the memory was even more potent and affecting. He was thirty-seven years old now; his oldest son, Wilder Jr., was ten. He was no longer a junior surgeon waiting in line, but a smart, young "comer"—a catch for the Royal Victoria Hospital. Even so, as a new chapter in his life opened up, his first, private reaction was doubt that he would be a match for its challenges.

"I must be a different fellow in Montreal than I have ever been before—and can I?" So he had written to his mother from the *pension* in Obernigk. Behind was the security of being a cog in a big hospital machine, with the best medical men in his field within calling distance in an emergency. Behind was the orderly pattern of ascendancy through the ranks, from the charity cases of the public wards to the wealthy patients in New York, "that city of millionaires." And behind now, too, were the easy friendships, many of them stretching back to college days, which, thinking of the city from this new perspective, made New York seem suddenly like home.

Settled in a room at the Château Frontenac while waiting for the train, he dashed off a letter to his mother.

"Canada! I've suddenly realized what the British flag here means. I never gave it a thought in England, as I was a foreigner there. Here, I am an immigrant....

"I'm a little frightened today, to tell you the truth. To build up a clinic and practice in the most narrow of all specialties, here in the Province of Quebec, where the majority are French Catholics seems to me a doubtful undertaking....

"Oh it will turn out all right of course. It is a great challenge and I'm on my own now—but in a smaller world. New York is so huge and the U.S. so powerful and rich it makes me feel as though I'm going into exile."

It was hardly a very risky exile, however. The terms he had negotiated included an appointment as Professor of Neurosurgery at McGill University, along with an appointment as Surgeon-in-Charge of Neurosurgery at the Royal Victoria Hospital. The wealthy Montreal allies of Edward Archibald had agreed to make up the difference between Penfield's actual earnings and $10,000 per year during the three-year trial period, and they had paid for the equipment he and Cone needed for their lab in Montreal.

For Cone there was a salary of $4,000 as Chief of the Laboratory of Neuropathology. In addition, Cone would share a percentage of their joint practice, albeit a smaller share, commensurate with his junior status.

But aside from these guarantees, the board was not offering Wilder a sinecure. To build up his private practice, it was clear that he would have to barnstorm around the country, speak at conferences and attend meetings to convince doctors to refer patients to him for brain surgery. And though Archibald had been a staunch and effective ally, as his protégé Wilder inherited some of the enmity he had accrued. Already the hospital had withdrawn its promised support of the laboratory ($2,000 per year toward the salary of a technician to run it), on some pretext or other, but in fact because of the antipathy of the hospital president, Sir Vincent Meredith, toward Archibald and all his undertakings. Once again Archibald's allies had stepped in and made up the difference privately, but it irked Wilder to have the lab dependent on charity.

Still, he and Helen had at least one friend in Montreal. Three weeks before, the Penfields had been riding about Vienna in the top of a bus discussing their future home when a woman in the seat ahead of them turned and said, "Excuse me, but I couldn't help overhearing. Are you Dr. and Mrs. Penfield?" Startled, they admitted they were, and she went on to say that she was from Montreal and had heard all about them. News that an American neurosurgeon was coming to Montreal had travelled widely. Her name was Mrs. Hugh Russel, and a friendship was struck at once.

On learning that the Penfields hadn't found a place to stay in Montreal, she told them she was returning in a few days and would take care of it. True to her word, Mrs. Russel met them at the station in Montreal and took them to rooms she'd found on the second and third floors of one of the elegant Victorian houses that lined the south side of Sherbrooke Street. She did so much for them in the next few months, and did it so mysteriously, that they christened her "Aunt Ariel."

Wilder set out from the Sherbrooke Street rooms early the next morning to walk to the hospital, looking about him with the keen and curious eye of an immigrant. If he expected to hear French spoken as he struck out eastward along Sherbrooke Street, he was disappointed. Although four-fifths of the million or so inhabitants of Montreal in 1928 were French-speaking—making it the second largest French-speaking city in the world—the English and French lived in worlds apart. With the easy arrogance of power, the English as a rule learned only enough French to deal with porters and upstairs maids. For their part, the French, by and large, spoke such English as their employment required.

The geographic divisions reinforced the isolation: as the city's population spread uphill from the old city at the river's edge it met the steep shoulder of Mount Royal and divided: English to the west, French to the east. The no man's land surrounding the rough dividing line of St. Lawrence Boulevard was populated by those who were neither French nor English: Chinese stranded after the completion of the transcontinental railway, which their labour had built; successive waves from Central and Eastern Europe; Jews fleeing the pogroms in Russia.

Religion and education played a part in the isolation. French education in Quebec was the preserve of the Catholic Church, English Protestant education the responsibility of the government.

The divisions were more than crude demarcations of religion, language, education and geography. Every institution and organization had its counterpart: the exclusive Mount Royal Club, where Wilder had been a guest on his first trip to the city, had its equal in the Club St. Denis, a mile to the east; McGill University, past whose massive stone gates Wilder now walked on his way to the hospital, educated some 3,000 students a year in English, L'Université de Montréal twice that number in French.

The result, as Stephen Leacock observed some years later in his history of Montreal, is that each race "sees too well the faults, too dimly the merits, of the other. The English think that many of the French are priest-ridden; the French think that many of the English are badly in need of a priest. The English think that those of the French who are crooked are crooked in a selfish, petty way, using favouritism for little jobs. The French think that the English, when crooked, are crooked in a big, unselfish way, stealing a million out of a franchise and giving silver cups to golf clubs."

To hear French spoken Wilder would have had to continue along Sherbrooke Street for half a mile. Instead he turned north on University Street, past the eastern gates of the McGill campus and on up the hill to the turreted fortress of the Royal Victoria Hospital. There, in the rooms set aside for the laboratory, he found Bill Cone busy unpacking the specimens brought from New York and the rest of their equipment. For the next few weeks the lab would be primarily Cone's affair, as Wilder set about mending a few fences.

While his notions about expanding neurosurgery to include a laboratory of neuropathology and clinical neurology had won him support and admirers in the Montreal medical community, it had also put a few noses out of joint. One such nose belonged to Horst Oertel, head of the Pathological Institute, who had refused them space in his building for their lab. Since he and Cone had been made welcome in the University Clinic, Wilder could afford to ignore Oertel. Not so Colin Russel, brother-in-law of "Aunt Ariel," senior neurologist at McGill medical school and chief neurologist at the Royal Vic. During Wilder's exploratory trip, Russel had been "gruff and a good deal less than enthusiastic" about his plans.

Since neither the Montreal General Hospital nor the Royal Vic had a neurosurgeon, it had been agreed that Wilder could operate at both hospitals. But he would need the co-operation of the neurologists in both places, for their referrals as well as their consultation. With an amused detachment he certainly didn't feel at the time, Wilder described his predicament in *No Man Alone:*

"But how was I, a surgeon, to involve the neurologists of Montreal in our project? A surgeon must admit that any highly trained physician has still some reason to be 'proud.' Their predecessors looked down on the barber-surgeons of the old days and we, who are the surgeons of today, still have our inferiority complex. And they? Well, they sometimes betray evidence of the reverse inheritance. Or, perhaps it is only that they recall the fact that when they graduated in medicine, nearly all the bright students in the class became physicians. The others went in for surgery.

"It must have been apparent to Montreal neurologists that the newly-arrived neurosurgeons from New York pretended to have some knowledge of neurology as well as some familiarity with the basic neurological sciences. Did they—the surgeons—also propose to practise clinical neurology? And would they compete with the medical neurologists, whose bread and butter depended on their neurological expertise?"

It was Colin Russel who, with little delay put the question to Wilder. It would have been a very interesting showdown to witness: Penfield, the young tiger, and Russel, the old lion, circling each other warily. The outcome was critical: if Colin Russel decided not to cooperate, his influence would make sure that most of the other neurologists in the city could comfortably ignore Penfield, making his stay in Montreal brief and unpleasant. If, on the other hand, Russel could be won over, he would bring along with him the support that could guarantee Penfield's success.

It is a measure of Wilder's growing self-confidence that he reacted calmly. He decided to like Colin Russel in spite of their first wary encounter.

No, he insisted, they weren't going to encroach on Russel's or the other neurologists' territory, except for the patients that they, Penfield and Cone, alone could treat better through surgery, such as patients with tumours, and epileptics. They did, however, want to reserve the right to continue the neurological investigations they had begun in New York and for which they had fought so hard to have lab facilities in Montreal. "Our laboratory is your laboratory," he told Russel, "if you will join us. We want to join you in the 'rough and tumble' of the public clinics. The time has come when we could all join together to make a more scientific approach to the unsolved problems of the nervous system, and this should include psychiatrists as well."

Wilder then went on to describe to Russel the Wednesday clinical conferences that had become a tradition at the Vanderbilt Clinic in New York, where neurologists, psychiatrists and neurosurgeons gathered after working hours to examine patients with particularly baffling symptoms and offered their professional advice.

The idea appealed to Russel immediately, according to Wilder's account in *No Man Alone*.

"He jumped to his feet. 'By gad! I'd like that. That's just what I have always wanted to do.'" Russel went on excitedly to say that he had specimens to add to the collection in Penfield's and Cone's laboratory, as well as a lot of teaching slides which he would bring, along with his microscope, and join them.

Wilder interrupted to ask if the French-Canadian neurologists in the city would care to join them at the weekly conferences. Russel "shook his head. 'No, I don't think so.

"'The English neurologists will come. I'll see that they do. They'd jolly well better come. We have beautiful cases to discuss at the outpatient clinic at the "Vic." They have even more such cases at the General.

"'But no. We've never mixed that way with the French-Canadian neurologists. Their patients rarely come to our offices for consultation. They'd rather die.'

"He chuckled and stood before me with his feet wide apart in an attitude that was to become very familiar, a freshly lit cigarette in his hand, his left eyebrow elevated by the pull of a small scar in his forehead. 'Bless my soul! They're just as narrow-minded as we are in the other direction. We live here in separate and independent professional worlds.'"

Russel's words were a challenge, and Wilder set out to prove him wrong. It would be a meagre practice to share with Bill Cone if they could only draw on the 200,000 Anglo-Montrealers and those patients they could draw from outside.

His words also came as a surprise. Archibald had turned to Wilder and, as a parting comment after their first meeting a year earlier, said *"A Montréal on parle français. Vous parlez, n'est-ce pas?"* Wilder's *"Mais oui!"* had been more a statement of willingness to learn than of ability, and he had relished the idea of learning a new language and living in an exotic, bilingual city. Now he saw that Archibald was an anomaly: he spoke French easily, and flitted back and forth over the dividing wall to operate on chest patients at the Hôtel-Dieu and Nôtre-Dame Hospitals as willingly as at the Royal Victoria Hospital. But there were few like him.

Having none of the built-in prejudices and assumptions of Russel and his colleagues, Wilder arranged to meet the French doctors, and found them not only congenial and well-informed, but quite prepared to co-operate. They were flattered by Penfield's interest, and impressed when he launched into French lessons so that he could improve his halting command of the language. Soon he was being called for consultation on their cases, and he returned the favour. When he invited them to the Wednesday conferences, Russel and the others were astonished to see how willingly they came, and how enthusiastically they participated. Before long, though with a few grumbles, the English doctors were unlimbering their high school

French and making their way to the French hospitals on alternate Wednesdays as a regular rotation was established.

Throughout the fall of 1928 Helen unpacked crates and trunks and settled into the house she and Wilder had found with Aunt Ariel's help; the children made new friends and began school, and Wilder plunged into his new routine. He had courses to teach at the medical school, new equipment to try out, nurses to educate in his operating room procedures, short trips to make around eastern Canada to meet other doctors, and the task of keeping up his U.S. contacts by attending medical meetings there. In the evening when he was in town he would dash home to spend a few precious moments with the children before donning a dinner jacket, or tails and a silk top hat, *de rigeur* in Anglo-Montreal society, to go with Helen to cocktails or dinner or the theatre. The social world in which they now found themselves was rather intimidatingly populated by Lords and Ladies; titles that rang awkwardly on his midwestern tongue, and on hers, and made them both ill at ease. Montreal was turning out to be a far cry from New York: there as a junior neurosurgeon his friends were his own and social obligations few. Here he was Montreal's only neurosurgeon, a distinguished specialist in a city that accorded inordinate respect to medical men.

Yet the welcome was genuine, and after a while the awkwardness began to wear off. The house the Penfields moved to from their rented rooms was on the lower slope of Westmount; it was large and comfortable with a view of the mansions above them. Across the street was a park with what promised to be a good toboggan run, an added bonus once the snow fell.

Bill Cone was settling into the lab happily, and had been joined by Edward Dockrill. They had decided earlier to leave Edward behind in New York because of his surly temper, but he turned up in Montreal one day, cap in hand, meekly promising to mend his ways, and they had relented. With that the transplantation was complete.

In the midst of all this, late in November came a telegram from Wilder's mother in California saying that his sister Ruth was seriously ill. If they came to Montreal, would Wilder examine her and try to find out what was wrong?

∞∞ RUTH

When the news of Ruth's illness came Helen was sick with the mumps, in bed with a high fever. Wilder cabled back quickly to delay his mother and Ruth, but it was too late. Jack Inglis, Ruth's husband, wired on December 2 "They will arrive Thursday morning....Ruth's condition seems urgent."

The telegram was followed by a letter of explanation from Ruth's doctor in California; in the last ten years Ruth had had four epileptic attacks. During one, the convulsions lasted for forty-eight hours. The last attack was a few months earlier; she had gone into a coma and they had thought she would die. Since then there had been frequent small convulsions, terrible headaches and vomiting. After seeing a neurosurgeon in California, Jean insisted on bringing her to Wilder in Montreal.

Wilder was stricken. He searched back through his memory of Ruth: the headaches and dizzy spells as a little girl, and when he was thirteen and she nineteen, standing outside her bedroom door listening in terror to the awful sounds of an attack, peeking in to see her lying unconscious on the bed. Then it had been called "nerves"— the great catch-all for anything medicine could not fathom. Now he realized it must have been a major epileptic seizure. All those years as, slowly but surely, he narrowed down on epilepsy, first as a field of microscopic study and later as a possible neurosurgical specialty, he had not known about Ruth.

It needs an explanation. First, Ruth's condition was something he had grown up with, something mysterious but a part of Ruth that those around her accepted. After she married and moved to California, her fits were something too ugly to discuss in any detail, apparently not even in a letter to her brother. And yet he had known about Ruth's fits all his life. Was he never more curious for details, did he never offer advice?

The answer brings us to Jean Penfield, their mother. Three or four years earlier when the attacks grew more frequent, Jean had gone with Ruth to a Christian Science healer. Jean was having trouble with her legs, but the real reason for her visit to the healer was her desperation at Ruth's condition. Mother and daughter had both converted on the spot, and Jean had sent Wilder pamphlets and written enthusiastically about the miraculous change Christian Science had wrought.

Wilder was not amused, and his dismissal of Christian Science as hocus-pocus had caused the first real strain in their relationship. In a rare letter from Ruth in 1926, wishing him happy birthday, she concluded an enthusiastic account of the improvement in her own and Jean's health with an apology "for this long discourse. I had no intention of dwelling upon this, or preaching any kind of a sermon...but it just came out. I'm like mother. She said one day 'I have tried to be very careful and not talk Science to Wilder, but in every letter he gives me some kind of a dig. So I'm not going to be careful anymore, but just be natural, and say what I feel like saying. If he persists in fishing in this pool, I shall rise to his bait.'"

It was likely his mother's touchiness more than anything else that kept Wilder from taking an active professional interest in his sister's illness. That, and the fact that by now it was quite simply a part of his perception of Ruth. And doctors are trained to believe they should never "doctor" members of their own family. If Wilder believed she was in good professional hands in California, he would not have felt it his place to interfere—especially since it would mean a battle with his mother on the subject of Christian Science.

On the Thursday morning of the first week of December, Wilder met his mother and sister at Windsor Station in Montreal. His mother's hair was now white, but she seemed calm and determined. She admitted to him, out of Ruth's hearing, that she had been afraid the whole way that Ruth would have a fit on the train. Ruth smiled to see him, but appeared dazed. He brought them home, and while they were still unpacking and getting ready for breakfast, Wilder decided he could wait no longer. He went up to Ruth's room and gently told her he wanted to examine her eyes. She stood patiently while he peered through the lens of the opthalmoscope, held a few inches away. There it was, the sign of a tumour growing behind her forehead. The head of the optic nerve was dreadfully swollen, with little red haemorrhages extending out over the surface of the surrounding retina: signs of the enormous pressure building up in the skull. She could be blind, permanently, in a day or two.

His knees grew weak and he thought he might fall. He put his hand on Ruth's shoulder to steady himself, pretending to continue the examination. When he had recovered, he led her down to breakfast, telling her jokes to make her laugh.

Colin Russel came by after breakfast to examine Ruth. The three of them then drove to the Royal Vic for X-rays. Bill Cone joined them. The radiologist looked at the X-rays and shook his head. There was a tumour there, but without surgery it was impossible to say how big it was or if it was malignant. They brought Ruth back to the house, and were joined by Dr. Archibald, who examined her as well. Then they gave her something for her headache and packed her off to bed.

The consultation began: Bill Cone, Colin Russel, Edward Archibald and Wilder, who had already made up his mind to do the operation himself. The alternative to Wilder operating was to send

Ruth to Harvey Cushing, but the low mortality rate Cushing had established in Boston, admirable though it was, had a lot to do with his caution in the operating room. Faced with a tumour in one of the frontal lobes, like Ruth's, that caution would mean that Cushing wouldn't dare risk a major removal.

So little was known of the frontal lobes in 1928. They were part of the 'new brain' that had evolved in humans—slowly enlarging the area over the eyes until that unique characteristic among the animals had formed; a skull deformed by a forehead which bulged up around the frontal lobes. That much they knew, and it was enough to cause the frontal lobes to be treated with almost superstitious awe: here were what neurologists called "the higher brain functions"— planning, initiative, morality, emotions, abstraction were all said to be located there.

And yet, Wilder wondered, if that was true, then what about his patient William Hamilton? Wilder had risked a large removal of the boy's frontal lobes—larger than any he or the other doctors in New York had ever heard of—and Hamilton had recovered without any detectable loss of "mentality." If it had worked with Hamilton, might he not dare to make such a large removal in Ruth's case if it might mean saving her sight and perhaps her life? The surgeon who operated on Ruth would have to be willing to take such risks, and no one else would. What's more, Jean had not brought Ruth all this way, admitting the failure of her beloved Christian Science, so that Wilder could send her along to some other surgeon. Still, he would need the professional sanction of the others gathered for his consultation before operating on someone so close to him.

He described Ruth's history for Cone, Archibald and Russel, and then, according to his version in *No Man Alone,* summed up as follows:

"My sister has had a brain tumour for almost thirty years. I'd like to think it is benign and encapsulated. But the fact that it seems to have begun to grow rapidly in these last months suggests that it may have become malignant, even if it was benign at the start. Surgical removal, which might have been relatively easy once, is difficult and dangerous now. But if I were in her place, I would ask for a radical attempt to remove the whole growth, however dangerous it might be to my life. But I would not want to be paralyzed. I'd rather die. If it can't be removed completely, then I would ask the surgeon to be as radical as he can be, short of paralysis. I would hope then for a year or so of useful life before the beginning of the end.

"She has many things to do that are important as mother and wife." he went on. "The two youngest children are boys, about six to eight years old. Carl Rand might have done the operation in Los Angeles. But it was my mother, I think, who insisted on bringing her here.

"We could probably take her to Cushing or to someone else and get her there before she goes blind. But we will have to hurry. Please, make this decision as if this woman were not my sister. I must not influence your thinking in any way. When you want me, you will find me with Helen upstairs."

With that, Wilder left the room.

It seemed a very long time before Bill Cone came to fetch him back, but when he re-entered the room Archibald simply asked, presumably for the record, "If you were to do this operation, could you do it as if she were not your sister?" When Wilder answered Yes, they agreed that he should go ahead with the operation the next day. Later that night Wilder cabled Ruth's husband: "Tumour in right frontal lobe of brain...probably removable by difficult operation. Shall I take her to another city or do it myself?" Jack replied, "Do what you consider best."

Two days later, Wilder found himself in the operating room looking at his sister's brain, exposed by the careful removal of a piece of her skull. He had taken all possible precautions, and Bill Cone was beside him, along with Miss Ann Penland, the expert anaesthetist from the Presbyterian Hospital in New York who had worked with him in the operation on William Hamilton. She had arrived the day before in response to Wilder's urgent summons. The procedure had been carefully rehearsed with the instruments nurse, and Wilder's modification of the protective screen he had seen Foerster using in Breslau that summer was getting its trial run. The screen had been devised by Foerster to permit careful observation of the conscious patient during long operations using only a local anaesthetic. This unusual set-up involved suturing a sterile sheet to the patient's shaven scalp to form a protective wall between the head and the surgeon on one side, and the patient and the nurses and doctors, who would carefully monitor her and provide comfort, on the other.

While Wilder probed, Ruth talked, telling him stories of her children until, at length, he begged her to stop so he could concentrate. They worked for hours. The tumour was, as they suspected, in the right frontal lobe, and they removed as much of the tumour as they could, back to the motor gyrus, and then paused for a moment. "This was already the largest brain removal I had ever made," Wilder wrote. "But, to my dismay, the growth was not all out. It extended underneath—gray, firm, malignant-looking tissue on the floor of the skull. Enormous veins came up through the tissue. They must connect directly with the venous sinuses in the dura beneath. The sinuses were capable of very rapidly bleeding, which would be very difficult to control."

This was the critical moment. Should he go on and risk severing the veins or stop, knowing that the tumour would go on growing and would certainly, in time, kill Ruth? At this point, Wilder looked at Bill Cone.

"He shook his head. 'Don't chance it, Wide.' I hesitated, arguing silently within myself with that other fellow, that daimon. There is a daimon that goes about with one and tries to keep him out of trouble. He was telling me now that Bill was right. 'But,' I argued within myself, 'I undertook this operation because I was afraid another surgeon would turn back too soon, not knowing how much she had to live for.'"

The discovery that there was more of the tumour extending toward the mid-line, so he wrote to Jack Inglis two days later, "filled me with a sort of frenzy, and I fear I was rather reckless." However, he managed to remove more of the tumour, despite the danger, giving Ruth three successive blood transfusions when the heavy bleeding suddenly began. But he dared not risk removing it all when he saw that it extended even to the left hemisphere. It was perhaps at this moment that, as he admitted in his report to Jack but omitted from the later account in *No Man Alone*, "for about fifteen minutes...I could not carry on and Dr. Cone, my assistant, stepped into the breach."

After they replaced the trap door that had been cut in the skull and sutured the scalp, Wilder stood for a moment beside Ruth with his finger on her pulse. She was awake and smiled, and apologized for the trouble she had caused them all.

Wilder left the operating room and went to the dressing-room alone, struggling with a sense of failure. Although the pressure would now be gone and her eyesight saved, there was little doubt that what he had left behind would kill Ruth in the end. An analysis of the tumour tissue would reveal the length of reprieve he had secured her, but there was the question, still unanswered, of how such radical removal in the right frontal lobe would affect Ruth's personality. For the moment, at least, there was cause to rejoice, for Ruth's recovery was rapid and there was, as yet, no sign that the removal had affected her behaviour or her ability to reason. The tumour appeared slow-growing and Wilder hoped that X-ray treatment would help retard the growth.

"It seems to me quite within the range of possibility that fifteen years may elapse before the thing grows large enough to demand attention again," he wrote in his letter to Jack. "If it should grow more rapidly at any time, she could be re-operated upon." Her convulsions would likely disappear, for a while at any rate. He advised Jack to keep the information to himself, and as far as Ruth and the family were concerned "assume that Ruth's trouble is over."

And that is what Ruth assumed, when she left on February 26, 1929, to return to her family. Aside from his carefully optimistic note to Jack, Wilder kept his thoughts much to himself.

Three weeks after Ruth left for home, she wrote two separate letters to Wilder and Helen thanking them for everything. One, which Wilder quotes from at some length in *No Man Alone*, is a gay and gracefully written note, testifying to the "miracle" that had occurred. "Of course no one can know what it means to be back in my own little corner and to feel I'm really needed. You'd be delighted to hear people exclaim over how well I look and didn't I put on weight, etc. My one pound gain must have gone to my face just as Wide wanted it to." The letter went on to say, quite gleefully, "The first Monday after arriving Jack took me to a dinner and dance for Rotary ladies night. It was such fun. Everyone seemed so surprised that I could dance and seem as well as ever. Perhaps they felt I should be in a wheel chair. I wore a tight blue hat that I had last summer with my blue dress."

This was the kind of follow-up report, wrote Wilder in *No Man Alone*, that a surgeon likes best.

The second letter, however, clearly was not—so much so that he omitted any reference to it. And yet in his office files under his sister's name was a small, rectangular piece of cardboard, and in Ruth's handwriting a note bearing the same date as the first letter, February 24. The first letter was addressed, like the other letters in the file "Dear Helen and Wide," but this one began "My dear Dr. and Mrs. Penfield." It continues in the same polite, remote tone and ends on this chilling note: "I must add a word of appreciation to Dr. Penfield for setting my brains in order. I must say I have not missed what he took out, not even have I felt light-headed, and if he has the little fungus pickled as a memento of my visit he is very welcome to it. I hope all future patients pay better than I."

It was signed R. P. Inglis—not "Ruth."

Was this an attempt at humour that missed the mark? Or a first sign of some change in her behaviour? Wilder himself was puzzled. He had pencilled on the piece of cardboard the question that must have echoed in his mind many times over the years: "After Operation. Is this a joke?"

All through 1929 Ruth seemed her old self—better, in fact, than she had been for twenty years. The epileptic fits were gone, as were the headaches and, most important, the constant insecurity of never knowing when or where the next one will occur. Her letters were reassuring and full of joy and thanks, and yet there was a faint disturbing note. Ruth found she couldn't do some things as well as before. Letters, however clear they sounded, took longer to write, sometimes weeks. "I have trouble getting organized," she wrote.

He made a brief visit to California that year, and Ruth planned a dinner for him. He arrived shortly before dinner and was alarmed to find the house messy, the children running about uncontrolled, the table not set and, in the kitchen surrounded by a great confusion of unprepared food, Ruth in tears. He immediately comforted and reassured her and helped her put the roast in the oven and make the salad, but as he did so his heart must have sunk as he saw the changes he had made in the abilities of this once-meticulous and organized housekeeper by the large frontal lobe removal. She could have done one thing or the other, but she could not concentrate enough to organize dinner, calm the children, tidy the house, set the table—all the demands of so familiar a sequence were too much for her to handle.

However, the crisis passed and she wrote gamely some months later "I am trying to be more alert. Sometimes it seems to be very slow progress. If you have any advice to offer as to how to learn to think, how to get something of an education when old, it will be gratefully received."

Then, in May of 1930, a year and a half after the operation, Ruth had a relapse and several severe epileptic fits. Four months later Wilder met his sister and mother in Boston, where Harvey Cushing had agreed to perform a second operation to remove more of the tumour. Again, Ruth recovered for a while, but the old fear was back, and six months later the fits reappeared.

On July 14, 1931, a telegram arrived from Jack saying simply "Ruth passed away at 1 P.M. Mother all right." Wilder called Helen from the hospital, and after they had talked, he wrote back offering what solace he could, ending sadly, "I did want to change the writing on the wall."

∞∞ EPILEPSY

Though there had been advances in the last ten years, these were still disheartening times for brain surgeons everywhere. Their cases were likely to consist of accident victims, whom they could patch up in the hope that the damage was not too severe, babies with birth deformities like hydrocephalus, in which the odds of surgery improving their condition were very low, and tumour cases like Ruth's.

Ruth's case was a classic. Hoping that the tumour was benign, a surgeon in those days would remove as much of the tumour as he dared, trying, with his sketchy knowledge of the brain, to steer clear of the most important brain functions. The more he removed, the more he risked a nasty surprise later. But Ruth had gained a year or more of relatively normal and happy life, and to both the patient and the surgeon, the operation seemed worthwhile.

That was Harvey Cushing's rationale and it accounted in some measure for then current attitudes: his reputation and influence were such that brain surgery was regarded as tumour surgery, with Cushing the high priest. Nonetheless, many doctors, partly from simple fear of meddling with the brain and partly from a realistic assessment of the temporary benefits of neurosurgery, were inclined to counsel resignation rather than an operation.

But Wilder had no patience for this narrow view of his profession, and he was temperamentally unwilling to plug along obediently in Cushing's wake as a mere tumour specialist. He wanted to prove that other kinds of brain surgery were warranted at the hands of a skilful neurosurgeon—and he wanted a specialty of his own.

What Cushing had done a generation earlier to make tumour surgery respectable, Wilder was determined to do for a procedure he felt held considerably more promise: surgery to relieve epilepsy. His interest in the disease had grown year by year during his time in New York. From seeing it as a field of laboratory study—and a particularly thorny one at that, until he mastered the Spanish cell-staining techniques—he had graduated to a faith in surgery as a cure for many sufferers of the ancient "falling sickness." Foerster had paved the way with his operations to remove brain scars on German veterans of the Great War. Wilder had made up his mind to make the next step.

Epileptic fits, he knew, were simply massive electrical discharges in the brain which electrocuted the patient into temporary unconsciousness. In certain cases, while the fit was going on the patient could continue to perform simple mechanical functions. If the fit occurred while the epileptic was driving a car, he could continue to drive, stopping at stop lights, and proceeding again when the light turned green. But if a seizure occurred in the midst of a conversation with a passenger the victim would be struck dumb—would become a 'zombie.' Some part of the brain was functioning, directing the simple and familiar action of driving a car, but the rest of the brain was shut down for the duration of the fit. Other, less fortunate patients, reacted to a seizure by going into spasms, as various of their muscular controls were caught up in the fury of the epileptic hurricane sweeping across the brain.

More often than not, the symptoms of an epileptic seizure were consistent from patient to patient; one would simply become unconscious each time it struck; another would have the same sequence of epileptic spasms each time. And in the symptoms lay clues to the source of the epileptic fit. Although in many cases the cause of the fit was simply a mystery—part of the general mystery of the brain—in other cases the fit was caused by a scar or a tumour or a malformation irritating or pressing against the brain and somehow triggering the electrical discharge. Because these fits had an originating focus, or point, the condition was called "focal epilepsy."

Although surgeons in the past had operated to remove scars causing epileptic fits, in many cases the excision caused another scar to form, and the fits continued or even accelerated. Most neurosurgeons weighed in the balance the perils of infection and surgical error, which in those days accompanied the simplest surgery, then rejected the operation as not worth the risk.

In 1927, however, Wilder had pointed out in an article in *Brain*, the prestigious British journal of neurology, some of the reasons for the recurrence of epileptic fits after such operations. First, surgeons were being too conservative: remove all of the damaged tissue and as much of the surrounding tissue as you can safely remove, Wilder suggested. If that apparently healthy tissue is in fact damaged as well, though as yet invisibly, it will in time cause the fits to recur. Secondly, leave the cavity, produced by excising a part of the brain, empty rather than filling it with fat or fascia or some other "foreign material," (as was then the habit). The cavity will fill up with the fluids of the brain, which in fact provide better protection for the healing tissues.

In Montreal in 1930 he followed up these radical suggestions in the Canadian Medical Association *Journal* with a summary of four cases of his, in which the epileptic patients had been freed of their fits. One of the four was William Hamilton: thirty months later he was back at work and showing no signs of mental deficiency, despite the large amount of brain tissue removed.

Predictably, the reaction to Wilder's stance on surgery for epilepsy was mixed. Some doctors shook their heads and warned it was too soon to tell if he was right, and too great a risk to take if he wasn't.

Others were cautiously optimistic and a few were enthusiastic. Before long, however, critics and supporters were referring to the operation as "the Montreal Procedure," and patients began coming there in the hope that Wilder Penfield and his co-workers could cure them.

It was a long and gruelling operation, one that demanded great physical endurance and exceptional skill from the surgeon, as well as great faith and fortitude from the patient. Since the patient would be conscious and actively helping guide the surgeon, trust was essential.

Wilder was a master at gaining the confidence of his patients; his files are full of letters of gratitude: "He was so unbelievably kind, warm-hearted, steadfast, gentle, quick to perceive and to respond," one patient wrote in a letter to Mrs. Penfield. "And he got to the heart of the matter immediately, with few words, usually with a smile, a sparkle in his eye, & that unequalled quiet humour....After two hideously unsuccessful operations in New York, six years of resignation to my fate and total disillusionment with all hospitals and neurosurgeons, I knew at once that he was of a different order."

Over a span of thirty years Wilder operated on more than 750 patients suffering from epilepsy. Despite extraordinary developments in diagnostic and supportive equipment, and innumerable important refinements in technique, it is remarkable how little the operation itself actually changed during that period—from either the surgeon's or the patient's point of view.

For the patient, the procedure begins with having one's head shaved bald then being wheeled into the operating room and placed on one's side on the table. The patient's head is then settled on a metal frame to hold it in place. Orderlies and nurses dressed in green move in and out of the field of vision, unveiling mysterious pieces of equipment and moving them into place, talking quietly under their masks.

The surgeon, or the surgeon's assistant, sketches the outline of the trap door that will be cut into the skull, then gives the patient a local anaesthetic. The brain tissue itself, though it readily recognizes pain messages brought to it along the web of nerves from the rest of the body, has no sensations. The surgeon now cuts through the scalp along the line that has been drawn, pulling back and clipping the skin to hold it in place, exposing the skull. With a hand or electric drill, five or six holes are made through the hard bone at each corner of the drawing. Then the surgeon passes a thin, flexible sawtoothed blade known as a Gigli saw down through one hole and threads it through and back up another. That done, the incision is completed and the trap door in the skull is removed. The three protective layers of tissue between the skull and the brain are cut and pulled away, exposing, at last, the surface of the brain.

The probing begins. Taking up a slender wire carrying a mild electrical current, the surgeon begins mapping the surface of the brain. Beside the patient is an assistant who acts as a relay to the surgeon above and behind, out of the patient's sight. Repeatedly touching the wire to the cortex (the surface of the brain), the surgeon looks for the points that control various functions: smell, sight, speech, the motor reflexes of arms and legs, etc.

"What do you feel now?" the surgeon asks.

"I feel a tingling in my left hand," the patient answers. Now that the surgeon knows where the left hand is represented on the cortex, a small ticket with a number is placed on that spot, and a note is dictated to the secretary in the observation gallery. And so it goes for the next hour, or more. Sometimes the surgeon won't need the patient's comment, as when the foot suddenly jerks of its own accord. Flashing lights and stars mean that the area concerned with vision has been found. A sudden inability to speak, or answer the surgeon's questions, means the centre of speech has been pinpointed.

For the surgeon undertaking this operation on a patient with focal epilepsy, the probe serves two purposes. First of all, when the patient's symptoms are discussed earlier, close attention is paid to the sensations that precede the onslaught of a fit, the "aura," as it is called. For one patient the signal might be a sudden strong smell, for another a twitching in the forearm, for yet another pinwheels of light across the field of vision. The aura offers a good indication of where in the brain the fit originates; thus if it begins with a visual distortion, the surgeon will look first in the sight area for the focus of the epileptic seizure.

The probing also serves another, vital, function. As the surgeon maps the brain to discover the exact location of the various functions, he isolates those parts that should not be tampered with for fear of leaving the patient blind, mute or paralyzed. Sometimes, a surgeon will gamble that cutting out a scar or tumour in one part of the brain will only result in a small impairment in, say, the left hand. But it is always a gamble.

When the focus of the seizure has been located—let us say it's a scar—the procedure for removing it begins. In the old days, until 1938 or so, this was done often with a noose of silk thread. Now surgeons use a sophisticated suction device. The blood is cleared away from the area with a "sucker," and the surgeon probes the area around the scar to see if any of the surrounding brain has been affected. If there is uncertainty about whether the focus has actually been found, the surgeon might touch the spot with the probe, increasing the charge to see if it brings on an epileptic fit right there in the operating room. Before the electroencephalograph, or "EEG," and various other devices made the whole procedure a great deal more accurate, this was really the only way a surgeon could make sure he had removed the cause of the patient's fits.

After removal of the damaged tissue, if the surrounding area seems healthy, the long surgical process is reversed. The layers of tissue are replaced one by one and stitched into position, then the trap door, and lastly the layers of the scalp. When that's done, the operation is over and the patient is wheeled away to the recovery room.

A fundamental part of Wilder's defence of surgery for focal epilepsy was that the neurosurgeon must be a trained neurologist as well. He must be familiar with the geography of the brain, and its way of functioning in healthy as well as damaged states, in order to use the probe effectively and draw the right conclusions before cutting into the brain tissue. This was not an attitude calculated to endear him to very many neurologists. Suspicious and, as often as not, contemptuous of neurosurgeons and their fledgling craft, many neurologists regarded such a notion as both heretical and impertinent. It also sounded as though Penfield was suggesting that properly trained neurosurgeons would make neurologists unnecessary.

The whole controversy was aired in an exchange of letters between Wilder and British neurologist F. M. R. Walshe in 1930. Walshe was a disciple of the premier British neurologist Gordon Holmes, with whom Wilder had studied briefly in London in 1920. Penfield and Walshe had not taken to each other for some reason— perhaps a rivalry as students of the same master lay between them. In any case, in this exchange Walshe was speaking for a large number of more restrained critics in British neurology who were contemptuous of "American notions." Walshe wrote: "I had an opportunity of seeing a few years ago in America...the way this admirable notion of the surgeon neurologist actually works out....If the unhappy patient happened to have paralysis agitans or epilepsy, that was his misfortune. If he had a vast glioma filling one hemisphere, then the hemisphere came out. I must admit it was so skilfully removed that the wretched victim of this surgical ecstasy survived—a bedridden, demented hemiplegic with a head like three-quarters of a watermelon, draped with a sagging scalp. Nevertheless, he continued to breathe, eat, make noises, and wet his bed for many months longer than life would have been possible had he not been mutilated, and he was therefore a neurological success...."

Although the attack was not on Wilder personally, and was more in the nature of a criticism of the young brain surgeon who, Walshe went on, "expects with no preliminary training to spring Minerva-like from the head of Cushing, full-armed and with nothing to learn, after a single year's gestation," Wilder took it rather personally. In his retort, Wilder agreed that the notion of the surgeon-scientist pushing back the frontiers of knowledge and treatment of the brain worked only when the surgeon was a well-trained neurologist. However, sensing in Walshe's attack another example of British disdain for surgeons and mistrust of brain surgery, Wilder responded vehemently: "But while I'm at it I should like to criticize neurosurgery as practised in Boston, Baltimore and at Queen Square. I refer to the attitude that neurosurgery means tumour-surgery. Brain tumour-surgery is hardly half of what neurosurgery should cover and it is the least encouraging and least stimulating half."

There was the heart of the matter. There were so many neurological problems that the weight of conservative opinion had labelled out of bounds for a brain surgeon—problems Wilder Penfield believed surgery might at least help if neurologists would stop treating neurosurgery as a bastard child and work *with* neurosurgeons.

In Montreal, with Colin Russel as an ally and the others won over by his and Cone's meticulous operating techniques and sound neurological training, Penfield's approach was beginning to work. Instead of taking patients away from the city's neurologists, the influx of patients drawn to the newly arrived neurosurgeons meant plenty of work for everyone.

As relations with the French-Canadian neurologists developed, they began to send their patients to Penfield and Cone. As well, Wilder's considerable talent for self-promotion bore fruit wherever he travelled and met with doctors and spoke at conferences around the country. The traffic between eastern Canada and Cushing's operating room in Boston began to dry up, and it wasn't long before Penfield and Cone had more patients in Montreal than they could handle.

But Wilder was still not satisfied. The slow progress they were making toward understanding how the brain worked made him impatient: what *caused* diseases like epilepsy? what *caused* tumours to grow? Every time he went to a conference or read a medical journal he discovered new studies, proposals for treatment, theories to account for one brain function or another—but all of it random and, to him at least, disconnected. He could no longer afford the time to drop everything and head off to Germany or Spain in pursuit of each new idea. The study of the brain was growing more and more complex every day. The impossibility of one practitioner keeping up with everything new and exciting was brought home every time he found himself in the operating room, forced to proceed by guesswork; trying to recall what so-and-so in Munich or London or Baltimore had written about some aspect of the problem. Everyone could afford to be phlegmatic about the pace of progress except the surgeon and his patient.

Just how impatient Wilder was, became clear to his sponsor, Edward Archibald, one day in January, 1929. Just five months after arriving in Montreal, Penfield placed a plan for a seven-storey neurological institute on Archibald's desk with a note of explanation: "The enclosed plan...may take you somewhat by surprise. The idea and the plans have been slowly taking form in my mind." The plan included a rough sketch of an institute that would have accommodation for forty bed-patients and seventeen laboratory rooms in a building attached to the Royal Victoria Hospital. Wilder proposed to take his scheme to the Rockefeller Foundation on his own and make a bid for financial support. He estimated the initial costs for building and equipment at around $650,000 and projected that the yearly scientific expenditure would run around $35,000.

The plan did take Archibald by surprise. Penfield had just arrived and already he was planning a major project. However, Archibald must have had some idea of the impulsive nature of his protégé, and they had in fact discussed the idea in more general terms in New York a year before. He guessed, perhaps, that Ruth's operation had had something to do with the precipitousness of the proposal.

Archibald approved the plan and suggested Wilder talk with Charles Martin, the dean of McGill, who looked it over and added his blessing to Archibald's.

So, on January 30, Wilder wrote to Dr. Richard M. Pearce, in charge of medical grants at the Rockefeller Foundation: "Would you be good enough to give me an interview if I came down to New York sometime in the near future? I should like to submit to you a plan for the development of an Institute for Neurological Investigation here in Montreal....I have been here long enough to work out the details of such an undertaking at McGill....

"The institute as planned would continue to form an integral part of the Royal Victoria Hospital without losing contact with general medicine and surgery, but with concentration of all the methods of treatment and investigation of neurological cases...."

Pearce agreed to listen to the proposal, and two weeks later in New York they had their interview. As Wilder wrote later, "I think it may have been one of the most successful applications that was ever refused."

However, the interview was not a total loss by any means. Wilder discovered that similar plans had been submitted to the Rockefeller Foundation from Philadelphia and from Cushing in Boston. As Wilder reported to his mother with pleased surprise in the weekly letter, written a month or so after the interview, "He said he had watched my work for a long time and would like to back it. He also told me he did not expect me to remain at McGill."

For almost two years Wilder had no correspondence with the Rockefeller Foundation about the Institute proposal. He turned his attention to his patients and to developing the small team at hand, still cherishing, he wrote, "the blind hope that the money for expansion of our work would come from somewhere."

∞ PUTTING DOWN ROOTS

Although the prospects for a neurological institute in Montreal seemed as remote as ever by the time the three-year wait-and-see period was up, there was at least one reason for the Penfields to want to stay there.

On one of his first mornings in Montreal Wilder had stopped on his walk to the Royal Vic to watch an automobile with a huge moose head and antlers strapped to the hood pull up in front of one of the Sherbrooke Street houses. He paused in astonishment as the driver and a white-coated houseman, who rushed out to meet the car, carried the trophy inside. The sight reminded him how close the wilderness was to Montreal, and that started him thinking about buying some land and building a cottage for his family. During the seven years the family had lived in New York they had spent the summer, or a month of it at least, camping in tents. He had enjoyed setting up a "model campsite," with tents for cooking and sleeping, and the gadgetry of outdoor cooking, and animal- and insect-proofing. And in the wilderness he felt an unspoken kinship with his father, otherwise so much an enigma. Helen, "my campfire queen," enjoyed the country as much as he did.

Now, for the first time in their lives, they actually had a savings account—containing the tidy sum of $10,000, the remainder of the recent indemnity payment awarded Wilder for his injury on board the *Sussex* during the war.

Early in March, 1929, six months after their arrival in Montreal, Helen spotted an advertisement in the Montreal *Star:* "Manning Farm for sale on Sargent's Bay." Sargent's Bay, she discovered, was a deep wooded inlet of Lake Memphremagog, where that summer the father of a patient, Howard Murray, had agreed to rent them a campsite and a small cottage.

Helen and the children went out to the site in the middle of July and settled in. Several weeks later, Wilder tidied up his desk, made a final round of his patients and set off to join them for a month. The first thing he did on arrival was erect a tent in which he could work on his papers—and then promptly ignored them in the pleasure of relaxing and fishing and swimming in the lake.

Lake Memphremagog, they discovered, stretched thirty-six miles from the town of Magog, Quebec, in the north to Newport, Vermont, in the south. Scattered about on the sloping rises from the lake there were cottages, some of them owned by wealthy Montreal Scottish and English businessmen and their families and, down across the invisible border, by wealthy American families from as far away as Boston and New York. Elsewhere, the lake was dotted with wooded islands. Several miles down, Owl's Head Mountain rose several thousand feet from the water.

At the end of the summer a Johns Hopkins classmate, Martha Eliot, arrived from Boston to stay at her family's cottage on the lake. One afternoon she took the Penfields for a ride in her motor boat and Helen asked if they could go into Sargent's Bay and explore. They landed on a beautiful sandy beach with stands of birch and cedar running up the slope behind it. Two farms bisected the beach, both abandoned. One belonged to the Fosters, who lived twenty miles away in Knowlton; the other was the Manning farm, which Helen had seen advertised for sale in the spring.

Returning to the cottage where they were staying, Wilder and Helen made a few inquiries and found that one of the farms, including 233 acres and three-quarters of a mile of lakefront along a steep point crowned with enormous pines was up for public auction in a few weeks. Before leaving for Montreal Wilder phoned a "gentleman farmer," Eric Fisher, who lived across the bay. The latter, obviously delighted at the prospect of new neighbours came right over in his motor boat, ferried Helen and Wilder back to his house and packed them into the car to take them over by road. The roads around there were in terrible condition; rutted, narrow and steep, which accounted for the fact that there had been no buyers yet. "That finished me," Wilder wrote to his mother in mid-September from Montreal. "Wild trout streams, little mountains, 80 miles to Montreal. The vision came to me of our children growing up there in a cottage on the shore."

That afternoon Helen, Wilder and Eric Fisher tramped all over the property and talked to the tenants of the dilapidated farmhouse, which faced an enormous barn across the narrow road. Then they investigated the adjacent farm and found that it had a road leading down to a ramshackle clapboard cottage right on the water. The farmhouse there, an ugly, squat building with a flat roof, a false front, and peeling paint also had a splendid view down the bay and over the rolling hills to the distant mountains.

Driving back with their host in the dusk, Wilder and Helen made up their minds. They would take the first farm at least. The next day they returned by themselves and staked out three sites by the lake, "one for us, and one for each of two married children!" A few days later in Montreal the owner's representative met with them and they bought the Foster farm for $2,500 "without the stock and implements." Wilder laid out their plans to his mother: "Now! we shall have to get a farmer on the place, try not to lose too much money on it, and gradually, as we can, build a road to the shore and a cottage there."

Helen's joy in their new acquisition was as great as Wilder's. Early in October his weekly letter notes that Helen was off to the lake again that weekend, taking Wilder Jr., Ruthmary, Priscilla and a friend. "She is almost three hours later than expected, and not back yet. She phoned that she had been held up by an aviation meet at St. Hubert airport for 2½ hours! She loves the place down there and so do the children. We have made no mistake in settling there."

A farmer named Jackson was hired and installed in the farmhouse. He began repairing the house and barn and started looking for horses and a few cows. By spring Wilder had bought the Manning farm as well, and was reporting optimistically to his mother: "Combining the usable land of the two farms makes a good cattle and sheep ranch, or farm. With 60 sheep and 18 cows the farm will pay for itself." He went on to reel off his careful calculations, presumably obtained from farmer Jackson, as to the various merits of sheep and cattle, the cost of hay and grain, and so on. On his last trip, he reported, he had performed his first rural medicine—trying to get a peanut out of the windpipe of Jackson's two-year-old son. Over the next twenty or thirty years Wilder would perform many such services and to this day it is almost impossible to mention his name within ten miles and not hear a story of how, in 1938, or '43, or '51, he delivered so-and-so's baby, or operated on someone, or bandaged up a hand caught in a thresher.

It was during a winter holiday at the end of 1930 that Wilder paused briefly in the headlong pace of his life to consider seriously his and the family's position in Montreal. After Christmas they had all gone out on the train to South Bolton, where they were met by Jackson, the farmer, driving the heavy plow team hitched to a box sleigh. For a week Wilder relaxed and played with the children, made an inventory of what the farm operation was costing and thought about the work they were doing at the hospital. "I have never seen the lake more beautiful—snow storms, mists over the mountains, deep, blue sky and sparkling sun, at different times.

"Last night a north wind shook the house and blew through all the cracks. This morning the sun rose red over the lake and we found a pipe frozen, but no harm done. We have had trouble with water supply, furnace and various things, but they are gradually straightening out.... Today Jackson, Helen, [Aunt] Ariel and I drove off in the bobsled in the morning and came back at dusk with a beautiful chestnut pony, a saddle on his back, leading behind us. Priscilla saw us from the hill where she had been contentedly sliding on a little toboggan. She told us in rapture that a little horse was following us! Ruthmary and her friend rode the pony over to the barn...."

Sitting at his desk looking out over the lake, listening to the children laughing and playing in the snow and the murmur of voices from downstairs, where Helen and Ariel were relaxing, he thought with mixed feelings about the situation in Montreal. The stock market crash of 1929 had plunged the world into a depression, and money was tight all over. The laboratory at the Royal Vic was still being supported for routine purposes by the anonymous friends of Edward Archibald, and by a small additional stipend from Jonathan Meakins, professor of surgery at McGill. But there would be no increases for some time. Still, though the laboratory didn't present a very impressive exterior, there was a spirited atmosphere inside. One room had been partitioned off to make an office for Bill Cone and a room for Edward Dockrill, the colourful Cockney technician. The second room at the end of the narrow hall in the University clinic contained a closet-size office for Wilder with a desk, microscope, shelves and a big window, and an outer office for the secretary. In the third room graduate fellows worked at benches shoulder to shoulder, and the room doubled as the neuropathology conference room. French- and English-speaking pathologists and clinicians came to this room and worked beside foreign visitors of all nationalities.

With special permission from her Mother Superior, the French-speaking nun who was chief technician in the laboratory of the Hôtel-Dieu came, to learn the Spanish method of staining cells with silver. At Friday afternoon conferences the room was crowded. Those who came brought microscopes; cases were reviewed and diagnoses made or checked by study of the tissue samples. "Cone and I took opposite sides on some point or other in almost every case," Wilder wrote, "and our heated disagreements became famous. I suppose most of those present realized that, after hearing other points of view, we staged those arguments for teaching purposes. Few, perhaps, perceived how much Bill and I enjoyed them and how close we were in understanding and affection. We used to laugh and carry on the business of the day with recurring reconciliations, knowing that it is far better to be wrong than to be without an opinion."

The laboratory and the men and women who worked there were, in Wilder's musings, the embryo of the institute he wished to build—but where was the money to come from? And where, if not in Montreal, should it be built? The children and Helen were happy in Montreal, though she was beginning to resent the pace he was setting for their lives. He was restless and, despite the farm, feeling somewhat rootless. To pass the time and calm (in his words) "the devil of unrest," he had set to work on another appeal to the Rockefeller Foundation, though he had no clear idea of what to do with it. Pearce, his contact at the Foundation, had died unexpectedly in 1930 and, so far, no successor had been appointed.

Then, on February 4, 1931, a letter came from Charles P. Howland, one of the trustees of the Rockefeller Foundation and father of one of Wilder's patients. This unexpected communication informed Wilder that Alan Gregg, from whose Paris office Wilder had received a fellowship to survey the neurological clinics of Europe in 1928, would be replacing Pearce as head of the Division of Medical Education at the Foundation. Howland reported, "Gregg means to go over the ground with you. I suggest you make a note on your calendar to bring it up about May first, if you have not heard from him by then."

But Wilder was reluctant to wait: "Time was passing and money was running out." Since he and Helen had already planned a short holiday in New York in early March, he decided to casually call Gregg up and see if he could drop by and see him. He needed to know what kind of a man Gregg was, what his interests were and what it would take to inspire him.

Wilder came away from the interview much taken by Gregg, aware of the limits of his budget, and convinced that Gregg would have to be wooed and primed with a rhetoric for defending to his board so massive an expenditure in Montreal for investigation of the brain. As he was aware, there were other, similar proposals; one from a group in Philadelphia, and one from Cushing in Boston. Gregg did not want to consider the matter until the fall, so Wilder hit on the idea of sending him the exchange of letters with F. M. R. Walshe with a note: "Because of our discussion of the situation in England, I am enclosing a copy of some of the letters that passed between F. M. R. Walshe and myself this winter, thinking you will find them amusing."

While Gregg was settling into his new job and, if he thought about Penfield at all, digesting the exchange of letters, Wilder and Helen learned that the house they had been renting was to be sold. Although the three-year trial period in Montreal was almost at an end, they had made friends and become attached to the city, and to having the farm so close by. Nonetheless, they had already resolved to go elsewhere, perhaps back to the U.S., if the Rockefeller Foundation decided against his proposal.

There had been rumours that Wilder was being considered for appointments in other centres but no firm offers had been made. The closest to an invitation had come a year before from the University of Pennsylvania in Philadelphia. At a medical conference one of the professors had taken him aside to mention that the professor of neurology was retiring, and had hinted that Wilder was being considered as a candidate. But Wilder had heard nothing from Philadelphia since then, and had assumed they had reconsidered—if they were ever seriously thinking of him.

The Penfields had made up their minds to look for another house to rent when out of the blue they received a call from a friend, Mrs. H. B. McKenzie. Her husband had died recently, her house was for sale, and she wanted them to have it. Helen and Wilder fell in love with it at first sight. It was a brick, colonial-style house on the steep slope of Westmount on Montrose Avenue, with a large, pleasant garden on a lower level. Inside, it was the home that Wilder had dreamed about ever since his Oxford days. The elegance and grace of the Oslers' house had stayed in his memory and become the model for a home of his own. Fifteen years later, there it was at 4302 Montrose Avenue.

From the main hall there opened to the left a small study with French windows, and a bathroom. Behind and facing the garden with a view past the St. Lawrence River to the distant mountains of the Eastern Townships, was an elegant walnut-panelled dining room. On the other side of the hall, running from the front to the back of the house, was a graceful living room, with windows on three sides and a marble fireplace. Upstairs there were six bedrooms on two floors, and in the basement a complete apartment for servants.

At first they said no. Mrs. McKenzie wanted to sell; they had planned to rent. But that evening, bringing the two older children, Wilder Jr. and Ruthmary, with them, they walked back up the hill from their house on Côte Saint Antoine Road. On the way home they decided to buy it after all, and the deal was made.

Then, in the midst of packing and moving, a letter arrived from the University of Pennsylvania, saying that a delegate was coming to discuss a job offer. It was too late to pull out of buying the house. The day after the move was accomplished, the delegate arrived with an offer of the professorship of the combined departments of neurology and neurosurgery; the faculty had a large endowment and Wilder would be given a free hand.

It was an enormously flattering offer. "Your plan," Wilder wrote to the University, "is almost exactly the [revised] plan that I have outlined in an application that I had thought to send to the Rockefeller Foundation. For a moment I wondered if you had seen it. It has never been sent. It lies hidden in my desk at home.—" In his weekly letter to his mother he reported, "I insisted they talk it over with Bill Cone as well." He and Bill were willing to discuss the matter and perhaps make an exploratory trip to Philadelphia, but in the meantime they wanted the offer kept secret. Gregg had promised to visit in the fall, and if he wasn't interested in the plan for an institute in Montreal, they would seriously consider moving to Philadelphia.

As unsure as Wilder was about settling in Montreal, the prospect of a move back to the U.S. had little appeal. He went to Philadelphia for more talks, but the city struck him as noisy and frenetic. And from a letter he wrote to Helen from there, it is obvious that the pressure of making a decision was taking its toll on their relationship as well:

"Dear Girl: Just because we are always together, is that any reason why I can't write you a love letter? Is it too silly to fold it up in my pocket and take it to you?

"I'm a terrible bachelor. I've been marooned here 24 hours and have been to New York and back but I'm very lonely. I don't think I can leave you long enough to go abroad this summer [to the first meeting of the International Neurological Congress].

"Don't you hope we aren't forced to leave Montreal, our home and farm there, and come here? It's hot here and there is noise and trip hammers.

"Does it matter such a terrible lot if we squabble occasionally? It's so absurd. Let's stop going at such a frightful speed. I care nothing for fame. I only want to fulfill—what is it? to find the secrets that

God meant me to find. I can do it better perhaps in lower gear. You gear down too, will you? I want more of you, want to seize the children before they slip through my fingers....I want to be very near you as the years roll around and you don't know how much I need you near me."

THE MONTREAL NEUROLOGICAL INSTITUTE

A visit from Alan Gregg was still to come, and in the meantime Wilder went to Switzerland for the International Neurological Congress, where he found that the secret of his offer from Philadelphia was on everyone's tongue. All urged him to take it. Consequently, he returned to Montreal to prepare for the meeting with Gregg in some considerable confusion about what he ought to do, and impatient to hear what Gregg would have to say.

The interview with Gregg on October 10, 1931, is the climax of *No Man Alone*, and of Wilder's dream of one day being master of his own neurological institute.

The two men met in Wilder's study in the new house in Westmount. Wilder collected Gregg at the railway station and brought him back for breakfast with Helen and the children. After breakfast, the two secluded themselves, and for an account of this interview we must draw entirely on Wilder's memory of it, as recorded first in his biography of Gregg, written some thirty years later, then in *No Man Alone*, written a decade after that. The accounts are substantially the same, although in the biography of Gregg, Wilder, after briefly giving his identity, refers to himself as "Associate Professor" or "A.P." throughout, with an uncharacteristic authorial shyness.

According to the account in *No Man Alone*, Gregg began the interview by drawing from his briefcase a folder of papers and slapping them down on the coffee table. "'This,' Gregg said, turning to me, 'is exactly the sort of thing for which we are always searching at the Rockefeller Foundation. I have the application you made to Pearce. I think I understand what you want to do. You have a plan that gives real promise in a field that is calling desperately for exploration. We can do no more than provide you with the optimum environment. You will have to direct the work. We want to see it go on and on, following the leads that come to you. Don't ever thank us. We thank you. You will be helping us when you do your job.'"

For the rest of that Saturday morning and the following day, the two men sat in front of the fire in Wilder's study while Wilder, prompted by Gregg, talked about the origins of the idea and his dreams for the bright future of the institute, already going up brick by brick and room by room in his restless imagination. Gregg, for his part, listened, nodding occasionally, trying to find out all he could about this man whose proposal he was preparing to take to the trustees of the Rockefeller Foundation. After interviews with the Dean of Medicine and others at McGill and the Royal Vic, Gregg boarded the train for New York, promising to let Wilder know as soon as the trustees should come to their decision.

The long wait was not yet over—not quite. Gregg had made no promise other than to help Wilder prepare the application for the Rockefeller trustees, but first Wilder had to decide where he would like the institute to be built. Gregg had meant it when he said he was prepared to back the right sort of man; Gregg would support Wilder's application if it came from Montreal or Philadelphia or elsewhere, though those two cities were at the moment the only serious contenders.

Gregg's *carte blanche* placed Wilder in a very favourable position. If Philadelphia could woo him away from Montreal, they would get not only Penfield but, in all likelihood, major financial backing from the Rockefeller Foundation. Following one of its guiding principles, the Rockefeller Foundation was not prepared to pay for everything. Before approving the plan they required a commitment from local sources to pay the cost of maintaining an institute. The Foundation would then cover the cost of the building and endow the institute with enough money to finance the basic research.

The University of Pennsylvania already had the matching funds in hand, but in the space of only three weeks, as Wilder's weekly letter reveals, Charles Martin, the Dean of Medicine at McGill, had already lined up the local endowments required by the Rockefeller Foundation.

One thing seemed certain in all the indecision: Cone and Penfield would stick together. But the fact that Cone was not present during the interview with Gregg was significant, as Wilder admitted many years later in writing the story of the Institute. "He was loyal to my projects in a more personal way, always the Good Samaritan, the tireless, selfless physician, taking a keen delight in serving the sick. But in spite of this and his brilliant and retentive mind and his loyalty to the ideas of scientific perfection, I suppose Bill Cone never quite understood the hopes and the thinking at the back of my mind."

The pattern of their relationship seemed outwardly to have changed little from the days in New York: Wilder was the leader, the public figure, the "front man." Cone was interested only in their scientific research and their patients. And although changes were coming, for the moment Penfield and Cone were content with their respective roles.

After discussing the plans and the possibility of moving to Philadelphia at length, Wilder and Cone made a second exploratory trip to Philadelphia. The University of Pennsylvania already housed an extremely distinguished group of neurologists and neurosurgeons, several of them long-time friends. By contrast, if Wilder and Cone chose Montreal, they would have to import the rest of their team for the proposed institute. Nevertheless, both of them wanted to stay in Montreal if at all possible.

Finally, on November 23, 1931, Wilder cabled Gregg: "Have thrown in my lot with McGill. We expect to have application in your hands by Saturday." Gregg replied that the trustees did not meet until April, and there would be no decision one way or the other until then. In Wilder's letters through January and February there are faint notes of discontent at the delays in agreeing on a site, the necessity of repeatedly redrawing the plans, and the lobbying that was taking place in Montreal. In the March letters there is complete silence on the subject.

Then, in April came the announcement that the Rockefeller Foundation had awarded McGill a grant of $1,232,000 for the creation of a neurological institute. The Montreal medical community was ecstatic at the news. The Montreal newspapers made much of the grant, and of their brilliant, young surgeon and scientist, who would make Montreal a world centre for brain research. On the morning of the announcement, Wilder slipped out of town. He left for Chicago, ostensibly to attend a meeting but actually, as he admitted to his mother, "to avoid the fuss and to get a chance to think about plans alone, before I'm asked about them."

The number of things that suddenly had to be done was appalling. The grant had been made on the basis of a rough sketch; now an architect had to be hired and a building designed. Equipment had to be ordered and a staff assembled. Diplomatic liaison had to be maintained between McGill, the Institute's 'owner,' and the Royal Victoria Hospital, to which the Institute would be attached and which would provide it with basic services.

Straightening out the various responsibilities of each institution took until July, and only then was Wilder free to tour U.S. medical facilities with the architect to gather ideas for the design of the Institute. Into the autumn, Wilder, the architects, the engineers, Bill Cone, Colin Russel and others worked over the building plans, floor by floor.

Wilder had his hand (and often his way) in every decision, no matter how small. If the debate was over the size of broom closets, he would take fifteen minutes that night to measure the brooms and mops in the closet at home, and appear the next day having calculated the exact size the Institute's closets ought to be.

In the fall, Wilder and Helen set off for Europe, he to attend a series of medical conferences and she for her first long holiday in fourteen years, since Wilder Jr. was born, both of them relieved to be escaping the scene of all this unending activity and negotiation and planning. After the conference in London they travelled in a roundabout way to Madrid to visit with Hortega. In London Wilder had tried to woo a New Zealander named Denny-Brown, who had worked with Sherrington at Oxford, to come to Montreal as neurologist at the Institute. Denny-Brown refused, to Wilder's disappointment. Then, in Madrid, Wilder came to an important decision about choosing the team of workers for his Institute. According to a letter to his mother he and Helen were listening to a concert to which Hortega had taken them:

"The orchestra was all Spanish, and here cut off by the Pyrenees it was playing lovely Spanish music that made me thrill. At one high point a sigh passed like a wind through the responsive listeners. Suddenly it dawned on me that it was so well done because it was themselves doing it on their own. I thought in a flash of the good English, good Dutch, good French, good Portuguese and good Spanish clinics I had seen, and I knew that I must give up transplanting anyone and build up a school of Canadians in Montreal, for Montreal, and do it all on our own and from our own students. Since then I haven't hesitated for a moment about that decision. If it is not possible to do it with Canadians it must be done by those who want to become Canadians, so that eventually there may grow up a local school of Neurology."

There would be problems with the plan, and he could see some of them developing already: "It means, I suppose, that I shall have to take a wider responsibility and perhaps retire into more of a professorial aloofness, which I dislike. Even in the past two years I have regretted very much the loss of some of the spontaneous contacts with the fellows, and have resented the increase in respectful distance between us."

All along there had been problems brewing with McGill, the official owner of the institute-to-be. By the end of 1932, the project was running $100,000 over budget and Sir Arthur Currie, Principal of McGill, was worried that McGill's contribution would grow to dangerous proportions. It was now the bottom of the Great

Depression, and Sir Arthur Currie, who had been commander in chief of the Canadian combat forces during World War I, was neither financier nor politician. The problems came to a head one afternoon late in January when Sir Arthur called a meeting on the campus and summoned Wilder from the bedside of a patient.

When Wilder arrived, Currie had in his hands a set of plans omitting two of the eight and a half floors of the Institute. "We must cut the coat," he said firmly, "to fit the cloth." So Wilder wrote to his mother, recording as well his own angry retort: "No one wants such a coat!" Then Wilder calmed down somewhat and went on to assure Currie, with some haughtiness, that the Institute would be able to pay its own way on the basis of the good work that would be done there and its recognition by medical benefactors. "Currie," Wilder continued in his account in *No Man Alone,* "brought his enormous closed fist crashing down on the table. 'Damn it! They told me you would say just that. Well, I've made up my mind what I would say in case you did.' He laughed and then added, 'We can't go on without you whether we like it or not. The university will have to take a chance that you know what you're talking about, and that you and Cone and Russel and the others can run your own show and keep us out of debt after the building is built.'" That explosive encounter, according to Wilder, ended the friction with McGill.

In June, 1933, the final building plans were accepted, and four months later, in October, came the laying of the cornerstone with all due pomp and ceremony, organized by Sir Arthur Currie to coincide with McGill's Founder's Day, on the sixth. On hearing of Currie's elaborate plans, Wilder wrote in his next letter to his mother, "I don't care what they do. Such occasions are just flourish and empty vainglory...the cornerstone laying is for the builders — the opening will be for us who know its meaning and who will enter its walls as a monastery to disappear, I hope, from public attention." After the ceremony on the sixth of October, Wilder reported, "Currie talked for some time and the Bishop blessed everything and I had a desire to weep and run away."

At Christmas, 1933, Helen fell ill with lobar pneumonia, and for close to three weeks her life hung by a thread.

On the thirty-first of December, Wilder wrote from Green Point Farm, as their country retreat was now called, and explained to his mother that Helen had come down to the farm with the children and servants on Wednesday of that week. Wilder was to join them on the weekend. When she left Montreal she had seemed to have a little cold, and that night she went to bed early with a chill. When Wilder called from Montreal the next evening, Thursday, he discovered Wilder Jr. had been trying anxiously to reach him by phone. "High temperature, pain in her side and rapid breathing was enough. It was too late for the night train and I found every road completely blocked with snow and impassable. So I collected many necessaries and caught the morning train to Magog. There a good fast team and a cutter met me. It was 35° below in Magog and said to be 42° below in South Bolton. The coldest day since we came to Canada. What a 14 mile drive!"

The fever continued to worsen and Helen became delirious. From Montreal, in response to Wilder's appeal for help, came an instant reply. A doctor and a special nurse from Magog were joined by specialists from the Montreal General Hospital and the Royal Victoria and more nurses. Bill Cone chartered a plane equipped with skis and landed on frozen Lake Memphremagog, floundered up the long hill through the deep snow, took some blood samples and headed back to have them analyzed. (There was even a futile attempt to put skis on one of the hospital's ambulances.) Meanwhile the telephone rang so steadily with offers of assistance from the local neighbours, they had to be asked to stop so that the party line could be used to keep in constant touch with other specialists in Montreal.

For nineteen days the fever continued. Wilder could do nothing but sit by Helen's bed, stroking her brow and listening to her rambling, incoherent whimpers. The younger children and their nanny, Fräulein Bergmann, were sent back to Montreal. Wilder Jr. stayed on to help stoke the furnace and keep the house warm. All the necessary and latest equipment was brought in on Jackson's sleigh.

Then, just before dawn on the nineteenth day, while Wilder was sitting by her bed, Helen began to recover. "She looked at me as she lay in bed and I thought I saw the beginning of understanding in her eyes, the eyes that had turned to me as to a stranger for so long.

"'Are you,' she asked, 'my father? Or, or my, or my husband?'

"Her brow felt cool again for the first time in so long. I hurried off to awaken Professor Meakins.

"'I think the time has come.'

"He rushed to her in his pajamas, thermometer in hand, and I followed. We waited two long minutes for the thermometer to register.

"'Sure enough,' he whispered to me. 'The crisis has come. She is going to get by.'"

That evening Wilder sat down and wrote his mother. "Helen is getting well. What words those are! Sometimes during the past 18 days I have faced the meaning of other words. Once, while I was nursing her at night, I looked out over the moonlit snow to the little burying ground on Royea's land where I could see the stones black against the snow and faced what it meant. I should have sold the farm, of course, and what would the children do? After that, for days and nights I did not dare to look out in that direction. I didn't even look out the windows."

Three days later, on a bobsled that had been rigged up into a covered ambulance by their tenant farmer, Jackson, Helen was brought to South Bolton. By stretcher, she was placed aboard the train to Montreal, and, on arriving, taken directly to the hospital.

At home Wilder found such an outpouring of concern and sympathy that he was astonished. Sixty-four calls from forty-two people in the first few days, according to Ruthmary, who was keeping count, and over a hundred letters and telegrams from all over. With Helen still in hospital recovering, Wilder went before a judge and became a Canadian citizen. That done, he accepted a long-standing invitation to become an elder of the Presbyterian Church. The first action acknowledged and expressed his gratitude for the temporal help of his Canadian friends, the second gave thanks for God's intervention in Helen's recovery.

By summer, with Helen completely well again and making plans for renovations at the farm, Wilder was once more in the midst of a crisis. Even as the Institute was nearing completion, Bill Cone was being wooed by a seductive offer from his alma mater, the University of Iowa.

"What will Bill do?" Wilder wrote in the weekly letter, dated June 29. "He has not told me but Prof. Bye was here from Iowa yesterday to see him. Their offer is complete charge of neurosurgery at Iowa and a double professorship—one in neurosurgery and one in neurology. He is to get $4,000 salary and they tell him he will make $10,000 in practice the first year, and $20,000 the second. It is his home and Avis' home—how can he refuse it? What is there here for him that is comparable? I offer him eventually an equal share in the clinic and whatever he can make. He may believe that some day, by some stroke of legerdemain the opportunity will come for us to build the greatest of all centres of neurological thought, to do something that neither of us alone could do. What is that fancy against supremacy and easy living in the home town?

"The trouble is he has left a facet on me that will be hard to hide. Laboratory detail I have let go since he came. The best thing is to get along without building the clinic and quietly work on epilepsy. There is so much to do on it, and life is so short, and I take upon myself so many other foolish unworthy loads."

Bill Cone left for a month to return to Iowa and make up his mind—though Wilder obviously felt that the decision had already been made. Then one afternoon while Wilder was working through the endless pile of letters and reports on his desk in the laboratory, he heard Bill's deep, rumbling laugh in the anteroom. The secretary came rushing in to announce that Bill was back with good news.

"'I've made up my mind, Wide, to stay with you. We've come a long way together. You've been a straight-shooter. I need your help to do what I want to do in life, and you can't get along very well without me here.'"

There was to be one more battle, one more crisis before the Institute opened. The plans for the building included a bridge that was to join it to the Royal Vic with a corridor over University Avenue. It would have meant reorganizing one of the wards at the hospital's end to have clear passage from one building to the other, and W. R. Chenoweth, Superintendent of the Royal Vic, had objected vigorously. But Wilder had been adamant: the Institute was there to serve the patients in the Royal Vic, and if they didn't have the bridge, patients, doctors and visitors would have to travel a long complicated route through a corridor in the basement.

The first round of this battle had been fought a year earlier, when some of the governors of the hospital saw the blueprints for the first time, though the hospital and the university had both formally approved the plans long since. Sir Herbert Holt, president of the hospital and a governor of the university, had promised to contribute $100,000 of his own money to help with the construction and endowment of the Institute. When he had seen the plans, however, he had sent Wilder a message through the Superintendent that ran something like, "If they build a goddamn bridge across University Street into our hospital, I won't give a cent to construction." Wilder was sure the message had actually come from Chenoweth. Nevertheless, Wilder held firm on his plan for the bridge. Construction went ahead, and when the time came Holt paid over the money.

Then, late in July with the bridge already built, Chenoweth informed Wilder that the hospital refused direct passage from the bridge to their main corridor. Wilder fell into a fury. He told Chenoweth he would write to the Rockefeller Foundation not to pay a cent to the hospital until and unless direct passage was granted. However, the board of the hospital held firm, and when Wilder appealed to the university to intercede, Edward Beatty, Chancellor of McGill, became angry and called Wilder "an obstinate devil."

And so the battle ended with a standoff: Wilder had his bridge going across University Avenue, but the other end was effectively blocked to traffic. So it remained for quite a few years, until a wealthy patient at the Institute asked his private nurse why she took so long to get back from lunch in the Royal Vic cafeteria. When she explained that it was a half-hour round trip via the basement corridor and up through the Royal Vic, the patient wrote out a cheque for the renovations to allow the bridge to open. Wilder was still so angry with the hospital superintendent, whom he held personally to blame, that when recounting the incident in *No Man Alone*, it took him three or four drafts to cool his temper—forty years later.

The official opening was set, finally, for September 27, 1934. It was now six years since the Penfields arrived in Montreal, and with the Institute to keep Wilder there, it would remain their home despite the many tempting offers that came in the future.

In the final weeks before the opening, there had not been a moment's pause: equipment ordered months before was late arriving, the accommodations for out-of-town guests had to be arranged, a speech of acknowledgment and purpose had to be written, and a hundred and one other details needed Wilder's personal attention.

Yet as Wilder had walked through the corridors and rooms of the new building, dodging workmen and technicians and listening to them exchange orders and arguments, a feeling of awe and a tremendous sense of fulfilment replaced his dread of the impending formalities and speeches. When he had set out so long ago to bring surgeons and scientists together under one roof, others had told him it couldn't be done, and now he had proved them wrong. For ten years he had dreamed of such an Institute, and for three years he had watched it rise, floor after floor, across the road from the Royal Victoria Hospital, with the whole city of Montreal spread out below. He had personally supervised every detail, arguing doggedly with the architects and engineers until they threw up their hands and gave in. He had drawn endless diagrams and sketches of this piece of equipment or that arrangement of lighting. His search for the latest and best ideas, the ideal layout, had taken him across the continent and around Europe. Six or seven complete blueprints had been done before the design was good enough to satisfy him. But that was over, for the most part, and the Institute was almost finished: eight and a half storeys of laboratories, operating rooms, teaching amphitheatres, wards and offices—even a squash court where the staff could smash out their frustrations.

The exterior of the Institute had been designed to harmonize with the limestone turrets and battlements of the Royal Vic across the way, whose fortress-like appearance was so beloved by the Scottish merchant princes who had built it. But the interior was ultra-modern in every respect. On the second and third floors the public wards were designed so that the lighting came entirely from windows placed at either end. The beds were placed crosswise to the long axis of the room, making the light, reflected from the cream coloured ceiling, fall evenly on every patient. In contrast to the effect created by the usual arrangement of windows by each bed, here there was no direct glare on the patients' eyes, and no drafts.

In the middle of each ward of twelve beds projected a glass booth from which the nurses could watch every bed at all times, even at night, when floor lights served to outline the beds without disturbing the patients.

The main operating amphitheatre on the fifth floor was equipped with a viewing gallery of such a height that those in the front row were quite close to the operator's shoulder, though separated by sloping plate glass, thus eliminating the danger of contamination and saving visitors the bother of wearing masks and gowns. In the operating rooms the temperature and moisture were automatically controlled, and the rooms were ventilated with thoroughly washed air, further reducing the danger of wound contamination by making it unnecessary to open the windows. The floor was of black linoleum, the walls a dark green; only the ceiling was white. The walls and the dark green sheets minimized eye-strain among the operators during long operations.

Beneath the viewing gallery was a small photographic cellar with a window placed behind the surgeon's back. The photographer entered by a ladder from the viewing gallery, and could open the window if necessary. Above the operating table was a photographic mirror whose angle the photographer could adjust by remote control.

Perhaps the most important innovation of all, and the most revealing of this Institute's purpose, was a series of operating room buzzers that rang in the fellows' laboratories. "It is essential," Wilder emphasized, "that each research fellow working in the laboratory may be able to get a clear view of every pathological condition exposed by the operator if he so desires and return to his proper work without loss of time." So the bells were installed to notify the research fellows when the brain had been exposed and the surgeon was about to begin.

But the Institute was to be more than a sophisticated and unique research and treatment centre—Wilder had planned it to be a temple dedicated to science. The lobby was the centrepiece. Frescoed upon the ceiling were the neuroglia cells in their proper layers within the cerebellum, after a drawing by the great Italian neurologist Camillo Golgi. In the centre of the ceiling was the head of Aries the Ram, the astrological symbol controlling the brain, and about the ram's head were four hieroglyphic figures which, according to a papyrus dating from 3000 B.C., are the four symbols that, in combination, represent the brain. The treasured papyrus is the earliest reference to the brain anywhere in human records.

In an outer circle surrounding the head of Aries and the hieroglyphics was a quotation in Greek from the second-century physician Galen. Galen considered himself a disciple of Hippocrates, but he took exception to the latter's statement that a wound involving the brain is invariably fatal. The inscription was his objection: "But I have seen a severely wounded brain heal."

Carved into the walls were the names of Wilder's heroes, the great scientific pioneers of the study of the brain and nervous system: Sherrington, Cajal, Pavlov and a half dozen more. Around the lobby, the floor tiles, the tables, the lamps, even the radiator grills were modelled on the complex structure of the brain and nervous system. For the place of honour in front of the doorway, Wilder had chosen a copy of a statue he had seen at the University of Paris, called *La Nature se dévoilant devant la Science*—Nature Unveiling Before Science. The statue was the figure of a young woman, heavily cloaked, with only her face, downcast eyes and part of her breasts visible, her arms parting the material demurely. When a wealthy Montreal doctor made a private donation toward the cost of building the Institute, Wilder had commissioned a sculptor to make a copy of the original out of white Carrara marble.

Wilder's mark was visible on the outside of the building as well. Carved into a slab of stone by the main entrance were the words:

DEDICATED
TO
RELIEF OF
SICKNESS
AND PAIN
AND
TO THE STUDY OF
NEUROLOGY.

Over the door was carved a brain, and elsewhere, in positions where the architectural design called for ornamentation, were various forms of trephine—an instrument used to make a hole in the skull. The trephines included primitive, rod-like augers, more complicated augers rotated by the string of a bow, and the more artistic bit and brace of the great sixteenth-century French military surgeon Ambroise Paré.

During the final week before the opening, even as the painters and electricians were putting on the finishing touches, Wilder performed his first operation in the new amphitheatre, on a man who had been rushed to the Institute in an ambulance after falling down an elevator shaft and cracking his skull.

With the kitchen equipment still being unpacked, five patients were admitted into the public ward—patients whose condition was too urgent to wait on speeches and formalities. They were only the first small trickle in the flood that was about to inundate the Institute. Across the continent and around the world in hospitals, clinics and consulting rooms, patients with brain tumours or suspected brain tumours, spinal disorders, head injuries, strange headaches and mysterious dizzy spells, and epilepsy, the "falling sickness," were being told that perhaps Wilder Penfield and his colleagues in Montreal could help them.

Finally the day of the opening came. At ten minutes past three on September 27, the procession of dignitaries, including the mayor of Montreal, the minister of health for Quebec and the dean of the University, set out from the medical school two hundred yards away to walk to the Montreal Neurological Institute. They were, Wilder would recall, "gowned in robes as splendid as anything the Middle Ages could have produced,...a splendor that, nowadays, only a university can bring forth to astonish the beholder."

No sooner had they reached the street when the skies opened, thunder crashed, lightning lit up the street and the rain came down in torrents. Back into the medical school they hurried, muttering about omens, their robes bedraggled, to wait for a fleet of taxis.

At last the dedication began, and Edward Archibald, who had lured Wilder to Montreal six years earlier, stood up before the assembled scientists and politicians and dignitaries, and spoke words that might as easily have served to summarize Wilder's own position as to mark the opening of the Institute:

"As the old Latin tag has it the end crowns the work. But *finis* is not written here. It marks truly the end of one stage, but it marks also the beginning of another."

CHAPTER SEVEN

Cursed with Success

∞ THE CHIEF

To a casual observer, the next five years would have seemed a busy, fruitful and very satisfying period in Wilder's life. In the quarter of a century since he entered medical school, the study and treatment of the brain had become the most exciting and challenging medical specialty. Every day new discoveries were being recorded and added to the growing volume of information about this five-pound, two-sided mystery of gray matter. Neurosurgery had made great strides. Mortality rates had dropped as surgical and antiseptic techniques improved, and neurosurgery was proving its value in treating a rapidly growing number of neurological problems.

Wilder Penfield had come a long way, too, from the days when he was a fledgling neurosurgeon, despairing of his "terrible profession." He had written those words late one night only thirteen years earlier, and already there had been changes he could never have imagined. And his own part in the changes had been handsomely acknowledged: within his profession, his star had risen with startling speed. At forty-three, he was director of one of the foremost neurological institutes in the world, and a surgeon whose reputation for innovative and radical treatments drew patients from great distances. At the opening ceremonies, the most eminent scientists and surgeons in the field had risen in the crowded auditorium to speak his praise, and to paint glowing pictures of the future of the 'Montreal Neuro' under his leadership. And they had been proven right almost immediately: no sooner did the Insitute open its doors than every bed was filled, and still urgent requests for treatment poured in from as far away as Europe and South America.

He had assembled a first-rate group of co-workers: neurosurgeons, neurologists, neuropathologists, neurophysiologists, and researchers whose explorations would take them into fields as yet unnamed. Their presence was testimony that Wilder's dream of so many years to unite science and surgery, operators and laboratory researchers, under one roof, had finally come true.

In addition, the facilities at the Institute were among the best in the world, and everyone on staff, from surgeons to nurses, was aware of the envy with which they were regarded by their colleagues at other hospitals in Montreal and beyond. Morale was high and as the fame of the Institute spread, requests flooded in not just from patients, but from medical people working elsewhere.

There was a certain magnetic quality about "the Chief", this tall, lean figure with deep-sunken, penetrating blue eyes, prematurely bald and looking older than his years. And yet for all his air of unquestioned authority, there was in his athletic stride and sudden smile something boyish and charming.

He could be arbitrary and domineering. He could be, in almost the same instant, both inspiring and infuriating—more than one young resident or research fellow came and left in a hurry, shaking his head and muttering about "Penfield's One-Man Show." He was very demanding, and he insisted on utter loyalty from those who worked under him—loyalty to the cause, to the Montreal Neurological Institute and to him.

Yet he attracted people to the Institute and kept them there because he had an uncanny knack for sparking enthusiasm and bringing out the best in people. When he was around, the building seemed to reverberate with his presence. One former nurse describes how she arrived at work one morning while he was still supposedly away on a trip. Before she got to the elevator she knew he was back—just from the atmosphere in the halls.

No one can properly explain how he did it but it was a way he had of expecting—demanding—the absolute best of everyone, from the porters to the scientists. Praise he could extend with a nod, a smile or a quiet word. When people were not doing their best, somehow he would know and they would encounter that puzzled, eloquent stare: "If you're not doing your best, what are you doing here?"

Somehow that was worse than his periodic furies, when, in a gesture that quickly became his trademark, he would whip off his glasses, and, glowering from icy blue eyes, wither the offender with a few darkly contemptuous words. And yet the waiting list of young surgeons and scientists anxious to train at the Institute—with the *best* scientists and surgeons and the latest equipment—grew longer every year.

Other scientists had to choose between working in a scientific environment and conducting experiments far removed from the hard, stimulating reality of suffering patients, or working in a hospital lab where experimental work would be permitted if it aimed at an immediate therapeutic treatment. But at Penfield's Institute a scientist could do both. Wilder's interest in the work—and Wilder was sure to be *very* interested—was both a blessing and a curse. Into the lab he would walk, asking questions, wanting to know what was going on, what that experiment was all about, making suggestions, inspiring each researcher with his excitement in the research and where it might lead, frustrating the experimenter by his habit of leaping ahead to conclusions that were not yet evident, and by the pressure of his expectations.

For the 'pure' scientists, the initiation rite at the Institute was a trip to the operating theatre while an operation was underway—an intimidating experience for many of them who had never seen the inside of an operating room let alone the exposed brain of a human patient. It was not necessarily a calculated gesture on Wilder's part, but the experience served them all as a powerful reminder of the order of their priorities, as they were chiselled into the granite slab at the entrance to the building: DEDICATED TO RELIEF OF SICKNESS AND PAIN AND TO THE STUDY OF NEUROLOGY. All roads at the Institute led, ultimately, to the operating room and the patient, and to Wilder Penfield. The operating room was his laboratory. In a way the whole Institute, from germinal idea to detailed execution, grew out of his determination to have the best resources and the best people at his beck and call during the long operations for which he was famous.

Between 1935 and 1939, Wilder wrote or co-authored some two dozen scientific papers: on intractable headaches and a revolutionary surgical treatment; on tumours and blood circulation and nerve fibres; on the surgical treatment of epilepsy and the new knowledge of brain function revealed by the operations. During those years, he also found time to write half a dozen papers of a more general kind, biographical sketches, and to translate a number of papers into French as his command of the language improved. Despite the Depression his private practice also flourished in the years following the Institute's opening. In fact Wilder's share, once Bill Cone had taken his and the office expenses had been subtracted, rarely dropped below $25,000 and some years was much higher.

And yet, beneath the surface of success and growing fame, something was seriously amiss. Wilder would fall into periods of depression and unhappy self-examination, and could only bring himself back to the endless demands of his busy life with great effort.

This malaise had to do in part with the difficulty of adjusting to the reality of the Institute. The pattern of striving for something with all his might, and then, when it was in his hand, eyeing it with suspicion, doubting its value—and, not incidentally, his own—was already well fixed by now. How could the drudgery of administration compare to the intense pleasure of watching the blueprints, *his* blueprints, become mortar and brick, rising storey by storey? Or the delight in seeing sketches of new instruments translated into shiny, tangible reality? Now he had to spend hours listening to pleas for research funds, new equipment, always more space, just one more assistant, all demanded in the name of science or better patient care. Being 'Chief' soon lost some of its glamour.

The worst of his doubts stemmed from a firm belief that if he were only a better man he would be able to juggle all the demands on him effortlessly. Returning from a film about Louis Pasteur which was playing at a local theatre, he wrote mournfully:

"The picture of a logical simple mind and a man who ignored non-essentials makes me see my own littleness and failure. What am I doing today? Making rounds to teach the staff and hold them together, operating, seeing dull patients in my office who pay fees, writing long letters to many doctors about their patients so they will send more cases to us and writing, writing to doctors who want advice and patients who want their epilepsy cured—how much would I charge for my brand of cure—going out with Helen or seeing a little of the children because I love her and them with a selfish sort of love and they balance everything else and need me.

"On my desk lie unfinished papers—husks of jobs that are done. If I can steal time before falling asleep from fatigue I polish up these papers for publication. But I don't think about those problems. With all of this when do I think about the problems for which the Institute was built, for which I went into neurology? Once in a while on rounds at the bedside, rarely during an operation when the brain lies exposed and the patient talks. Once in a great while when writing the first draft of a paper or perhaps the second draft. Most often perhaps in the solitude of a thundering train when no one speaks to me and I can write. Writing does help me to think, that's why I'm writing now....

"I am trying to do by organizing what would take care of itself if I were a man big enough to have an institute and fill all of its workers with driving force, with ideas."

Wilder was going through a mid-life crisis of a kind. He was no longer the young challenger; no longer the zealot impatient with bureaucrats, but the bureaucrat himself. Somehow he had not imagined that success would be like this.

In addition, though his general health was good and his vigour unimpaired, the long brain operations were taking their toll. He had developed varicose veins in his feet, and near the close of a ten- or twelve-hour operation his "Sussex knee" would develop a painful ache. Such physical strains were not unusual among surgeons. According to Foerster, both his legs went completely numb before the end of an operation, and Cushing had "lost a toe or two and goes about in a wheelchair." Wilder found a solution in the heavy rubber support stockings he began to wear in the operating room. He remained a ferociously competitive tennis and squash player and skier, but now he took every fall, blunder or foul as a personal insult, gloomy evidence of incipient old age. His periods of forgetfulness (always an accurate measure of the extent to which he was overworked) grew: briefcases left in train stations, letters never mailed, birthdays forgotten. Each of these occurrences prompted a resentful outpouring in the pages of his diary.

Into the midst of this growing malaise, early in May, 1935, came deep sorrow. He, Helen and the children were at the farm for a brief holiday when an urgent cable came from Herbert: "Mother passed away quietly at 10:30 nothing you can do." For twenty-four hours Wilder was in a daze. Then on the evening of the second day he sat down at the desk in his bedroom and began to write, struggling to capture her life on paper and reduce the loss to tolerable proportions in the flow of words that covered page after page.

From his reservoir of childhood memories Wilder plucked half-forgotten fragments: listening in the darkened hallway of the house in Spokane as she sobbed alone in her bedroom; her special sanctuary in the woods surrounding the summer tent-camps that his father would set up, then abandon for Spokane and the company of men, and her habit of placing a stick across the path so that the children would know she wished to be left alone for a while; her dreams for him and her devotion, made more precious by his knowledge of her grief at Charles' betrayals, grief that burned into his young mind, though she tried to conceal it from him.

Desperate with sorrow, he relentlessly examined each fragment, discarded a few, and marshalled the rest to create a coherent picture of their two lives. On his annual visits of the last four years he had found her bedridden and failing in health, but strong of will and mind. During these brief visits "she harked back in her conversation with me not to Galahad nor to Hudson but to Spokane. She puzzled over the failure of her married life and seemed comforted when I made her realize how much she had done for her children by leading them back out of the Spokane environment. And yet the ghosts of those days were very much with her.

"Idealist she was always," he concluded. "A mind too penetrating and intolerant to lend itself to the purposes of a pliant wife. She could not give Father what he required, no doubt. And although I do not understand her and probably never will—she understood me completely, at every stage, and gave me everything I needed in sympathy and love for 44 years."

Wilder's long, handwritten eulogy was, in a way, the final payment on his debt of gratitude to his mother for all she had done. Her death brought to an abrupt end the Sunday letters. But there was still the urge to write about his life and the things that pleased or troubled him, the writing that had always been his way of coming to a decision, or simply of understanding.

In the years ahead, this impulse found an outlet in a motley collection of notebooks, children's exercise books and elegant gold-lettered diaries, in which he wrote when the mood was on him.

There were other problems. Most serious was Helen's growing jealousy at his preoccupation with work. One of the consequences of his and the Institute's growing fame was an endless series of invitations to speak at medical and scientific conferences around the world, invitations he often felt he could not refuse, since they fed the Institute with patients and funds, and attracted eager and talented people to come and work there. Hardly a month went by between 1934 and 1939 when he was not on a train for Chicago, New York, Philadelphia or somewhere even further afield. And when he was in Montreal his work at the Institute kept him away until late, or called him away from a dinner party or a table in a restaurant. Before going to the theatre he always left word where he would be and, on entering, pointed out to the usher where he would be seated, just in case.

Wilder was acutely aware of Helen's resentment and, though it helped little, sympathetic. When he was away he wrote daily letters full of love; when the resentment she felt erupted into serious arguments he tried to placate her with flowers and self-criticism and romantic, stolen weekends at hotels in Quebec City or Toronto or the Laurentians.

Despite his attempts to be father and husband on the one hand and Institute director on the other, he felt all too often that he was failing at both, and dreaded the day when he might have to choose between them. The choice, he wrote, would mean throwing over the Institute and its demands. "I thought it over and over as in a merry-go-round with horrid repeated music one weekend when I went duck shooting and had the trip out and back alone. The conclusion in my own mind was that I would not give ground, that I would succeed, would lead, would deserve the respect and the love that I could not demand."

Witholding her love was the only way Helen could shake him from his preoccupations long enough to give her the attention she wanted. Though their relationship had always had a stormy side, during this period it took less and less provocation to spark off violent quarrels after which Helen displayed a devastating, glacial calm, increasing Wilder's misery and confusion.

In mid-July, 1935, after just such a bitter quarrel, Wilder set off from Quebec City, bound for England and Germany. He had applied for a D.Sc. degree from Oxford and was going over for the ceremony, then to Brussels to deliver a paper and on to Breslau to visit his old friend and mentor Otfrid Foerster. On the way back to Canada three weeks later he took time to record the events of the trip in his diary. The quarrel with Helen, he recalled, left him "with a stone on my heart." On board he had met an English girl, with whom he had struck up a conversation. Learning that she had been to school at Oxford, he suggested that she come up and spend a day with him while he was there. He admitted to his diary, "it seems women are just naturally better companions than men. No doubt there is consciousness of something else that forms an unexplained background." However, no sooner was the invitation out of his mouth and accepted, than he realized that strolling about Oxford with an attractive young woman on his arm might raise a few eyebrows. They agreed to luncheon in London instead.

Left to his own devices, "I grow very easily lonely and have little capacity for enjoyment alone and so my mind turns to levels where it does not belong. How can a real bachelor tolerate his solitude?"

One night alone in Brussels he found his way to an Italian restaurant and bought a half-bottle of Asti to drink with his solitary dinner. "I left some," the diary continues, "but all the same it blurred my vision... so I walked off through the shouting and din of merry-makers and ended by trying various side shows including snakes, tricksters and naked bathing girls and so home to the club in a jangling streetcar."

From Brussels he took the train to Breslau to see Foerster. Foerster had greeted Wilder warmly whenever they had met at neurological conferences over the years, and Wilder had been sadly aware that each interval had marked another stage in the gradual dimming of the aging man's brilliance. Returning now to Breslau, he suddenly realized that Foerster had also to contend with a new and ominous reality. Foerster's wife was partly Jewish, and in the new Germany he had reason to fear for her and for his children. And ancient, elegant Breslau had changed, as Wilder discovered:

"At the entrance to the hospital, a new surgical building had gone up in bright new brick. Once in the court all looked the same. A news bulletin had been erected and on it some papers and a picture of Spain with arms and legs in bandages—soon finished. As I approached Abteilung #8 a great square building blocked the way, new red brick and square windows. On its front written something which meant devotion to *patriae* and *scientiae*, the *patriae* coming above just as photos of Hindenburg & Hitler were larger and above all the other photos back of Foerster's own desk. I tried to enter the front door of the *Neuroligishes Forshungs* Institute but it was locked and deserted."

When he finally did find a way in through the back, and was ushered into Foerster's office, he found the last few years had left their mark. "Of course he has aged. He walks with a cane and his face is drawn. Yet the change is not all in that. The change was some inward thing that made him look out the window while he talked as though his thoughts too slipped out on some other errand."

In Berlin two days later Wilder observed, "Hitler's face everywhere, a complete despotism but that is nothing very new; absolute monarchs are an old story and I cannot conceive of any other way of dealing with so pig-headed a lot of men. Everything was parcelled out, just barely enough & a sin to waste. All convinced they are so much better off. Uniformed and drilled. Walking outside of Carlsruhe we saw men marching in perfect order down a country road with shovels (!) over their shoulders."

The atmosphere of menace in Germany added to Wilder's general state of self-doubt and unhappiness, causing him to question his motive for the trip and the value of his contribution to neurology. On his way home he confided to his diary, "Of course I applied for that degree. I always envied the red & grey gown and it is said to be about as hard to get as F.R.S. Eng. But I am a little ashamed to have applied for it as that implies that I think I deserve it. It is one of the things I have always hoped for. What my work is worth I really have no idea. Perhaps the headaches and the...nerve fibres are good but the latter I simply told Edward to stain feeling sure it could be done. The headaches was the result of a chance operation. It was not a preconceived theory. Neuroglia was nothing but steadfast study and description of simple obvious things all of which should have been seen by someone else somehow. The cytology was a good idea & it is useful but that was only editorship not science. Tumours?—I've covered the field but have only described obvious features. My attempts at hydrocephalus are a failure. Now it's epilepsy and other forms of headache.

"The surgical treatment of epilepsy is justified the first five years. Will I think so after 10 & 15 years? The physiological mechanisms of the attack is what I wish I could discover. It is doubtless simple. Many men saw an apple fall before Newton visualized the mechanism of gravity responsible for it.

"But so far I have worked hard—that is about all that can be said, and with an unwavering purpose."

To the list of woes that plagued him were added in 1936 and 1937 several patient deaths that he was convinced ought not to have happened. Thinking that somewhere in the operating and postoperative procedure infection was creeping in, Wilder and the other surgeons desperately analyzed and studied their technique, even bringing in a surgeon from the outside "to spy out our faults." To no avail it seemed, and for a period the scribbled entries in his diary were a litany of despair:

"St. Denis is dead. I took out a scar from his brain. I watched the brain while he had a fit but I couldn't see the underlying mechanism and a staphylococcus either introduced at his accident two years before or by our careless technique has closed his chapter—His wife with a baby of two months—thanks me for what? All dressed in black and hoping the baby will grow up like his father.

"Chester Ames wanted to be free of his epilepsy and wanted a stronger right hand so he could milk better. I watched his brain while he had his fits and did a gross, crude removal of scar and brain without knowing why or what was happening when the fit took place under my eyes. As death drew near to him he used to tell me how much he appreciated the time I gave him and how my fame would grow when he told the people down in Vermont what a wonderful man I was!

"I've been haunted by him at night but there is no time to study his problem."

Although the entries are not an altogether accurate reflection of his life during these years, and there were unquestionably many happier moments, the diaries go some way toward explaining the fact that by 1939 he was seriously considering leaving the field of medicine for good. The unexplained deaths, the incurable patients, the pressure of administration and surgery that kept him from doing much more than nibble at the edges of the mountains of data on the brain accumulating in the Institute, the death of his mother and the feeling of being cut loose that ensued, the periodic struggles with Helen: all these made him want to seize the opportunity that dropped into his lap one evening in late August of 1939.

Wilder was dining at the Mount Royal Club when George MacDonald, a governor of McGill University, stopped to talk with him. Before the conversation was over he had asked if Wilder would consider becoming Principal of McGill.

Penfield's reputation as a forceful leader and effective administrator had obviously been widely broadcast in the five short years since the Institute opened. The suggestion was also an indication of how warmly the exclusive Anglo-Montreal Establishment—whose members could trace their ancestry in the city back six or seven generations—now regarded this recent arrival in their midst. Aware of what a compliment he was being paid, Wilder was both flattered—and sorely tempted. "It was the end of summer. I had a taste of glorious holiday at Lake Memphremagog and it seemed very distasteful to return to surgery and administration of the M.N.I. For that reason or because of a love of change and adventure or for some other reason which I do not myself understand the suggestion thrilled me. It seemed the thing I wanted to do and my other life seemed stale."

Wilder promised to consider the proposal, and hurried out to the farm to discuss it with Helen. From there he went to New York to talk to Alan Gregg and solicit his opinion, and then to Philadelphia to ask Professor Aydellotte (who had once tried to lure him to that city), for his opinion. Perhaps all this consultation was already an indication that in his heart of hearts he knew he would merely be running away from one job that had become wearisome to another that would be less demanding of him—and significantly, of his relationship with Helen. There is no record of her counsel, but Gregg said "No" and Aydellotte said "Yes," and Wilder was searching his mind for a rationale for the move. "I asked myself if I would do anything from 48 to 60 that would be worthwhile scientifically and wouldn't my contribution be greater from 48-65 as Principal."

Then, suddenly, the outside world came crashing in and brought an end to such idle dreams. At the farm the morning of September 4th, Wilder was in the midst of shaving when he heard a radio news report that German soldiers had marched into Poland. War seemed inevitable and the decision was suddenly obvious. "I am a surgeon and if Canada wants to use it I have some capacity to patch up injured men. So I must put aside any temptation to lead an academic life and must offer my services."

The note of relief that seems to ring through those words is reinforced by what followed. The governors of McGill, determined to make him an offer he couldn't refuse, suggested that Penfield accept the post on the understanding that the vice-principal would act in his stead during the war years. He refused.

The decision made, he went on to muse, "I am wondering if the Institute staff could not serve both here and abroad. Would they want to use us as a unit? Could we co-ordinate the treatment of head injuries, nerve injuries, brain lacerations that may lead to post-traumatic epilepsy and even to psychoneurosis? Some of these things must be treated in general hospitals. Others should be segregated and treated in a special unit abroad. That unit abroad should be co-ordinated with a unit back here, perhaps at the M.N.I. so that records & treatments there would co-ordinate with the same here.

"I'm not sure whether I should take the initiative," he concluded, "and who I should write to."

Meanwhile the summer was drawing quickly to a close, and with the time to relax and the future, at least for a while, blessed with a purpose, Wilder noted that the last two weeks at the farm were "the happiest period I can remember. Helen has sailed with me in the races each Sunday and we have been very close. She is such a brick."

∞ WAR YEARS

Getting into the war proved a great deal more difficult than Wilder could have imagined in 1939, when he decided to offer his services and speculated about forming a neurological unit to go overseas with the troops.

On February 3, 1941, he noted in his diary, "It is 17 months now since war was declared and I'm still living the same life at the M.N.I. and Bill Cone and Colin Russel, not I, have been in service."

Before the war was a week old, while Penfield was pondering who to approach with his proposal, Colin Russel, a former army medical officer, contacted the authorities in Ottawa with a similar plan. It was approved and he was directed to proceed with the formation of "No. 1 Neurological Hospital."

Wilder accepted with good grace that Russel had beaten him to it, but he was disappointed when Russel chose Bill Cone to be surgical chief instead of him, and noted pointedly in his diary that Russel chose some of the other men for the unit unwisely. It was arranged that Wilder would continue to support the Penfield-Cone joint practice, and that at the end of a year he would change places with

Cone. Wilder was privately relieved not to be leaving Helen and the children behind, at least for a while, and willing to accept the argument that he was needed more at the Institute than in uniform.

Before the No. 1 Neurological Hospital team could leave, however, Lord Tweedsmuir, then Governor General, suffered a severe concussion in a fall at Government House in Ottawa, and for a week Penfield, Cone, Russel and the Institute were the centre of attention across the country and beyond.

During his five years as Governor-General, John Buchan (the title Lord Tweedsmuir had been conferred on him by George V) had set out to meet Canadians who could not count themselves among the powerful, and this had endeared him to a great many people across the nation. In addition, his fame as a novelist and his adventurous expedition to the Canadian Arctic stood out in contrast to the behaviour of his more staid predecessors.

On the morning of February 6, 1940, Tweedsmuir was about to step into his bath when he had a mild stroke and fainted, hitting his head on the edge of the bathtub as he fell.

He was discovered lying unconscious on the floor of his bathroom an hour later. What at first appeared to be a simple concussion quickly became more complicated, as Tweedsmuir was not in good health, and Penfield, Russel (now Lieutenant Colonel, R.C.A.M.C.), and Cone were summoned from Montreal.

For four days Tweedsmuir lay unconscious as his condition gradually worsened and the specialists, not wishing to further endanger his life, stood by periodically releasing bulletins to a public hungry for news. Finally on February 9, they decided to operate in an attempt to relieve the pressure on Tweedsmuir's brain. The operation, which took place in an improvised emergency operating room set up at Government House, was at least a temporary success. Then a decision was made to move him to the Institute. Several hours after the operation a special train left Ottawa and raced to Montreal, stopping beside a specially erected platform near the foot of Mountain Street. From there, Tweedsmuir was rushed to the Institute by ambulance.

The entire Institute had been mobilized for the crisis, and one entire floor cleared for the vice-regal party. For the next four days the lobby overflowed with reporters and well-wishers while Penfield and Cone operated three different times. On the tenth of February, following two operations the night before, Tweedsmuir seemed to improve and showed signs of returning to consciousness. On the eleventh he suffered a relapse. Again they operated, and again he seemed to rally.

Then, just before six o'clock on February 11, a clot which had formed in his leg led to a pulmonary embolism and his heart stopped beating. For over an hour the surgical team tried desperately to resuscitate him but without success. The final official bulletin, released at 7:20 P.M. stated simply, "The Governor General died at 7:13 P.M." It was signed by the five doctors who had been with the patient almost constantly since he arrived Friday morning: Penfield, Cone, Meakins, Russel, and Dr. Gordon Gunn, Tweedsmuir's personal physician.

At the Institute, despite the fact that everything possible had been done for Tweedsmuir, depression set in.

A year later, commenting on the affairs of the Institute in his diary, Wilder noted with some satisfaction that he had succeeded in stirring the staff out of the emotional slump that had begun with Tweedsmuir's death and had deepened inevitably as others went off to the war while they became the "stay-at-homes."

As the initial conviction that Germany would be defeated in a matter of months was replaced by the gloomy realization that the war could last for years, the Institute switched to a war footing. Before long a temporary military annex had been thrown up behind the building to accommodate wounded soldiers, and in every lab peacetime research problems were ignored as the staff threw themselves into trying to solve problems brought on by the war.

The research at the Institute was conducted on half a dozen different fronts. A team led by two recent recruits, Herbert Jasper, a promising young neurophysiologist, and Andy Cipriani, a brilliant biomedical engineer, began a series of studies for the Air Force on the cause of pilot "blackouts." Trying to develop an "anti-G suit" pilots could wear to withstand the air pressures at high altitudes, they built in the basement a large centrifuge upon which they could spin monkeys to simulate the centrifugal forces in dive bombing. The suit they developed was adopted by the Canadian Air Force, and a similar one they helped develop was soon in use by U.S. Navy pilots.

There were, as well, experiments on the treatment of burns, studies of nerve injuries, tests to measure the reaction of the brain to newly developed antibiotics, and a series designed to prove to the conservative Army medical authorities that patients with head injuries could safely be transported by air at high altitudes. For that purpose a part of the seventh floor of the Institute was cleared to make way for a decompression chamber in which to simulate high-altitude flying.

While all this was going on at home, overseas the No. 1 Neurological Hospital was struggling with mixed success against the combined Canadian-British bureaucracy to achieve something worthwhile. Bill Cone had written, much depressed, that in close to nine months in England the unit had operated on only eight cases, and that without any real operating room. The inactivity was owing in part to the fact that the ratio of head injuries to other injuries was well below that of the last war: when bombs landed people were either killed outright or only mildly hurt.

The Canadian unit had been relegated to doing civil work for one county, Hampshire, and while it was stuck in one spot, the British had a small fleet of mobile head-injury units with fully equipped trucks capable of moving to a location, setting up and operating in very short order. The invasion of Britain, which seemed imminent in the dark winter of 1941, could come anytime, anywhere, but No. 1 Neurological Hospital would have no way of moving to the battlefield.

"It seems to me that the conception (of) No. 1 is wrong for this war," Wilder reflected. "They need the Neurological Hospital but not the neurosurgical. Either that unit should be ready to send mobile operating units to the scene of the push...or we should provide each Canadian base with one really good neurosurgeon so that support may be given where it is needed."

Despite the evidence that little was being achieved by the unit, Wilder was anxious to go overseas—though he worried about leaving Helen and the children and doubted that Cone would be able to maintain their joint practice single-handed. But each time Wilder had written Cone and Russel to make arrangements, both attempted to discourage him with reports of their inactivity and argued that he could be more useful back in Canada keeping the Institute running efficiently. Wilder chafed, and grew impatient: "I have a feeling there must be something really effective that I could do. Perhaps that is because of an absurd idea of my own ability...I seem to be sitting in an empty hallway...There are many doors but I don't picture anything worthwhile behind any one of them. Am I too old to be of use?"

Even as President of the Royal College of Physicians and Surgeons of Canada he had been unable to accomplish much that would satisfy his urge to pitch in and help—although he had written a letter to the six hundred members in June of 1940 urging them to write to their U.S. medical brothers that they might use their influence to bring the U.S. into the war. "In any letter you write," he advised them, "do not adopt a defeatist attitude. Point out that we feel here that Britain can defend herself with the help of the Dominions and can hold the sea. If the United States will join the rest of the English-speaking world without too great a delay the war can be won and an international police force established capable of guaranteeing peace and freedom to those people who desire it."

As a propagandist, as Wilder himself admitted, he was strictly an amateur, and it was time for him to go overseas and at last see things for himself.

On July 24, 1941, Wilder Penfield was huddled on a pile of mattresses in the deafeningly noisy interior of a four-engine bomber, shivering as he wrote in a brand new diary purchased for the trip. He was finally on his way to England, but not in uniform. His attempts to enlist had been doomed from the start. He failed the common-to-all-arms paper on his first attempt, though he subsequently passed — thus reaffirming the pattern of his life-long relationship to exams.

Following that embarrassment, it was agreed that he would go over in April or May, and he was told to buy the uniform of a Lieutenant Colonel, having received his commission ten months earlier. A week before he was scheduled to leave a second physical exam was conducted and chest X-rays were taken and sent to Ottawa, where the medical examiners found traces of an old tuberculous infection. Although a number of further tests indicated the scarring on his lungs was unlikely to cause future problems, a medical board and an army specialist refused to recommend Penfield's admission to the army. "That ends my military career," Wilder wrote in his diary when he was informed of his rejection, adding "I am quite honestly relieved."

As soon as he was turned down by the army Wilder went to the National Research Council, and told them he wanted to make a report to the Council on the surgical treatment of war wounds. He then went to the army and told them he wanted to study the handling of head cases by the Canadian medical corps. Both agreed at once, though, as Wilder recorded from his perch in the bomber as the trip neared an end, the president of the N.R.C. said "he would not urge it or recommend it because of the risks....He still regrets and grieves over the death of [Sir Frederick] Banting who died on just such a trip as this two months ago."

Despite the bitter cold and the discomfort of the nineteen-and-a-half-hour transatlantic trip, Wilder was filled with excitement at finding himself on his way to some serious, war-directed research at last, aboard a B-24 *Liberator* travelling at the awesome speed of 175 m.p.h. All night, by a dim light from an adjacent compartment Wilder scribbled away, exercising his fictive eye, with descriptions of his fellow passengers, the bomber's interior and the coast of Scotland, that finally appeared below the clouds. From the air the British Isles looked peaceful and undisturbed, Wilder observed, looking down nostalgically on the pleasant pattern of hedgerows, and the red roofs, from which rose the idling smoke of peat fires. Visible against the green countryside were white clusters of grazing cattle. From the air, the only jarring notes were a submarine leaving a long trail of white against the water, and a burned-out factory with only a smoke stack left standing.

The plane landed in Glasgow and Wilder caught the first train to Edinburgh, where he was met by J. R. Learmouth, Professor of Surgery at the University, and brought home for a late breakfast. There the true face of the siege of Britain slowly became apparent: every inch of the glorious flower garden Wilder recalled from earlier visits was planted over with vegetables; there were no servants in sight, and of breakfast he wrote: "Porridge, with a little sugar offered in a brave manner. Marmalade made from some lemons they got by standing in a queue some time ago." At the university, he wrote, there were no young men and at Learmouth's clinic at the Royal Infirmary, just one resident and some third-year medical students acting as dressers. The windows at the clinic were sandbagged below and painted over a yellow-red so the blue light they operated by would not show through.

From Edinburgh, Wilder travelled to London on the train and laid plans for the next two months. Between the beginning of August and late September he visited one hospital, military base and medical-research centre after another, taking copious notes, asking questions and planning dozens of ways Canadian and U.S. medical and scientific resources could help in particular situations. He sat in on endless committee meetings, taking part in the discussion of numerous problems: the proper way to ventilate and light the instrument panels of tanks; how to insulate helmets; how to improve blood-transfusion techniques and burn treatments; how to condense food and design clothing for the troops. He returned to London from his forays into the countryside to fill dozens and dozens of dictaphone cylinders at the Canadian High Commission offices. At day's end he would return wearily to his bedroom at the Mirabel Hotel to try to sleep despite the music that floated up from the band playing in the dining-room below. Any spare moments he used to visit with his friends among the British scientists in London and out at Oxford and Cambridge.

Bill Cone travelled up to London to talk with him early in August, and Wilder found him both "happy and unhappy," totally involved in his work but frustrated at how little the unit seemed able to achieve. A week later Wilder paid a visit to Basingstoke, where No. 1 Neurological Hospital was based. It gave him a curious feeling to see all of his old friends and colleagues, nurses and doctors alike, in uniform while he was in civvies, and he did not return.

Somehow it did not help matters that everyone he spoke to raved about Bill Cone. Colin Russel, he reported, "is ecstatic about the work Bill has done and can do and wants everyone to recognize it. In a year if he remains he says Bill will be the best known surgeon in England." Gordon Holmes took Wilder aside and said that Cone must not leave the unit because he had the confidence of all the people in the other hospitals. Even Geoffrey Jefferson, whom Wilder had visited at Manchester University where he was in charge of research—and whom Wilder admired and liked above all others—remarked, "I can't make out whether Bill Cone is the greatest surgeon I ever met or whether I am just a damn fool."

Why should so much appreciation of Cone disturb Wilder—as it apparently did? There are only a few clues in his diary. Likely, a combination of things caused Wilder's mixed feelings. There was the fact that Colin Russel had chosen Cone and not Penfield as surgical chief of the army medical unit. Wilder had been rejected by the army, but Bill was in uniform. The near-adulation of Cone that Wilder had been hearing since coming to Europe may have caused him to feel like a teacher who has been surpassed by a favourite disciple. As well, there were signs that, before taking charge of the medical unit, Cone had been less willing to accept the subordinate role in their professional relationship, reflected in the division of responsibilities at the Institute and income from their joint practice.

Cone's lower public profile had much to do with the fact that Penfield's position at the Institute demanded a constant stream of books, articles and reports, many of them summaries of work done jointly with Cone and other staff members, while Cone had been fully occupied in caring for the patients, operating, and continuing the research—to him, more important tasks than spreading the news about discoveries made and conclusions reached. Yet, although they both chafed from time to time at the bonds that kept them together, they recognized their need of each other: without those bonds Bill would not have been free to do what he liked best, nor would Wilder.

In addition to the fundamental affection he felt for Cone, and the essential practicality he saw in their relationship despite the strains, there were other sources of reassurance on this trip. In Glasgow, he noted the contrast between the time of his first visit there, when he was treated as just another wide-eyed medical student, and now, when he was regarded as an elder statesman in the field, one that every young neurologist would do well to emulate. And Geoffrey Jefferson, after his high praise of Bill Cone, had gone on to speak admiringly of Wilder's prewar reports of the results of his surgical procedure for epileptics. The observations Wilder had made about brain function, from operating on conscious patients, moved Jefferson to say that he wanted to do a study of the seat of consciousness which "begins with Descartes and ends with Wilder Penfield." As well, Helen had been writing cheery letters and sending parcels of food, clothing and other items in short supply in Britain to friends and soldiers from Montreal, so that everywhere that Wilder went he met with gratitude for her thoughtfulness.

There were moments of acute loneliness in the two months he spent in England, moments when he missed Helen and the children and the farm terribly. When his tour finally came to an end his return home took him, via Lisbon, to Estoril and Horta in the Azores. There his return was delayed for several weeks by foul weather and a shortage of space on transatlantic flights.

The delay proved to be, as he wrote in his diary on October 6, "a curious interlude in a busy life. As though one were suddenly picked up at his desk and dropped in a desert island." In his room at the half-empty and somewhat forlorn Hotel Palacio in Estoril, he sat by the window editing his reports, occasionally glancing out over the palm trees and smooth white beaches, relishing the soft breezes that blew in from the ocean.

After a week of hard work Wilder recorded that he had just finished his fifty-fourth report. "I must now write an interpretational analysis, the only thing any one will read, I suppose. I've been very superficial and have missed a lot that I ought to have seen, but I have the picture and I know where the blanks are."

With the bulk of his reports in hand he turned instead to his diary to write, lying on the window ledge "practically naked" in the sun, and watching the little children run about in the park below.

Reflecting on the people he had met during the frantic months now passed, he noted: "Times like this I always turn most toward women." As always he found in the company of women the warmth and comfortable conversation he needed. He went on to write a series of thumbnail sketches of the women he had met, for the most part the wives of his medical colleagues, admiring this one, expressing heartfelt thanks he didn't have to live with that one. When he came to the secretary who had been assigned to him in London, it was clear that she was special—"a good companion who laughs at the things I laugh at and remains silent about the things I would ignore, 29 years younger than I, the age of Ruthmary and yet loving my company as I hers."

This line of thought led to his recalling a visit to a woman, a sister-in-law of one of the Montreal surgeons, with whom an innocent indiscretion had caused a certain amount of embarrassment some years earlier. The recollection, in turn, raised the question of his susceptibility generally. When he visited the woman at her home near Basingstoke there was, he wrote somewhat ruefully, "No sign that we were once very good friends, no more sign that there ever was for there never was anything between us except matter of fact chatter and yet my stupidity in walking with her from the Institute over the mountain to her brother's home while the Resident was moving heaven and earth to find me led Helen to fear I was more fond of her than I should have been. I was, no doubt. I shall always be fond of some understanding woman but never love in the sense of my love for Helen. I am happiest if I can take her with me and I had thought never to go away from home without her. Does a man become more dependent on a woman's understanding and companionship as the years pass? I got on quite well with no such companionship in the days of my engagement while up at Oxford. Curiously enough I should not like to have Helen read this and yet it has helped me to write about it. I have always been puzzled that I can not ignore the women about me. If I were a real scientist & really engrossed in great undertakings surely I'd never notice smiles and eyes and hair and grace. Well.—quite enough of this.—back to the best method of lighting the instrument panel of an airplane."

He made a few other entries in his diary before his plane finally left Horta. Soothed now as always by the exercise of writing, he decided that he was well off not to be in Bill Cone's place, "slowly losing my reason—probably not so slowly. I have been too long master of a unit and it would have been very hard to take orders from superiors in the Army." He might even, he concluded, "have found some outlet writing a novel or worse."

For a while after his return, Wilder was ready to strike a temporary truce with routine.

Two years before he and a colleague at the Institute, Theodore Erickson, had completed a twelve-hundred-page book on epilepsy, the definitive work on the subject. They had only set out to write about focal epilepsy, but in their enthusiasm had drifted into an encyclopedia that covered the history of the disease back to the ancient Egyptians, its symptoms, causes and treatments, both medical and surgical.

Now the book was on the market and getting very favourable reaction from all quarters. The Yale library asked for the manuscript for the university archives, and while Wilder agreed with pleasure, he noted in his diary that the final manuscript "is nothing. The first draft is something alive, an old scarred friend, an opponent I wrestled with, a record of labour, comparison and happy discovery and occasionally I know there are pages which wrote themselves as though the writer's hand was on a wigi [sic] board and I was sometimes excited then as though after toil and thirst I had blundered into a land of discovery but always it was only for a moment and then came more toil with always the hope of arrival again."

"Kipling," he continued, "must have felt that way when he wrote. Otherwise he would not have written 'The Explorer.'"

Again and again through his life, from the time he first read the poem at Galahad School, to his last days, he would look to it as his battle cry. Kipling, the poet of Empire and White Man's Burden, had written about exploration on the frontiers in a way that no one had written about science—and yet for Wilder the reasons for being a scientist, the thrill of scientific exploration, *were* matters for poetry. And it is no coincidence that as he grew older he came to see this as the only neutral ground that lay between him and his father. Here he was the son of no weak philanderer, but a scientist whose father had ranged through mountain passes in search of the most elusive big game; both he and Charles had been pioneers in their own ways.

In many of the verses of Kipling's poem something chimed with Wilder's idea of destiny:

> "There's no sense in going further—it's the edge of cultivation,"
> So they said and, I believed it—broke my land and sowed my crop —
> Built my barns and strung my fences in the little border station
> Tucked away below the foothills where the trails run out and stop.
>
> Till a voice, as bad as Conscience, rang interminable changes
> On one everlasting Whisper day and night repeated—so:
> "Something hidden. Go and find it. Go and look behind the Ranges—
> "Something lost behind the Ranges. Lost and waiting for you. Go!"
>
> So I went worn out of patience; never told my nearest neighbours—
> Stole away with pack and ponies—left 'em drinking in the town;

And the faith that moveth mountains didn't seem to help my labours
As I faced the sheer main-ranges, whipping up and leading down.

March by march I puzzled through 'em, turning flanks and dodging shoulders,
Hurried on in hope of water, headed back for lack of grass:
Till I camped above the tree-line—drifted snow and naked boulders—
Felt free air astir to windward—knew I'd stumbled on the Pass.
....

Well I know who'll take the credit—all the clever chaps that followed—
Came, a dozen men together—never knew my desert fears;
Tracked me by the camps I'd quitted, used the water-holes I'd hollowed.
They'll go back and do the talking. *They'll* be called the Pioneers!
....

Have I named one single river? Have I claimed one single acre?
Have I kept one single nugget—(barring samples)? No, not I!
Because my price was paid me ten times over by my Maker.
But you wouldn't understand it. You go up and occupy.

Ores you'll find there; wood and cattle; water-transit sure and steady
(That should keep the railway rates down), coal and iron at your doors.
God took care to hide that country till He judged His people ready,
Then he chose me for His Whisper, and I've found it, and it's yours!

Yes, your "Never-never country"—yes, your "edge of cultivation"
And no sense in "going further"—till I crossed the range to see.
God forgive me! No, *I* didn't. It's God's present to our nation.
Anybody might have found it but—His Whisper came to Me!

As much as the poem spoke to him of his heritage and of the higher calling of science, it was becoming more and more an eloquent summary both of his own restlessness in his scientific pursuits, and of a more general impatience with whatever was at hand. It was always what lay ahead that interested Wilder and spurred him on—the urge to try something different, to break new ground, somewhere. It was a compulsion that would dog him all his life.

Along with the book on epilepsy, a handbook of neurosurgery (which he had finished just before going to England) was also on its way to medical schools and libraries. The Institute was sailing along quite smoothly, leaving him time, should he choose, to turn to research. And yet he was strangely reluctant to take up his old habits, finding in the war a handy and at least partially convincing scapegoat for his reluctance to engage in new experiments.

At the end of the first week in December, Bill Cone suddenly returned. "It is good to have him here," Wilder wrote, and went on to note the changes in Cone, remarking that Cone's interests had expanded "only clinically, not into intellectual or spiritual fields, nor political. Well, I don't think my own understanding goes very far. But I must become oriented to changed circumstances, for a rather different man has returned, one who has been surgical chief 2 years." A few weeks later, referring to these same changes, he wrote a touch resentfully that Cone was working ferverishly on new clinical problems "and is more jealous than he was of priority in his work and yet is no more ready to write about it."

Writing about it was half the fun of research, as far as Wilder was concerned. He loved the cut and thrust of scientific debate; writing up conclusions was a way of issuing a challenge. He saw writing as a responsibility to let others know what you were up to, and allow them to dispute it if they wished. Publishing scientific papers was also good publicity for the Montreal Neurological Institute.

Through the National Research Council in Ottawa, there were now subcommittees assigned to various aspects of war work, but there was as yet no organized approach to the problems of wartime surgery. Wilder's report on the surgical techniques being used for war injuries in Britain had received wide circulation, as had his observations regarding the problems modern warfare was presenting to surgeons.

Throughout the fall and early winter of 1941 Wilder lobbied the National Research Council to create a separate subcommittee on surgery, and when it was finally done early in 1942, he was appointed chairman. The function of the committee was primarily to review all the data on surgery coming in from the Front and from the Allies' hospitals in Europe, and to act as a resource for the various branches of the armed services in developing more appropriate surgery for war wounds. Throughout 1942 the members of the subcommittee met and debated surgical treatment of burns, bone grafting, amputation, various ways of speeding up wound healing, the problems of ruptured discs, early diagnosis of nerve injury, and a host of other specific problems.

In addition, at the end of January, 1942, Wilder was made chairman of a committee formed to try and find a cure for seasickness. The problem was obviously important to the navy: Sailors who couldn't develop an immunity to seasickness had to be transferred to some other branch of the armed services. Though not so obviously, the problem was equally serious for the army. Soldiers were expected to spend hours tossing on heavy seas in landing craft and assault boats, and then go immediately into action when they landed.

The first problem of the committee was to develop a machine to simulate a ship's movement and produce motion sickness. Wilder and a team from the M.N.I. paid a visit to an amusement park near Montreal and persuaded the manager to let them spend the afternoon taking free and prolonged turns on the Ferris wheel, "Shoot-the-Chute," "Flip-Over," "Loop-the-Loop," and other rides. Wan and bedraggled by the end of the day, they now had some idea of the type, degree and frequency of oscillation that most rapidly produced motion sickness.

The next step involved the construction of a machine large enough to take a volunteer. There was no room in the flimsy wartime annex and no room in the Institute itself except in the squash court, so it was there that the machine—christened "the good ship Mal de mer"—was installed.

There, for the next six months, pink-faced recruits who had "volunteered" for the experiment entered the squash court in the morning, and, green-faced, stumbled out again at night. The result, after much trial and error, and further experiments on real ships in heavy seas, was a little pink pill containing a thiobarbiturate called V-12 which was issued first to sailors of the Royal Canadian Navy and later, to soldiers during the invasion of Europe.

Throughout the year 1942, committee work and war research filled up much of the time left over from administering the Institute and operating. Wilder, like everyone else, followed the news of the war anxiously. In February, after a dinner party with a few friends in Montreal, the assembled guests filled out predictions concerning the course of the war, and placed them in envelopes marked "to be opened Feb. 24, 1943—War Predictions."

"Will Britain have launched a continental invasion? Will the Germans have been expelled from Russia? Will the Germans have launched an invasion against England? Will the Japanese have made a landing on the N. American continent? How long will the war last?"

Wilder fared rather well, only three wrong out of ten; better than Helen by one and better than most of the others. The war would end in 1945, he calculated, and no, the Japanese would not have made a landing in North America in a year's time.

Somehow the possibility of war in the Pacific seemed too remote then to take seriously. And so it was on December 7, ten months later. Even as Japanese fighters bombed Pearl Harbor, Wilder sat out on the porch in the unseasonably warm weather, recovering from a cold, looking down the long peaceful slope of Westmount, noting in his diary that the airplanes droning overhead and occasionally performing stunts were "the only evidence that we, too, are at war." A week later, again writing in his diary, he had much to say about the attack on Pearl Harbor and the news that the Japanese were nearing Singapore: it was most fortunate in some respects because it had precipitated America's involvement in the war, for one. Further, "one may hope for an international police force after Germany and Japan are crushed.... The English speaking countries will win," he continued, ignoring, in his enthusiasm, the other Allies, "because of their fortunate geographical location and, perhaps, because of strength of mind and spirit that is preserved by their way of life."

Wilder Jr., after graduating from Bishop's University, had spent the summer at the officers' training camp in Brockville, Ontario, and then enlisted in a tank corps. He was now twenty-four. Ruthmary, a year younger, still carried an American passport and had gone over in April to London to act as confidential secretary to Gil Winant, U.S. ambassador to the Court of St. James and a Princeton classmate of Wilder's. The two youngest were away at boarding school: Jeff, bursting up to new skinny heights, bounding exuberantly about the house on his visits from Trinity College School in Port Hope, Ontario, and Priscilla "in a schoolgirl haze" at Netherwood in the Maritimes. Helen, for her part, was busy with volunteer war work, and assiduously maintaining the flow of parcels and comforting letters to their friends overseas.

For all his committee work and other preoccupations Wilder was feeling left out. To make matters worse, two days after Christmas he stood on the platform at Windsor Station waving good-bye, as Wilder Jr. set off in a vast sea of servicemen. Towering above the crowd with his beret at a rakish angle, knapsack over one shoulder and swagger stick under his arm, he looked altogether so splendid and so young that his father dreaded how the boy might look the next time he saw him.

With their eldest son's departure hanging over Wilder and Helen like a shadow, the Christmas holidays had been short and precious. The family had gone up into the Laurentians for some "skiing in the sun, then tea at the club in a glow from the cold and climbing, and home in the car singing all the way."

"The young men go away," Wilder added gloomily, sitting alone in his study that night. "The old men, old women, children remain behind."

◊◊◊◊ AMBASSADOR FOR SCIENCE

If no one would call on him, perhaps it was time for him to take matters into his own hands. There must be more—even for a man of fifty-two—than committee work and waiting impatiently on the sidelines while the war was fought thousands of miles away. But what?

The answer came in a telegram on January 1, 1943, from the Director of the Institute for Investigation of the Nervous System in Moscow, Propper Graschenko. He had paid a visit to the M.N.I. before the war and had been much impressed; indeed he remarked later that in his opinion it was the best organized institute in the world. In the telegram, he sent his best wishes for the New Year and suggested cautiously that there was a change of heart in the upper echelons of the Soviet bureaucracy with regard to communication between Soviet scientists and those of the Allies. There was talk of inviting a delegation of medical men from Britain to come to the U.S.S.R. to discuss Soviet methods of dealing with the wounded. Would Penfield be interested in coming along, and could he arrange such a thing?

Nothing could have suited Wilder better. From the start of the war he had been arguing the need for open exchanges of information between the allied countries including Russia, a stand that had not made him very popular in some quarters. As usual, he had somewhat overstated his case. Troubled by the memory of Foerster's institute shuttered against the outside world, isolated by Germany's new leaders from the rest of the international scientific community, he had protested during a committee meeting in Ottawa that basic research results should not even be kept secret from the Germans.

Sir Frederick Banting, who was a member of that committee, reacted angrily. He retorted, according to Wilder's diary, in language the latter was unwilling even to record privately, "that he would not tell the ⸺ ⸺ Germans a word of what we were doing."

That was in the fall of 1939; by now Wilder had become more

willing to accept the restrictions of war, and the scientific community had become less feverishly patriotic. Nonetheless, Wilder had recently urged that more information from the so-called "war research" be passed along to the universities, where it could lead to non-military scientific advances. He then made matters worse by formulating his ideas in an article and sending it off to *Science Magazine*. Mainly because of the article, as he noted in his diary, "there had been some resistance in Toronto to letting me have information in regard to secret stuff!" The questioning of his reliability and discretion cut him to the quick, but only served to make him stick to his guns.

Now, the telegram from Graschenko seemed to offer not only an opportunity to prove his point about the free exchange of information, but a trip to the Soviet Union and a chance to contribute something worthwhile to the war effort, as well.

It took some delicate negotiating, and Wilder had to pull a few strings, but in the end it was arranged that Wilder would make the trip as a member of the British team of doctors. On May 25, he was at the Soviet Embassy in London getting his passport stamped along with the other six members of the now-designated "Russian Mission"—three from Britain, two from the U.S., and Wilder, informally representing Canada.

It had not been simple organizing this trip and countering all of the arguments of those in government opposed to the idea, and there would be many more skirmishes from embassy to embassy in London before the team could depart. The Foreign Offices and Intelligence Services of three countries had to be satisfied with the arrangements as well. But for Wilder the delay in London had several compensations. Within the space of a week in London, he went through the ceremonies of becoming an honorary member of the Royal College of Surgeons (Hon. F.R.C.S.), and a Fellow of the Royal Society (F.R.S.); and when the King's Birthday List came out on June 2, he found his name on it: Wilder Penfield, C.M.G. (Commander of St. Michael and St. George).

It was a heady experience. Membership in the Royal Society pleased him the most, not only because it carried the most prestige, but because the representatives of medicine in the Royal Society were usually physiologists and "other types of laboratory men." A few days after the formal signing of the members' book, adding his name to a list that included Newton, Huxley, Pepys, Sherrington, Pavlov and Darwin, he reflected that traditionally surgeons were considered beyond the pale, "not outcasts for they have never really been considered scientists.... Like the Kingdom of Heaven which we are given to understand has never had its quota of rich men, so the Royal Society seems to have managed very well with only an occasional surgeon who slips in—I don't know how. Perhaps it is by being something other than a surgeon." And since to be more than a surgeon had been Wilder's goal when he launched into his research at Queen Square a quarter of a century earlier, his election to the Royal Society was, more than anything else, formal acknowledgment that he had achieved his aim.

But his success had not by any means resolved the debate, or eliminated the superiority "scientists" felt towards "surgeons." In a revealing diary entry, Wilder described several of the serious problems faced by a surgeon-scientist, "...perhaps because he cannot control the conditions of his work well enough. He does experiment though he must not admit it unless the result is a happy one. After a series of unsuccessful experiments a surgeon is left not plotting an impersonal graph but facing a series of shades of people to whom he was attached, and what is even worse he must face the bereft wife, husband, mother, child." Furthermore the surgeon's attempts to publicize his work often miscarry, he noted, recalling that a paper he had delivered to a conference had resulted in a newspaper report that he claimed to be able to cure epilepsy with electricity. (A couple of days later a letter had arrived: "Dear Doc," it began, "I read your ad in the paper—How much do you charge?")

While the final arrangements for the trip to the Soviet Union were being made, Wilder worked on his Russian, with Ruthmary as the teacher to whom he was grateful for correcting him "very tactfully and wisely." He also tried to read up on medicine in the U.S.S.R. while he was waiting, but all he could find, and that in the basement of the library of the Royal Society of Medicine, was one small, dusty shelf of out-of-date journals. And so he waited and chafed until finally at midnight on June 28, after five weeks of delay, the Russian delegation took off in a Liberator bomber.

The northern route to the U.S.S.R. was closed, and the route they took was a long southern loop by way of Gibraltar, Tripoli, Cairo, Tehran and, finally, to Moscow, a journey of four days. It became immediately apparent on their arrival that the Soviet authorities were giving this delegation of Western medical and scientific experts high priority. During the next three weeks the delegates were whisked from one hospital to the next, to clinics and research institutes, to meetings with scientists and high government officials. And everywhere in spite of the general shortage of food, they found tables groaning with caviar and other delicacies, and endless bottles of vodka with which to pledge undying friendship.

And yet, despite the hospitality, there were sour notes. After a tour of one of the front-line hospitals, Wilder observed: "They feel rather superior to us.... They do not seem to be curious about what we think of their medicine or rather they are not curious about what we may know but are anxious to have the applause they know they deserve. They have no feeling of being cut off from the world. Rather, the world is here in the Soviet."

On another occasion the British and American delegations visited the clinic of Burdenko, the chief surgeon of the Red Army, head of the Medical Council, founder of the Russian School of Neurosurgery and director of the Neurosurgical Institute. This formidable-sounding personage turned out to be "a little squatty man who was stone deaf, talked with a jerky grunt or roar so that Russians obviously had trouble to understand him and who communicated chiefly by paper and pencil; who only shook hands, gave a vibrating bow and smiled suddenly." Burdenko performed two operations for the benefit of his visitors, and Wilder at least was not impressed: "The whole approach to a post-traumatic epileptic was 30 years behind good therapy. He grew suddenly tired and hot and cross. Wiped his brow on his assistant's shoulder, stamped his foot and glared at the nurse."

It became apparent to the members of the team that while the profession was keen for exchange of information on techniques, the authorities were more interested in good public relations, and were keeping a close watch on their own scientists, rarely leaving them alone with the visitors. "Col. Hill offered to take two of the Russians at our dinner home in his auto," Wilder explained. "He heard one say to the other—are you sure we will not get into trouble for riding with this foreigner? The other replied—but surely we are coming from an official dinner. That explains their great friendliness when all is in order, and the sudden shut down and disappearance of all these friends otherwise. It explains why they are never alone."

Between official visits, Wilder and his colleagues managed to get out into the streets of Moscow to see the people—who struck them as stern and preoccupied as they hurried about their business—and to stroll through Red Square and the streets near their hotel.

There were some amusing moments. While watching a long and rather tedious operation, Wilder decided he wanted to discuss something with one of the Russian doctors. Accordingly, he slipped up beside him and, in a whisper and with gestures, attempted to suggest that the two step outside into the hall for a moment. Somewhat puzzled at first, the Russian seemed finally to understand and the two of them left the operating room. Down the corridor, the Russian paused before a closed door and waved Wilder in, and the latter found himself all alone in a washroom, with only the dripping taps for company.

On all but one occasion Wilder managed to get through the interminable toasts that accompanied every meal by sipping port wine. However at one dinner he was seated next to a persistent Russian officer "who kept toasting me...and when I would not drink he would clink his glass against mine as it sat on the table. When I drank he made a deprecating gesture because I took so little out." This comical scene continued, with Wilder growing more and more irritated and doing his best to ignore his neighbour's attentions. Then came the final toast, or so it seemed, and Wilder drained his glass. "But there followed a superfine toast to victory or the Red Soldier, or British-American-Canadian and Russian doctors or some such important subject! Everyone stood. My glass was empty so a young man filled it from a carafe.

"It looked like water and I was glad to have it. The toast was interpreted and I downed the thing. It was vodka. I felt all right and danced with our interpreter Miss Marasova.

"Out into the night we went, with a flashlight ahead and a Russian officer holding the arm of each guest. The woods echoed with shrieks of laughter and shouts. Looking back the whole line was weaving back and forth, a strange sight. I tried to extricate myself from my captors' grip for I resented the assumption but without avail and of course we could not talk to each other. Arrived at the hut I watched my room mate being put to bed and realized that everything was whirling about and I'd better undress without getting up if I wished to keep up my bluff. When I closed my eyes everything whirled much worse and a great weight seemed to settle on my head so I kept awake long after everything was quiet until about one o'clock."

When it came time to leave, the delegates did so with regret, although with little idea of what had been achieved. Individually they had made friends and acquired some idea of how the Russians were dealing with war wounds of various kinds. Wilder discovered, to his delight, that although apparently only one copy of his and Erickson's book on epilepsy existed in the U.S.S.R., the Russians were impressed with his work, and he left behind an assortment of surgical instruments as gifts, and invitations to several of the Russian surgeons to pay a visit to the M.N.I. if they ever could.

More than anything else, it seemed a precedent had been set. That was the delegates' conclusion, and the conclusion of the British official who acted as their liaison and wrote the official report after their departure. He had wryly observed the cycle from being "full of enthusiasm" on arrival, to being "rather disgruntled" at the delays and red tape, to the final "most satisfactory" meeting with the People's Commissar for Health. "It is too early to say whether their efforts to establish medical liaison with the Soviet Union will bear fruit," he concluded, "but the preliminary indications are not discouraging."

They left just before daybreak on July 23 for Tehran, and eleven hours later Wilder was seated on the terrace of the British Legation there, drinking tea in the late afternoon sun, relishing the peace and quiet and feeling as though he had come back home. The others were indeed on their way home, but Wilder was going onward to China; in for a penny, in for a pound. The loss of the seaport cities to the Japanese had left the Chinese with but one of the original twenty-nine medical schools open before the war started. China obviously needed help from abroad, and before leaving London Wilder had arranged to make a visit to China and report on conditions there for the British and Canadian governments.

Aside from the hope that his report might bring real help to China, Wilder was eager to visit the Orient. He had always loved travelling and he was enjoying this trip immensely. "I can never hear a train or a boat whistle without wanting to pick up and go," he would say. Even the inevitable confusions and delays of travel had their advantages: they were beyond his control, however much he fumed or stormed, leaving him no alternative but to sit back and relax. Travelling also provided him with private moments alone to write in his diary. On this particular journey he filled half a dozen notebooks with a running account of his progress, the strange and wonderful landscapes, the strangers he met along the way.

On the twenty-sixth of July, he noted that because of delays in getting a space on an aircraft, in three days he had travelled only as far as the Royal Air Force base at Habbaniya, just outside of Baghdad. Writing in the cool of the evening, in the Senior Officer's Mess where he was staying, he noted that the blast of hot air that had hit him as he stepped off the plane had reminded him of "the blast of air that used to come up the big register of the Presbyterian church in Hudson, that ballooned the ladies' skirts in such a satisfactory manner....Strange how childhood memories come back in these completely new environments," he mused. "The hot ground & thirst reminds me of the harvest field at Roberts, Wisc. and a little boy who wore his shirt outside his overalls the way the men did and followed the reaper around the field...looking forward to the corner of the field beside the fence, next the wood where wild cucumbers grew upon the bushes & seemed to make a wall—the corner where a jug of oatmeal water was kept to quench thirst and which without anyone realizing the wisdom of the plan gave us sodium chloride...(this method of preventing sun stroke with water & salt has become very important out here. The past week has come close to their record for temperature out here—121.4° day before yesterday.)"

Wilder's plan had been to proceed, as soon as a space on a plane was available, to Karachi, and from there to Calcutta, where he could make a connection into Chungking. But the next day, word came from the Middle East Command in Cairo that he would have to wait where he was for ten days.

Rather than being angry at the delay, he was delighted. "When I started around the world," he noted in his diary, "I thought of...Mother at once. Now it so falls out that I am given a week in Mesopotamia of all places, a few miles from Babylon in the desert. Granted that it is in the summer's worst heat in an area that is regularly hotter than India....This time I shall dedicate to the memory of Mother."

The connection between Jean Penfield and Mesopotamia went back to her last—and like the others, unfinished—literary effort. On their final visit in California not long before her death, he found her fretting over the bundle of carefully typed pages she referred to as "The Story of Sarai." She had been working diligently at it for almost ten years; it was to be an instructive romance, full of sturdy Christian morals for young people and, as Wilder would put it in an uncharitable moment, "that large body of adults whose intellectual evolution lapses in early youth....She understood them and could write for them."

Much of the story was set in the ancient city of Ur, where Abraham spent his early years and where, according to Jean's version at any rate, his half-sister, Sarai, had come to visit and had fallen in love with her handsome half-brother. Jean had been having difficulty trying to picture Ur and the surrounding countryside; difficulty in fact with the story as a whole and her inability to finish it, and Wilder offered to finish it for her. She agreed to the co-authorship idea and he promised to send her whatever he wrote. She handed the manuscript over to him with relief. She died within the year and, after a cursory reading, Wilder put it away and turned to other things.

Eight years had passed, and now he found himself close by the excavations of the ancient city of Ur, with ten days on his hands. He approached the principal medical officer for Iraq and Iran, a group captain by the name of O'Neil, with his proposal to take a trip to Ur. "An Irishman who said my scheme was mad," as Wilder later recalled, O'Neil nonetheless agreed to make the arrangements and to accompany Wilder himself. Three days later Wilder was at the regimental staging post of Ur Junction—how queer it sounded!—at four in the morning, just as grey light edged the eastern horizon.

No matter how many times he would write of this first visit, the note of awe that runs through his first diary account would best capture his feelings and impressions.

"A thin red line appeared on the very brim of the flattest horizon I have ever seen. It grew wider. The fleecy clouds were splashed with yellow gold. My shadow extended a long way across the camp.... the Ziggurat lay ahead of us, reddish brown and seeming to stand on a ridge which was indeed the city of Ur....

"We climbed the steps straight up to the top of the Ziggurat. Sand grouse, big brown breasts & rapid wing flew by in flocks large & small—all going north to water...quite low, they pipe pitchou-pitcher-pitchou.... A hyena started up at the foot of the Ziggurat and I watched him gallop away, then stop, and gallop several times. Coming from the north a herd of camels passed east of us, drifting in stately manner, adult and baby camels, as though etched on the back of a Christmas card. The cloak of the Arab who followed flapped in the wind."

Below, he could make out the market place "where the priests bartered peace of mind and benediction for food, drink & ornament," and to the right of the steps, the temple of Ningal, wife of the Moon God. He and O'Neil walked back down and through the excavated town, down streets "the sides of which I could touch with either hand," and through doorways so low they had to stoop to pass through, Wilder wondering as he stepped over shards of broken pottery if this house or this might have been the house in which Abraham grew up. Time seemed to stand still as the two men walked through the queer, echoing ruins, Wilder peering and touching and racing back in his mind to how it might have been.

The wind grew stronger and blew up the dust in a haze, and when they stopped for a sip of water Wilder noticed that his companion didn't look well, so they headed back. While O'Neil slept, Wilder scribbled, and soon they were back at the base.

His imagination fired by the trip, Wilder went into Baghdad to visit the Museum of Archaeology and there he spent the time before the plane left, poring over the texts and examining artifacts that offered clues to the daily life of Ur thousands of years ago. By the time he set off on the next leg of his journey, he had decided to try his hand at rewriting his mother's story.

Baghdad to Basra, Basra to Karachi; Karachi to Gwalior, Gwalior to Calcutta: four days of delays, little sleep, stale sandwiches and lukewarm coffee brought Wilder on the ninth of August to the last leg of his journey. As daylight waned he found himself in the freight compartment of a DC-3 threading its way through the mountain passes and "over the hump" of the Himalayas into China, in the midst of a monsoon.

Every little while one of his companions on the Calcutta-Chungking flight would stand up, wipe the mist from the windows and peer out to see if anything was visible through the clouds and rain. They were flying less than ninety miles from the Japanese lines, and one of Wilder's companions, a Chinese newspaperman, informed him that they were very lucky that visibility was so bad: "These planes are very easy for a fighter to get—just like a fat pig!"

Wilder turned from this comforting thought to his diary and, recalling again the excitement of the dawn trip out to the Ziggurat looming reddish-brown out of the desert, recorded his determination to return when the war was over. Soon he could feel his ears popping, and he stirred from his reverie. The plane had passed over the mountains and the sky had cleared. As the aircraft sailed in low to Chungking, he craned his neck to look down and saw below the wide flood of the Yangtse "winding like an enormous tan snake through its gorges." Beyond as the sun set into great peaks of golden clouds, the lights of Chungking blinked on. China!

In August of 1943, when Wilder arrived in China, the Sino-Japanese war was dragging through its sixth inconclusive year. In the first push, the Japanese had driven Chiang Kai-shek and the Kuomintang government and armies out of north China and the coastal cities and into the hinterland in the south. In Chungking, generously supplied with American arms and money, Chiang set up base and marked time. The faltering alliance between the Kuomintang and the Communists—a marriage of convenience to defeat the Japanese—had broken down completely, and Chiang's conduct of the war had come under bitter attack in China and abroad. In many diplomatic quarters the Kuomintang government was regarded as weak, unrepresentative, oppressive and corrupt. Western representatives who had dealt personally with Chiang and the glamorous and influential Madame Chiang held them in the deepest contempt. General Stilwell, the American military advisor, referred to Chiang as "peanut." The name caught on among foreign attachés in China, to whom it was apparent that Chiang was callously reserving his best troops and material for the coming civil war with the Communists, calculating that the Allies could be counted upon to defeat the Japanese. Chiang's faith stemmed from the recent victories of the Allies in the Coral Sea, at Midway, Stalingrad and El Alamein. The stalemate that existed between Chinese forces and the Japanese invaders was mainly attributable to the Communist armies in the north, who, under Mao Tse-tung, continued to fight vigorously.

That Wilder was unaware of all this when he landed in China is apparent from his diaries, which are full of praise for "his Excellency Chiang Kai-shek, Generalissimo and most important popular hero of China," and for Madame Chiang "also reverenced by the people," who did "too much" for her country and thus unwittingly invited "the kind of slander the great inevitably receive."

It would be uncharitable to make too much of Wilder's blinkered view of the situation in China during his short visit there. If the long view of history has caused us to revise our opinions of Chiang Kai-shek and to regard this period as one of the sorriest in American foreign policy, there were few outside of China in 1943 who had any idea of what was going on inside the country. In fact Madame Chiang had recently returned from a triumphant visit to America where her poise, beauty and U.S.-educated English had completely bewitched an American (and Canadian) public already inclined to view the Nationalist Chinese as a heroic David battling the Japanese Goliath.

That, certainly, was Wilder's innocent view when he arrived for his fact-finding mission. A fairly astute judge of character, he would come away from his encounter with Madame Chiang aware that he had been (as President Roosevelt would later admit to having been) "vamped" by her beauty and charm. Like Roosevelt, he sensed the unbending steel and ambition that lay beneath. But Wilder's natural respect for authority would make him keep these unworthy thoughts to himself. In appraising the larger scene, his perception was limited not only by the fact that he was not much of a political observer, but by the fact that his tour was confined to the safe area around Chungking, far from the threat of the Japanese.

So, by the diary accounts, Wilder's unschooled eye saw little evidence of the enormous changes brewing in China in 1943, changes that would eventually force the Generalissimo to retreat from the mainland to the island of Taiwan and would make the name Mao Tse-tung reverberate around the world. Nowhere in his diaries is there a mention of the Communists or their uneasy alliance with the Kuomintang, and there was no visit to the ragged Communist armies in the north. Nor is there a mention of Norman Bethune, the Montreal doctor who accompanied Mao on the Long March and whose death in 1940 had made him a martyr. In Canada, the press reports of Bethune's death had been skimpy, and Wilder no less than the rest of the world would be stunned to discover twenty years later that to 800 million Chinese, Bethune's Chinese name—Pai-ch'iu-en—had a reverential lustre second only to that of Mao Tse-tung.

During his stay in Chungking Wilder was quartered in the United Church of Canada mission next door to the home of the Canadian representative in China, Major-General Odlum. And though he occasionally complained of feeling "like a poor relation to the embassy," everyone clearly went out of their way to help him enjoy his visit and get the information for which he had come. Odlum himself took charge of Wilder, who noted with some pride and amusement: "Apparently I am the first Canadian to come here & require care—and I require a lot of time, money and precious petrol."

He had much to do during his short visit, and so little time "to reflect and to catch on these pages the colour of first impression of a new nation, the greatest nation, from the point of view of numbers, in the world."

It was the numbers, the vastness, that stunned him. He spoke to a professor from the university at Chengtu who had taken a census in a few of the districts and calculated that the current estimate of 400 or 450 million was short by well over 100 million. Coming home from the embassy in a rickshaw through the crowded streets of Chungking, Wilder's impression of the country was a blur of infinite multitudes "sweating, straining, lifting, working...brown legs pulling and pushing, the grunts of the chair carriers that clear their path, great loads of grain creaking up the hill with four men pulling, rickshaws all in a line trotting along...junks being rowed by a dozen men with long oars in unison like the old galleys, and the captain standing behind with an unbelievably long oar steering," and of "men poling boats upstream, men carrying huge pails of water fastened to either end of thick pieces of split bamboo. It seemed to be toil and sweat in a heat that makes sweat break out all over you when you exert yourself the least bit." Here and there in the crowds a disturbing note: the children of the rich, "young people who are carried in chairs with an expression of utter langour."

In Chungking he first met with the Surgeon General of the Kuomintang Army and various government health officials, and after three days set off in the Canadian legation car to drive north to the city of Chengtu to visit the universities—what was left of them. His companions on the trip were a Canadian medical missionary, Dr. Kilbourn, a missionary by the name of Bell, a man named Patterson from the embassy, and a Russian driver "who speaks three languages," Wilder reported. It took two days to reach Chengtu, motoring north and west through Szechuan Province through the richest and most intensively tilled farming country he could recall seeing.

Along the highroad Wilder and Dr. Kilbourn passed a constant stream of rickshaws going at a run, and coolies carrying enormous loads, a hundred pounds and more, going at a trot they would keep up all day, covering upwards of thirty kilometres from sun-up to sundown.

At Chengtu there were more meetings, more and more information to assimilate for his report: the size of the Kuomintang army (five million, with four million more in the labour corps), their diet, the number of first aid stations, the equipment they were using. Everything was in short supply—where even to begin to help? Wilder had little time to digest what he had learned before heading back to Chungking for a meeting with Generalissimo Chiang Kai-shek and Madame Chiang.

The purpose of this meeting is unclear, and his detailed account is little help in that regard; perhaps it was simply a courteous gesture on Chiang's part to a friendly and possibly influential foreign visitor. The meeting took place over dinner at the small, Western-style house—nicknamed "peanut's palace" by Stilwell *et al*—where the Generalissimo lived. Wilder had come with Major-General Odlum. His diary account began with a description of their hosts:

"Madame entered first, black hair, black eyes, and smile. She looked at you long enough to take in anything of interest. After that she sometimes looked at you with just enough coquetry, occasionally serious and direct. The Generalissimo came in in black Chinese costume which hung to his feet, a man several inches shorter than I [height was always the first thing Wilder referred to in these thumbnail sketches of men] slender and straight. He smiled and nodded, and after shaking hands he put each hand in the opposite sleeve. Madame interpreted for us."

During dinner Chiang Kai-shek asked, through his wife, about Wilder's trip to Russia. "Apparently I did not hit a very high level, and she translated nothing to him and he was thinking of something else. Then she said, Tell us the most interesting experience you ever had. I said, Do you mean in surgery? Yes, she said, or anything. I felt my face grow red and could think of nothing so I went back to talking about Russian partisans."

At that point the conversation was interrupted by General Odlum, who had a bone to pick with Chiang Kai-shek on a matter that was irksome to all of the foreign government representatives in China at the time. Here is Wilder's report of the conversation that followed:

"Odlum began. 'Would the Generalissimo pardon me if I made a blunt statement?'

"'He is never anything else,' I told her [Madame Chiang]. Yes, the G. would be glad to hear and he smiled with his eyes and just a little with his lips in a way he has.

"General Odlum said, 'The Chinese soldiers are not well looked after. In every other country the soldiers are better cared for than civilians. Here it is just the opposite." Etc.

"She was not smiling now, but interpreting as fast as possible. I squirmed. The reply was, 'The Generalissimo says this is not true. We are a poor people. The ports are closed, and transportation is difficult. The poor people of the country do not have meat oftener than 2 or 3 times a year. Soldiers have meat twice a week.'"

With that dinner came to an end. They left the table, and Madame explained they were going down the hill below the house to a hall to see a Canadian movie, a Hollywood-made picture, Wilder wrote, in which "Redcoats, bad half-breeds and flaxen-haired heroines produced a fake war that had more of an atmosphere of Hollywood than Canada."

Eventually the movie dragged to its inevitable finish, and after a brief and "aloof" farewell, the Generalissimo and his wife departed.

Wilder left China in early September. His travels had exhausted him both physically and mentally and he was anxious to be home. He had been away since the last week of May, his longest separation from Helen since their marriage, and the travelling had begun to lose some of its allure.

Although the trip south to the city of Kunming had been a disappointment, with no one to meet him, no appointments set up and much confusion, his two weeks in China had provided enough material to write a lengthy report for the National Research Council. Since the Chinese had no proper research council and could not ensure that restricted documents sent into the country would be kept secret, there was no point in proposing the kind of open exchange Wilder hoped they could extend to the Soviet Union. There was a desperate need for all kinds of medical supplies and food, of course, but that was not the sphere of the National Research

Council. It would be best if they could send experts to consult with the Chinese on more technical matters: for instance, the making of surgical instruments and the manufacture of certain drugs. Also, Canada should offer to train Chinese doctors in large numbers, for even if they weren't much use during the rest of the war, Wilder noted in his report, "they will nevertheless help China greatly in the difficult period of reconstruction that lies ahead of her. As well as being a friendly act," he concluded, "it is obviously very much to our own advantage to help China pull herself together after the war."

Other than the general recommendations about the form medical assistance to China might take, Wilder's report to the National Research Council had little to add. His comments on the situation in China no doubt echoed what the Canadian government and the British government, who received a copy, had already heard through their official channels. Nonetheless, he worked hard on the report during the round-about return flight, and if no one else took it very seriously, at least he did. When he was interviewed, on his arrival, he steadfastly maintained, according to the article in the Montreal *Star*, "Whatever their difficulties...there was no talk of capitulation among the Chinese people...and no criticism was levelled against Generalissimo Chiang Kai-shek. The Chinese leader was the one great personality who united the people of the huge country and held them together to fight the superior forces of the Japanese, Dr. Penfield believed."

When he next travelled to China nineteen years later, Wilder would come bearing a film about Norman Bethune as a gift to the Chinese Communist leader Mao Tse-tung. And he would return to Canada with as much enthusiasm for Mao as he now showed for Mao's enemy, Chiang Kai-shek.

It was a great relief to be home, and Wilder would do no more junketing until the war ended, satisfying himself instead with committee work in Ottawa and running the Institute. He arrived at Dorval Airport in Montreal on September 6 to find Helen waiting, and after talking to the gathered reporters they set off on a leisurely drive to the farm—to, he observed contentedly, "coolness and wind, and a country green by no one's effort."

CHAPTER EIGHT

In Full Flight

∞∞ GREAT DISCOVERIES

On the sixth of August, 1945, an atomic bomb, developed in secrecy by American and European scientists, was dropped on the Japanese city of Hiroshima. The city was destroyed instantly. Of its two million inhabitants, seventy thousand were killed. Two days later the Soviet Union declared war on Japan and invaded Manchuria, and the following day an even more powerful atomic bomb was dropped on Nagasaki. The war was over.

A week later, waiting for the news of Japan's surrender to come over the radio, Wilder turned to his diary to collect his thoughts for the first time since returning from China in 1943. Gone was the sense of urgency and siege that had permeated Canada during the war, despite its distance from the battlefields. Gone too was Wilder's sense of purpose, given him by the knowledge that he was useful to the war effort in his own small way. Now, with his National Research Council committee work at an end, that anxiety momentarily returned and he observed ruefully, "During the 6 year war interlude, I have made no scientific contribution worth the name. I have contributed something to Research Council activity, have spent much time administering the Institute...but have gone from age 48 to 54 at a standstill—making a living and being a citizen."

Long ago he and Helen had decided to celebrate turning fifty by driving off a cliff; who wanted to be that old? Later, when little Ruthmary developed a passion for dissecting mice, frogs and beetles, Wilder brought her a bottle of chloroform from his lab and labelled it

"For Use on My 50th Birthday." Instead he had celebrated the occasion by skiing down the long hill below the farm house in fifty seconds.

The passing of his fiftieth birthday wasn't the only reminder that Wilder was no longer a young man. In April he had become a grandfather. Ruthmary had married an American intelligence officer named Crosby Lewis the year before, and the first grandchild, a girl named Catherine, was born in Wiesbaden (where they were stationed). The event had been greeted with much fanfare and publicity, since the baby was the first (legitimate) child born to a member of the American occupation force in Germany.

Recent news had come from Wilder Jr. that he too was about to get married. He had spent the last two years of the war as an officer in wireless intelligence in the Canadian army, and had met a young American girl while stationed in Holland. The girl's name was Berry Bonynge, her mother's family was Dutch, and she had spent two years driving heavy trucks in the evacuation of refugees in Holland, Wilder Jr. had explained in his most recent letter. Priscilla had gone off to Wells College, where she had done creditably (though she was "much worried about her ugly-duckling stage. The swan is emerging but she does not yet suspect it"). Jeff had graduated from Trinity College and, following in the footsteps of his father and brother, was heading off to Princeton in the fall.

The nest had emptied and Wilder thought "the new stage of solitary married life...very pleasant." In stolen moments over the last few years he had been working away at the novel on Abraham and Sarah started by his mother, though he was keeping it a secret from everyone but Helen. He had a plot now, and though he was often frustrated by his clumsy writing, there were moments when he found the process thrilling. When he came to a dead end, he would turn to Shakespeare and read a few pages, returning to his own writing with renewed enthusiasm. In the last two years he had even occasionally felt the urge to drop everything else and take up writing as a full-time career. However, an article he had written about his trip to China and sent off hopefully to *The Atlantic Monthly* had come back with a polite but firm rejection.

Now, with the war over except for the formalities, he was ready to plunge into the job of reorienting the Institute to normal life. In the weeks and months ahead, he suddenly found that everyone had a new research project, something vitally important that had been shunted onto the back burner at the outbreak of war, and everyone needed money, more space, another assistant. The staff's mood affected Wilder and charged him with an enthusiasm he hadn't felt for years. The temporary addition would have to go—it was too flimsy, and in its place, they would need to add a whole new wing to the Institute. He must start looking for money for that. Endowments for research had fallen way behind requirements, and he would have to go up to Ottawa and see if he could wrest some kind of yearly subsidy from the federal government, a task he wasn't looking forward to. As well there were researchers in other hospitals and laboratories that he'd had his eye on, and he would have to set aside some time to pay them a visit, talk about their work and see if they and their projects might fit in at the Institute.

Although he could be mulish in his resistance to new approaches that he did not trust, he was constantly searching for new people and new ideas that might advance the understanding and treatment of the brain. When he welcomed a researcher in some new field of study to the Institute, Wilder would add the prefix "neuro" to his or her specialty—with the flourish of King Arthur knighting the warriors who gathered at his round table.

According to K. A. C. Elliott, a research chemist and the first so christened, with Wilder Penfield everything was "neuro this and neuro that." Thus Elliott's specialty became Neurochemistry, and when photography was added to the resources at the M.N.I. it was dubbed Neurophotography. There was Neuropsychology, Neurocytology, Neuropathology and Neuroanatomy. In Wilder's view, titles were important: attach the prefix "neuro" to someone's field and the researcher would know that the Institute believed that the work could be bent to the common purpose. Who knew what wonderful thing might result? In Elliott's words, Wilder "had the hope that many people who are not in a [given] field have, the hope that this particular kind of scientist will pull a piece of magic. I mean he wouldn't say it like that, but he always had the hope that I would just discover a breakthrough."

And while Wilder was waiting, there was always something else that needed to be done. He had developed an extremely effective style of administration: "don't delay." His secretary Miss Dawson would present him with the matters she felt deserved the director's attention, and he would go through them methodically, shutting out everything else while he made a decision about the matter at hand and then pushing it out of his mind completely while he moved on to the next thing.

While Wilder was the Institute's head, Bill Cone was its heart. The Institute was Cone's whole life. Late at night he would be there, going down the darkened halls from bed to bed, checking up on his patients, washing and feeding them and doing jobs that, as far as

Wilder was concerned, were for nurses and orderlies. Sometimes it seemed Cone never left the building. He was developing a habit of performing his operations during the night, which placed a considerable strain on the residents, who had often spent the day in the operating room. But they rarely complained, and it was not because they feared a reproach, as they might have from Wilder under the same circumstances. Cone was as demanding, in his own way, but he made his demands quietly and he met complaints about his hours with a cheerful dismissiveness that was disarming: "Oh, come on now. I'm up, the patient has been prepared, let's get to it."

Cone also supervised the work in the pathology lab, and was taking on more and more of the surgery that came in to his and Wilder's joint practice. When he wasn't involved in any of these responsibilities, he was busy thinking up innovations to instruments and equipment to improve the comfort and care of the patients. He had developed a number of obsessions: one of them was to perfect a technique for stitching up incisions so that only a barely visible scar was left.

Cone had been growing more and more independent of Wilder since his return from England and the position of chief neurosurgeon to the No. 1 Neurological Hospital. And if Wilder occasionally sensed that Bill was jealous of the time he was spending with the various research fellows who came and went, he pretended not to notice and it soon seemed to pass.

But thanks to Bill's efforts, Wilder found himself at war's end with time to turn to research problems of his own that had, like everyone else's, been pushed to one side during the war years. In particular, he was keen to get back to the work begun with one of the most promising of the pre-war recruits, Herbert Jasper.

Curiously enough, despite Wilder's high expectations for the laboratory research being done in the new fields, such as neurochemistry, it was from the operating room that the most exciting discoveries were coming. In the years before the war, as they searched for the source of epileptic seizures, Wilder and Jasper had started using a new process for electrically measuring brain waves: electroencephalography, or EEG for short. They had little idea when they began that their postwar collaboration would, in a few short years, make the names Penfield and Jasper on a paper or a book the cause of a sudden, special interest among workers in the field of brain research. Nor did they suspect that it would bring reporters flocking to Montreal and make headlines around the world. With Cone busy with his own interests, Herbert Jasper would become Wilder's most important scientific collaborator.

Wilder and Herbert Jasper had met in the autumn of 1937 at Brown University in Rhode Island, where Wilder had gone to give a talk. The next morning he was told that a young man wanted to speak to him. He was led to a lab in the basement of one of the buildings, and into a room that was a maze of chicken wire, which was serving, he was told, as an electrical shield for some experiments. "Inside the maze," Wilder would recall fondly, "was a young man moving about like a bird in an aviary." Jasper invited him in and began to explain what he was doing.

A few years earlier in Paris, when Jasper was doing a doctoral thesis on the electrical activity of the nervous system of crustacea, he saw the first primitive EEG machine being used to measure the electrical output of the brain by means of electrodes attached to the skull. Hans Berger, a German psychiatrist, had pioneered the EEG in the 1920s in the face of much skepticism, which only abated in 1934 when two Cambridge scientists, one a Nobel Prize winner, had confirmed his results. Jasper was himself skeptical at first, but in his lab at Brown he had constructed an EEG machine of his own and begun doing tests. Two groups of volunteers were tested: normal people and epileptic patients. As he explained to Wilder, he could localize the focus of an epileptic seizure by the disturbance in the brain rhythms picked up by electrodes attached to the surface of the skull. By connecting the electrodes to especially constructed amplifiers and ink-writing oscillographs that moved up and down on a sheet of moving graph paper, he could show clearly the intensity and rhythm of the electrical output from each point of the brain. An abnormal portion of brain tissue, he explained, produced a different pattern from healthy brain tissue, a longer, spiky pattern. In the epileptic patients, he had discovered an area of the brain producing these unusual patterns, and he was convinced that this area was the source or "focus" of the epileptic fit.

At first Wilder simply didn't believe it. But Jasper was persuasive. He had two patients suffering from epilepsy in whom he believed he had located the source of the trouble, and he wanted to send them to Penfield in Montreal for operation. Wilder agreed, and their first meeting ended.

Two months later, while Jasper watched from the observation room, Wilder operated on the patients and discovered that Jasper's technique had in fact pinpointed the epileptic focus. Impressed, Wilder asked Jasper to do EEG readings on some of his epileptic patients. Jasper agreed, and proposed to commute back and forth from Rhode Island to Montreal with his EEG machine on the back seat of his car.

So, through the winter of 1938, Jasper would leave Rhode Island early Monday morning with his machine, arrive late at night and go to sleep in one of the residents' rooms at the Institute. The next morning, Wilder would operate on a patient with focal epilepsy and Jasper would take EEG readings. After the operation and often late into the night, they would go over the results. The same schedule would be repeated on Wednesday and occasionally on Thursday, and by Friday Jasper was back in Providence—trying to cram a full week's work into the weekend.

By May Wilder was not only convinced but excited. He decided he would have to find a way to bring Jasper to Montreal. They had calculated it would cost $66,000 to launch Jasper on a preliminary four-year EEG study of epilepsy and other diseases of the brain. After a desperate search for the funds, Wilder produced $16,000 from his own budget, then went to the Rockefeller Foundation again. Gregg agreed to recommend a grant of $25,000 toward building an addition to the M.N.I. to house the EEG set-up if Penfield could raise a matching grant from Montreal.

Wilder called J. W. McConnell, the publisher of the *Star*, who had already contributed generously to the building of the M.N.I. When Wilder explained that McConnell's money would be bringing a matching sum from the Rockefeller Foundation as well as bringing this new fellow whose work Penfield was so keen about, McConnell said "Why, of course! He must come. Go ahead." By the end of the summer of 1938, Herbert Jasper was on the staff of the Institute.

At the beginning Wilder saw the EEG primarily as a tool for locating the disturbance in the brain that was causing a patient's epileptic fits. Up until now, a surgeon had had to employ a number of not always satisfactory methods in the search. He would begin by going through the patient's account of the sensations that preceded a fit, looking for some clue. If it was a sound he heard, or a smell, or a tremor in the left hand, the fit might originate in the part of the cortex where that function was located. But not always: an epileptic brain is a brain periodically suffering from massive electrical disturbances, and a fit could begin in one spot and move quickly to a series of others. Still, it was a clue.

The surgeon could also take an X-ray of the brain, looking for the shadow of a scar or a tumour or a malformation, or, alternatively, use Dandy's ventriculogram for the same purpose. None of these methods was absolutely reliable; nor was the probing or simple observation of the exposed brain. The result for brain surgeons like Wilder was that unless they could either see the lesion in the spot indicated by the various pre-operative techniques or could induce either the preliminary aura or the fit itself with the electric probe, they could not justify excising a portion of the brain, however strong the suspicion that a particular area was the source of the disturbance. In one operation out of five during the first ten years of operating on focal epileptics in Montreal (1928-1937), the surgeons were obliged to simply close up the skull again and send the patient home, hoping for partial relief through the use of anti-convulsant drugs.

Between 1938, the year Jasper arrived, and 1947 that percentage of operations dropped from twenty per cent to five per cent, and by 1956 "negative explorations," as they were called, disappeared at the Institute, largely due to the EEG.

But as Wilder and Herbert Jasper had quickly discovered, the EEG could be put to other uses. During an operation they could continue reading the output of the brain, even as Wilder moved across its surface with his probe. In short order they were able to confirm what Wilder had suspected all along: that the "epileptic hurricane" spread out from the focus along established pathways; that in a sense the effect of the repeated discharges of the epileptic fits was to sensitize a particular pathway or series of pathways which the next fit would likely follow.

Now when he found the focus, a scar perhaps, Wilder could remove a bit of brain tissue, then check with Herbert to see what changes in the wave pattern the removal had made. If the abnormal discharge continued, he would remove another piece of tissue, then another until the EEG showed a normal reading. It was like looking through field glasses at the fuzzy outline of an airplane moving across the sky, and then having someone reach over and adjust the focus. Bingo! you were looking at a DC-3, reading the serial numbers on its wings. It meant that the surgeon could tell whether the apparently healthy tissue surrounding the epileptic focus was in fact damaged, and could avoid having to operate again later as a result of not removing enough epileptogenic tissue. However, as wonderful as the EEG was turning out to be as a surgical tool, its extraordinary potential had not even begun to be tapped. Penfield and Jasper discovered before long that if it were used in conjunction with the electric probe, the mapping of the brain took a great leap forward. Over the next few years, they confirmed many areas of function already recognized, and identified new ones. Most important of all these new pieces to the puzzle was a baffling series of responses coming from the temporal lobe, still unknown territory in those days. If you reach up and touch your temples, you are touching the skull directly outside the temporal lobes, the two extruding lobes of tissue that are the most distinctive anatomic feature of the brain.

It was here in the temporal lobe that Wilder came across peculiar instances of recalled memory. The first instance occurred in 1930. Wilder was probing the exposed brain of a middle-aged woman who was suffering from epileptic fits. When he touched the temporal lobe, she suddenly spoke: "I seem to see myself as I was when I was having my baby." Though surprised at her reaction, Wilder simply made a note of it and continued his probing elsewhere, thinking it could have resulted from the trauma of surgery, or the drugs, or any one of a number of other causes. But over the years the experience was repeated in a number of patients, and always when he was applying the probe to the temporal lobe.

In one case, Wilder was operating on a fourteen-year-old girl who suffered from epileptic seizures in which she became suddenly frightened and screamed and grabbed anyone who happened to be nearby for protection. When she was admitted to the M.N.I., Wilder questioned her carefully. He learned that the fright that distinguished her seizures was the recollection of something that had happened to her when she was seven. On a lovely day she was walking through a field of high grass, her brothers ahead, when a man came up from behind and said, "How would you like to get into this bag with the snakes?" Very frightened, she screamed to her brothers and they all ran home, where she told her mother about the experience. The terrifying event reappeared in her nightmares, and eventually became a part of her epileptic attacks. During the attacks, however, the girl remained conscious of her actual environment and could identify the people around her: she seemed to be thinking with two minds, one in real time and one reliving this memory from the past of walking through the meadow with her brothers.

During the operation, Wilder stimulated the girl's temporal lobe, and she suddenly cried out: "I saw someone coming toward me, as though he were going to hit me." A moment later she called: "Don't leave me." Wilder moved the probe along a bit further, and the girl cried out that she heard people shouting. "They are yelling at me for doing something wrong; everybody is yelling." Asked who was yelling, she said it was her mother and brothers. He stimulated another point and she said "I imagine I hear a lot of people shouting at me." Wilder repeated the stimulation three times without warning, and again the child heard people shouting. Touching yet another point caused her to cry out, "Oh, there it goes; everybody is yelling!"

Wilder decided to excise an abnormal part of the temporal cortex which had developed in infancy during the administration of an anaesthetic. He pinpointed with his probe the area causing the abnormal electrical discharges and removed it. When the girl recovered from the operation she was free of her seizures and of the intense hallucinations, although she could remember the man in the meadow and the fear associated with him.

In subsequent cases involving the temporal cortex, the probing produced a variety of hallucinations and perceptual illusions. When Wilder was stimulating the right temporal lobe of a young South African, the patient said, "Yes, Doctor! Yes, Doctor! Now I hear people laughing—my friends—in South Africa." A young French Canadian woman heard an orchestra playing a song, and if Wilder held the probe to the same spot she could hum along as the song progressed from verse to chorus. When he removed the probe, the song stopped abruptly. Each time he touched the spot the music was so clear and vivid she was quite sure someone had turned on a gramophone in the operating room. Not only could she hear the music, she felt the same excitement and pleasure as when she had heard the tune played in a concert hall.

In the nineteenth century, the distinguished English neurologist Hughlings Jackson had noted that patients with temporal-lobe epilepsy entered "dream states" during their seizures, and would have a sudden feeling of strangeness, of unexplained familiarity, occasionally re-experiencing a complicated scene from the past. Now, by probing the temporal lobe, Wilder was actually bringing on these vivid "dream state" experiences. With each incident his excitement grew. The probe's ability to evoke complicated and detailed scenes from the past made him wonder if he hadn't somehow stumbled on the brain's storehouse of memory.

As more and more patients with temporal-lobe epilepsy came to his operating room, more data about these strange experiences accumulated. Time during the stimulations was real time—witness the patient who could hum along with the music in the tempo in which she'd heard it played. The memories always moved forward, never backwards. They could be stopped by removing the probe, and often replayed at the same spot. The memories were evoked one at a time, all the others held back by some inhibitory mechanism.

When Penfield and Jasper considered their results, it appeared that the brain held an untold number of film clips, each with sound and picture, of vivid events from the patient's past. The replaying would evoke, as well, the emotions that accompanied the original experiences.

Exciting as this data was, there were problems with calling these experiences 'memories': they were too vivid to be like ordinary memories. They were also too fragmented, and the process of recollection too selective. Nevertheless a function that related to one specific area of the brain had been identified—nowhere else could the probe elicit these bizarre experiences—and in the late 1930s, when Wilder first reported his findings, that was startling news. The whole study of the human brain at that time was going through a period of transition from a general view of the brain as an organ whose various functions depended on the *amount* of cortex it contained, not on any anatomic specialization within one or another area of the brain, to an appreciation of the extent to which the human brain had specialized functions in different areas.

When conditioning rats, it was a matter of *how much* cortex there was, not *where* a function was located, that governed their ability to learn new things. The simplistic thinking that had resulted from work with rats—"big brain good, small brain bad," or rather "big brain smart, small brain dumb"—began to break down with Pavlov's work on dogs and later work with monkeys and chimpanzees, in which scientists discovered that areas of the brain became more specialized as the test animals climbed the mammalian scale.

Still, in the 1930s many scientists clung to the notion that the level of intelligence in an animal related directly to the amount of cortex present. And with this reverence for the cortex went another assumption. It was the prevailing notion at the time that this "new brain" ('new' in evolutionary terms)—this outsized development of cortical tissue, which included the frontal lobes—was what distinguished humans from lower species on the evolutionary ladder. Here, they assumed, were the "higher functions" that separated humans from beasts.

Then Wilder Penfield entered the discussion. As a brain surgeon operating on patients with focal epilepsy, he was in the unique position of being able to work directly with the *human* brain, whereas most other scientists had to draw their conclusions from laboratory animals. Those who questioned his results often did so with more than a touch of jealousy: as Sherrington remarked wistfully to Wilder "it must be wonderful to have your scientific 'preparations' actually speak to you."

But Wilder, as much as everyone else, was puzzled by the information being gleaned during these operations using the electric probe to stimulate the cortex. If the cortex was the highest level of brain function, then the probe should elicit the refined actions and sensations attributed to those highest levels. Instead, as he reported in a paper in 1936, stimulating the cortex with the electric probe could "produce no more evidence of a directed, purposeful, skilful movement than is to be found in the mockery of action produced by an epileptic cortical discharge."

As he moved across the surface of the brain using the probe, muscles would twitch depending on which part of the brain he touched: a foot would jerk, a hand would wave, the patient would make a strange groaning sound. In an analogy that Wilder used some years later: "action that is produced by electrical stimulation of the cortex is so gross, so lacking in dexterity, that it may be likened to the sound of piano when the keyboard is struck with the palm of the hand." Just as the 'memories' he could evoke from the cortex were disjointed, hallucinatory and difficult to analyze, so the motor and sensory responses he could elicit there were primitive and unimpressive.

Then how and from where in the brain did the concert pianist transform that crude action into the subtle, dextrous movements of a Mozart piano concerto? Or a ballerina transform the crude cortical reflex into the graceful *pointes* and *pirouettes* of the *Nutcracker Suite*? Somewhere in the brain, Wilder concluded, was "a discrete area... whose integrity is essential to the existence of conscious activity." Somewhere there was a transformer, or a "switchboard," and that somewhere would be found deep down in the "old brain," not in the cortex.

The idea that there was a process of integration of perception, memory, and behaviour taking place continually in the brain was not a new one. Hughlings Jackson in the nineteenth century had proposed the existence of such a "highest level of integration," and others had followed. However, no one had yet dared to go out on a limb and suggest that there was a specific mechanism or point to a possible location—and if they had they would probably have pointed to the cortex rather than to the brain stem.

His operations on patients who were fully conscious had given Wilder an opportunity not only to study the effects of electrical stimulation on conscious mental processes, but a chance to observe what happened when he removed large portions of the cerebral cortex. Even very large removals—in some cases including all of the cerebral cortex of one hemisphere—he discovered, did not cause the patient to lose consciousness.

Few among the scientists interested in how the brain integrates the various elements that go to make up conscious acts had the opportunity to be confronted by such forceful evidence of the cortex's limitations. On the other hand, it was common knowledge that relatively minor damage to the brain stem often resulted in sudden and prolonged periods of unconsciousness, or coma. There was also fairly recent evidence that the brain stem contained a system of neuronal pathways—separate from classical sensory and motor pathways—which were capable of controlling the electrical activity of both hemispheres. And since both hemispheres obviously were involved in conscious mental activity, the brain stem seemed to Wilder the obvious locale for the integration of higher functions.

There was a final piece of evidence that, more than anything else, convinced Wilder that there actually was an integrating mechanism, and that the cortex was the wrong place to look: the evidence was the strange "doubling of awareness" that occurred during his stimulation of the surface of the brain. Somehow the patients always knew they had not willed a leg to rise, or a sound to come from their throat, and when, in probing the temporal lobe Wilder caused them to re-experience moments from the past, the distance between the patient's response and the patient's awareness was even more striking. From somewhere else, or so it seemed to him, the patients were observing their brain being manipulated, while they or some aspect of themselves, remained apart—interested, but somehow remote.

This phenomenon fascinated Wilder. If there *was* a specific part of the brain that could be described as the seat of consciousness, think of what scientists might learn by actually exploring its workings. If they could identify the part of the brain responsible for "reasoning" and "thinking" then they might begin to discover why an individual thought or believed one thing instead of another. Might they not, some day, be able to describe in scientific terms what went on in the brain while, say, a composer was creating a piece of music or an inventor was formulating some new invention? The psychological, philosophical, and religious implications were stunning.

However, Wilder was not blind to the fact that this was treacherous territory for a scientist to venture into. As long as he stuck to simply describing the patients' responses to the probe and the results produced by the EEG, he was within the bounds of respectable scientific exploration. If his data presented a challenge to prevailing notions of brain function, the greatest risk was that he would be proven wrong. But the mere mention of the word 'mind' was enough to cause most scientists to raise disapproving eyebrows. That sort of thing was for psychologists and their ilk, and they, as everyone knew, were fuzzy-headed to begin with; certainly not *real* scientists, not in those days.

Wilder's retort, kept in check at first, was that any scientist worthy of the name followed scientific investigations wherever they led, even into this no man's land of mind and thoughts, and reported the findings and conclusions without fear or favour. That, in Wilder's view, was what being a scientific explorer was all about: venturing into unexplored country and returning with maps and charts so that others could follow. It was to explore this new country that he had gone into the study of the brain long ago, in Sherrington's lab at Oxford. And if he was not supposed to enter here, why had he been presented with the exciting discoveries that appeared to be the key to the door between the brain and the mind, between science and philosophy?

The answer was simply that philosophy was not regarded as a scientist's province. Science could only remain aloof from the muddle of human affairs and faiths by sticking to cold, hard clinical facts. For a time, with a mixture of reluctance and relief, Wilder satisfied his urge to push on from the data by prefacing his papers with challenges such as this one in 1938, speaking as much to himself as to his audience:

"A neurosurgeon has a unique opportunity for psychologic study when he exposes the brain of a conscious patient; no doubt it is his duty to give account of such observations on the brain to those more familiar with the mind. He may find it difficult to speak the language of psychology, but it is hoped that material of value to psychologists may be presented, the application being left to them. It seems quite proper that neurologists should push their investigations into the neurologic mechanism associated with consciousness and should inquire closely into the localization of that mechanism without apology and without undertaking responsibility for the theory of consciousness.

"To make such an inquiry is to ask a very old question, as is shown by the following quotation from...the Book of Job:

> Surely there is a vein for the silver
> And a place for the gold where they fine it.
> ....
> But where shall the wisdom be found?
> And where is the place of understanding?

For the moment, the first rumblings of interest and skepticism were interrupted by the war, and to a large extent, so were further investigations by Penfield and Jasper. But that paper was reprinted widely, and in 1946, Wilder was invited to elaborate his theories in the prestigious Ferrier Lecture to the Royal Society in London. It was a golden opportunity to present his views before an audience composed of the most distinguished scientists in the English-speaking world, and he accepted with delight.

With the war over and the house empty, there was no longer any reason for Helen to stay behind when Wilder travelled, and many good reasons for her to come: no more of the loneliness which caused his thoughts to roam at "levels where they don't belong," he decided. They would go via New York to see Wilder Jr. and meet his bride-to-be, and would include a trip to Germany in their itinerary to see Ruthmary and her husband, and of course Catherine, their first grandchild.

Accordingly, with the Institute running on an even keel, they set off for New York, where they met and approved Wilder Jr.'s choice, then boarded ship for Southampton.

The S.S. *Queen Mary*, on which they made the six-day crossing, was much the worse for her three years' war service, during which she carried more than one and a half million troops, usually unconvoyed after the first few miles from port because of her great speed. The cabins were badly scarred and damaged, doors had been removed and replaced with rough boards, and on deck the railings bore the initials and names of many a soldier and his sweetheart.

Still, the Penfields found a comfortable cabin waiting for them, and there, while Wilder worked on his speech, Helen began a travel diary, which continued for more than a month before it ended as abruptly as it began. Hers is not a very revealing account of the trip, but in several places the impersonal chronology of events blossoms into a characteristically wry observation about one of their fellow passengers. Mrs. So-and-so "told us she is fond of doing things with her hands...and says vaguely that she has so many interests that if she lived to be 180 years she would never be without something thrilling to do." But although Wilder, in his usual way, got into several heated arguments about the war, in public Helen was content to remain her husband's "echo—which I often find is the most comfortable attitude to take, since it avoids difficulty."

A week after leaving New York they arrived at the cottage in Farnham where Gordon Holmes, the eminent neurologist who had been Wilder's teacher in 1920, and his wife were living. With them came fourteen pieces of luggage, five of which were full of food and luxuries—like tennis shoes, chocolate and soap—in short supply in Europe, as presents for their friends and for Ruthmary. Gordon, now seventy, though still "very hale and hearty," was semi-retired, and he and his wife Rosalie were living happily in a pretty country house surrounded by three acres of gardens and orchards, which Gordon took great delight in tending. After several days, the Holmes' idyllic life moved Helen to note wistfully, "I wish we could retire in exactly the same way. But Wide would never tie himself to a garden."

During much of the time he and Helen spent with the Holmes,

Wilder and his former teacher closeted themselves in the study for long conversations about the address Wilder was shortly to give. Wilder argued that the time had come for him to state firmly his conclusion that a central co-ordinating mechanism existed in the brain, and perhaps even to go on and suggest where it might be found. Holmes admitted Wilder's data was exciting but felt he was getting carried away and urged caution: he had given the last Ferrier Lecture himself and knew that it was not the place for radical hypotheses. Reluctantly, Wilder accepted Holmes' advice and set about toning down the conclusions with which he had planned to end the address.

The title he chose was "Some Observations on the Cerebral Cortex of Man," and when the day finally came he began by remarking that "no greater honour could come to a Canadian surgeon than to be asked to give this lecture." It showed, he said, "a recognition that observations made in the operating room may have a value which is equal scientifically to those made in the laboratory." He was crowing, and justifiably. "The experimental 'preparation' of the physiologist can neither feel nor speak," he continued. "But the man who lies on the operating table under local anaesthesia while his brain is being explored is usually alert and acutely interested. If the surgeon will but listen, this observer from underneath the sterile coverings can tell us what he is made to feel, to see, to hear and to dream."

As the basis for these observations, Wilder had behind him 190 operations, performed during the last nine years, in which the brain was explored under local anaesthesia. He reported on the strange, fragmentary memories the probe had evoked in "10 cases in which stimulation produced an experience that might be considered similar to Jackson's 'dreamy state.'" And in all these cases the positive stimulation points were found on the temporal lobe.

Then he moved on to his main point, but instead of the bolder assertions he'd planned before talking to Holmes, he referred more moderately to "strong evidence in favour of the existence within the central nervous system of a place where neuronal circuits converge, thus making possible both sensory summation and the initiation of discriminative action." There was nothing to suggest that this place was in the cortex, he reiterated, and so far their exploration seemed to have reached no more than a "middle level" of elaboration in the total function of the brain.

Describing the occasion in his diary, Wilder wrote that when the lights came on after the lecture, he "saw a perfectly still audience [and] interested faces, [Sir Henry] Dale, [A. V.] Hill, Helen," and that he felt "glad to have done the whole thing" to know that he "had gone only as far as the evidence carried [him]." Wilder had played it safe, and seeing the crowd of scientists who gathered around the podium to discuss the speech excitedly and to ask questions warmed his heart.

The remainder of the trip, with the exception of a second lecture delivered at Oxford just prior to returning to Canada, was devoted to pleasure. In London he and Helen had an audience with the Queen (the King was away), and in Paris, on their way to see Ruthmary, they visited the old haunts remembered from their honeymoon in 1917. Characteristically, the nostalgic setting gave rise to mournful ruminations in Wilder's diary: "I've been wondering why I should have been interested in immortality on earth...no ordinary person can have that. But, if not, what is the joy that comes from scientific work well done and summarized and crystallized? Is it no more than a field harvested, with shocks of grain in orderly rows that a farmer turns and views with satisfaction as he trudges home to dinner?"

In Heidelberg Wilder and Helen found Ruthmary "happy and very much in love," and their first granddaughter "beguiling."

In mid-July, having visited their old friends as planned (among them Sir Charles Sherrington, now in a nursing home), they again boarded the *Queen Mary*, this time bound for Halifax with a last load of "service dependants": war brides and babies. The passage provided a chance to reflect on a trip that had been good for them both. The positive response to his Ferrier Lecture and the more recent lecture at Oxford was a feather in his cap. If he had soft-pedalled his views on the location of the "switchboard," his suggestion that such a mechanism existed had been surprisingly well-received, and so had his reports of the temporal lobe stimulations. The reaction convinced him that this was what he should devote himself to in the years ahead. Among the reflections in the diary is one in which he recalled that after his return from Oxford in 1921, he had chosen surgery at the Presbyterian Hospital over more scientific investigation in physiology with Cuthbert Bazett in Baltimore because of his family, his debts, "and perhaps a desire for practical treatment of people. I can't remember. But it was clear that if I had been a lone bachelor I'd have chosen physiology. Now I've come through long preparation and much surgery back to physiology."

Gordon Holmes wasn't around to urge caution when, some months after the Penfields' return, Wilder and Herbert Jasper decided the time had come to publicly state their conclusions. They were invited to write an article for the *Proceedings* of the Association for Research in Nervous and Mental Diseases in the U.S.. Herbert enjoyed issuing a challenge as much as Wilder, and they both believed that the results of their studies were convincing evidence of what they wished to propose. First, in the article called "Highest Level Seizures," they reported more instances of temporal lobe stimulations, and used the word 'memory' for the first time.

The thrust of the article was that the occurrence of hallucinations made up of remembered fragments "argues that the acquired pattern in the temporal lobe actually constitutes the record of such memory;" a record an individual would draw on voluntarily to recall a past experience, and the same record that could be activated by an epileptic fit. The existence of a memory storehouse in the temporal lobe, however, was still very much a matter of conjecture, and less interesting to the authors than their principal hypothesis: they proposed the existence of a "highest level of functional integration" and presented a diagram of how this mechanism might function. There was no firm anatomical basis for it; they had not actually found such a mechanism, but if their hypothesis was right, it would be found "within the diencephalon and mesencephalon" of the upper brain stem. Anticipating the reaction this would provoke, they offered as justification that though "such a diagram may well serve to expose [their] hypothetical thesis to easy criticism,...more advance may result from clear statement of an hypothesis, right or wrong, than from timid confusion of thought and expression."

The motor and the various sensory regions of the cortex were relegated, according to their "hypothetical thesis," to the role of "half-way stations," between "the periphery of the body" and "the older subcortical centres" of the brain where the integrating mechanism would be found. In other words, according to their theory, the cerebral cortex was simply receiving the signals from the eyes, the tongue, the hands, feet etc. and sending them along to the mechanism. It, in turn, sorted out the messages, constructed appropriate responses, and sent those signals back along the same route via the cortex.

If you happened to be driving along a highway and suddenly there was a car coming straight at you, your eye would send a message to the cortex and on down to the mechanism: "Alarm! Danger! Oncoming car!" The mechanism in the twinkling of an eye would sift through the store of past experience, and if you had been in this situation before, there would be a record. If, the last time, you slammed on the brake and swerved off the road and the oncoming car went by without hitting you, the mechanism would send off messages instructing the foot to quickly step on the brake pedal and the hands to turn the steering wheel. If there was no record of a similar crisis, the mechanism would send off a quick message to the "thinking" or "reasoning" part of the brain (which might or might not be in the cortex), requesting a suitable response, which it would then pass along to the foot and the hands controlling the car.

This analogy is, of course full of holes and shaky assumptions, and so, in 1947, was the proposal for the existence of such a mechanism. Although there was intriguing evidence for this radical theory, it was fundamentally an attempt to reason backward—from the evidence that somehow memory, reasoning and action are integrated every moment of our lives—to a model that would account for the evidence.

Though this theory would be attacked again and again, it proved to be a remarkably durable model. For many years, discoveries in other research centres would seem to support their model, and to the end of his life Wilder would be tinkering with it to account for each piece of conflicting data.

The constructing of models is both the pleasure and the danger of science. Without them new scientific data dangles, confusing and often meaningless. In making them, however, the scientist has to navigate cautiously between twin perils: fall victim to the first, and your analogy will be *too* simple, too pat, and tomorrow someone will make a discovery that makes your model look ridiculous; make it too complex, and it does not serve its function of providing a simple framework to explain your data.

There is a third peril, as dangerous as either of these and more insidious. It lurks in the very process of constructing a model, when its neatness and beauty is so mesmerizing that the creator begins, unconsciously at first, to distort the data to fit the model.

Mankind has always reached for metaphors, for analogies plucked from the familiar world, to explain the mysteries that are most perplexing. The metaphors chosen are illuminating. Our early forebears, puzzled by the stars twinkling in the night sky, chose an explanation beautiful in its simplicity and common sense. If you hold up a piece of fabric with holes pricked in it to the light, each little prick lets a small beam of light pass through, and since the visual effect of the stars in the night sky is the same, that, they decided, must be the explanation. This model was the more credible for suggesting an awesome and blinding light beyond the pinpricked fabric draped over the earth from horizon to horizon.

The first attempts to understand and explain non-physical components, the life force or spirit that moved in men, were no less reasonable. Aware of the complexity of the mechanism the spirit inhabits, early philosophers and scientists wondered how the spirit makes the mechanism work. Aristotle placed the spirit in the heart, considering that it pumped blood and life out to the limbs. Galen, in the second century A.D., moved the spirit up some eighteen inches, declaring that the reservoir of the soul's "animal spirits" was in the hollow chambers of the brain, the ventricles, which are filled with a watery fluid. These spirits in their watery solution, Galen declared, were pumped by the brain to all parts of the body. Fifteen hundred years later the first serious challenger to Galen, the anatomist and physician, Thomas Willis, said that the "animal spirits" were lodged in the brain's grey matter and travelled about the body through a network of nerve fibres.

Closer and closer: from mysterious incorporeal elements, the soul's "animal spirits" were identified by the first microscopists as the subtle juice they could see oozing from severed nerve fibres. As the theory of hydraulics developed, it was used for a time to explain the transmission of sensations from the sense organs to the brain. Then, in 1791, Luigi Galvani of Bologna noticed that when his wife hung dead frogs out on a copper wire in preparation for dinner, the legs twitched mysteriously. It was just a small step from there to an understanding that electrical currents run through the body and move the muscles, and with that understanding secure, "animal spirits" and hydraulic pressures went the way of the dodo.

As for the brain, once it was reluctantly recognized as the commanding organ, the metaphors used to describe it either slid into the 'magic black box' category, or reflected the most complicated inventions of the period. For the ancient Greeks and Romans, the system of brain and nerves was compared to the system of reservoirs, aqueducts and sewers, of which they were so proud. As various machines were invented to serve humanity, the most complex ones were chosen to explain the brain—a clock, for instance.

In the last hundred years or so, as the invention of one mechanical device led to another and another in quick succession, scientists studying the brain eyed the more sophisticated of these for their metaphorical possibilities. Sherrington drew a vivid picture of "myriads of twinkling stationary lights and myriads of trains of moving lights" as a metaphor for the firing of electrical impulses in the brain, evoking "an enchanted loom where millions of flashing shuttles weave a dissolving pattern, always a meaningful pattern though never an abiding one; a shifting harmony of subpatterns." For this image of the brain rousing from sleep he could have been attempting to describe the view at dusk high above a great city, as the lights of lamp posts, office towers, moving automobiles and commuter trains were lit against the darkness.

Probing and exploring the "shifting harmony of subpatterns" of the human brain has been one of the greatest challenges of modern science. And so it will remain, no doubt, for many years to come. Wilder believed his role as a scientist required that he not only summarize the startling evidence of brain function that he observed, but that he formulate as well a theory to account for it. In the case of the central integrating mechanism he believed would be found somewhere in the brain, the search for vivid metaphors to illustrate his theory would seduce him into comparing the mechanism to a telephone switchboard, with lines coming out. Later, when the computer was invented, Wilder and other scientists would seize on it as a metaphor for the brain. The analogies he would choose for the record of memory that could be switched on in the temporal lobe included a tape recorder, a library of film clips, and microfilm.

If it seems from all this that scientists continue to reach for what is familiar to them in order to explain the unknown, that is true. It should be equally obvious that attempts to explain the mystery of the brain will both depend on and provoke inventions and discoveries in the rest of the wide world of science and technology. And though that is the way that scientific theories evolve, sometimes the pursuit must seem as frustrating and foolish as a cat chasing its tail, around and around and around.

It would not seem so to Wilder Penfield, or not yet. In 1947, he and Herbert Jasper were making giant steps into new territory, not always with a sure footing, but deeply convinced of the rightness of the search and the correctness of at least the broad outlines of their theories of brain function. But already, in those exciting years of scientific discovery, there was a lingering, quiet doubt whether science would ever lead them to any final understanding of the brain and of man. For now, he was content to confine his doubt to the musings in his diary.

In 1948, riding back on the train from a hugely successful series of lectures in California while Helen slept beside him, he made the first such entry.

"The complexity of the mechanism seems to paralyze one's thought. We are like the ancient 'wise men' who looked at the heavens. Perhaps a century from now the physiologists will be as much closer to an understanding of the millions of neurons as the mathematical astronomer today is in comparison with the astronomer of old.

"For many centuries we shall probably come closer to the truth by jumping the whole physical complexity and inferring the existence of a soul and of a God—act of faith, perhaps.

"There must be a soul, somehow related to this extraordinary mechanism, and if there is a soul there is a God.... And now to bed."

∞∞ "THE GHOST IN THE MACHINE"

The evolution of Wilder Penfield, Canadian neurosurgeon, into the humanist-scientist-philosopher of world fame, happened because he was saying things people wanted to hear. Even when he was speaking cautiously about the broader implications of research on the brain, he did so in a way that made the audience feel that they shared something with him, despite his impressive scientific stature.

What he shared with them was an acknowledgment that he as well as they knew that there was more to humanity than hard scientific data would ever explain. Other scientists might insist on a purely materialistic explanation; he believed that Man contained a mystery that would never be explained.

This belief came from his faith in God, the God of his mother and the Presbyterian Church in Hudson. All his life he had felt guided by some power he could not perceive or really understand, but whose existence he never really doubted. When he struggled to bridge the gap between science and faith, he did so because he would have felt ashamed to deny his faith. If there was a conflict between science and faith—and there often was—that was one of the challenges in his life that he accepted. His uniqueness was not in being a scientist who believed in God—many scientists of his generation did, and many still do. But most take the easy and perhaps the most sensible way out, hanging up their faith when they put on their lab coat.

There were moments when he envied them, and tried to emulate them and simply couldn't. His faith was too strong. But so was his devotion to the rigorous principles of science, and he was an extraordinarily meticulous scientific observer. He could either let these two impulses war in him unchecked or he could try to reconcile them—and that is what he did. He reasoned, "I am a scientist and I believe in the soul, therefore there must be a scientific theory to account for the soul." That was the basis in faith of the centrencephalic system, the "switchboard" in the brain. Here, if anywhere, spirit met flesh and the two were joined. The idea was by no means just wishful thinking: there was what appeared to be impeccable evidence on which to base a theory of a switchboard mechanism. All that Wilder added—and he added it silently—was the missing element, the spirit.

Though his scientific papers were always models of restraint when it came to presenting his findings, when he came to interpretation he ended up using the language of faith, biblical references, references to Shakespeare and Kipling, to poets and philosophers, as though to say "look, we are not alone in this quest, we are like other men."

As news of Penfield's discoveries and theories seeped into public awareness, reporters began to turn up at the M.N.I., introducing another important element to his dilemma. It would be many years before over-exposure to science would make the general public cynical; the decade after the Second World War only confirmed their awe for the wonderful, terrible power of science and scientists. Public awe placed an added burden on scientists who took their duty to society seriously. If scientists were to be cast as the High Priests of the new era, weren't they obliged to seriously consider the hopes and fears of their flock and speak like High Priests?

Uneasiness with that public role and simple modesty were only two of the reasons Wilder was at first very reluctant to let reporters into the Institute. There was also the conviction that in presenting scientific data to their readers, reporters simplify to the point of distortion. And in part, Wilder's reaction was conditioned by the enormous publicity drawn to the M.N.I. when, in the early years of the war, Lord Tweedsmuir had been rushed there for treatment. For a week the building was infested with impertinent reporters camping out in the lobby, pestering anyone who came down the hall, from orderlies to the director himself. For a week the staff was the focus of public attention, making ordinary life and work impossible. Then, just as suddenly, when Tweedsmuir died the lobby emptied and the reporters vanished. Secret pleasure at being the centre of attention gave way to injured dignity at being so unceremoniously dumped.

And so Wilder and his colleagues at the M.N.I. were wary of the reporters who came to their door. To be sure, Montreal was kept well informed of Penfield's projects at the M.N.I.: J. W. McConnell, benefactor and publisher, saw to that. Every day a reporter from his paper, The Montreal *Star* would stop by the head nurse's office to see what was up, and anything that seemed newsworthy was duly reported. Wilder's personal comings and goings were also a regular feature of the *Star* and the Montreal *Gazette*: "Dr. Penfield Sails for

U.K.—Famed Neurosurgeon to Attend Paris Congress"—"World-Famous Neurosurgeon, Dr. W. Penfield, Presented with U.S. Medal of Freedom."

Most of all, though, Wilder and the M.N.I. staff were reluctant because of a lurking awareness of how the public might misconstrue their work: what we might call The Frankenstein Syndrome was every brain surgeon's nightmare. Patients who have been through a brain operation are often dazed and disoriented for days or weeks afterward, no matter how brilliantly successful the surgical procedure. As well, the patients have frightening-looking scars on their shaved heads to mark the surgeons' point of entry. Brain surgeons have good reason to be cautious about letting reporters see the fruits of their handiwork until the patients are reacting normally and their hair has begun to grow back.

The pilgrimage of journalists to the M.N.I. began in earnest with a 1948 item in *Time Magazine* reporting on the new hope for epileptics from the Institute's pioneering operations. The "soft-spoken" surgeon Wilder Penfield proved to be eminently quotable: "It is our task to accept the most desperate sufferers whether they come from farm, mine, factory, city street, the home or from other hospitals. We undertake apparently hopeless cases referred to us by doctors everywhere," the article ended.

The article in *Time* was followed in 1949 by a long feature in the *Saturday Evening Post* with pictures of operations under the headline "Now They're Exploring the Brain." The article went on to say, "During this amazing and painless operation, patients see stars, smell, move, talk—and dream. But it has produced some startling cures, even revealed the mechanism of the brain itself." After that there was no looking back. In the next ten years every major Canadian and American magazine and newspaper could claim to have "covered" Penfield. Feature spreads became commonplace. The level of reporting varied widely, from thorough and well-written articles in *Fortune* and *Maclean's* to a wide-eyed account in *Coronet*, a pulp digest that trumpeted from the magazine racks of supermarket checkout counters across the continent in 1951 "SCIENCE FINDS 'THE HUMAN SOUL.'"

These articles share one interesting feature. In each case the reporter was drawn by the discoveries or the radical treatment, and ended up writing an inordinate amount about Dr. Penfield himself. He was "distinguished," "soft-spoken," "brilliant" and "modest." His researches were "pushing back the frontiers of the human brain." He was "obviously revered" by his staff, who called him "The Chief." The "gentle giant from Spokane," as the jacket of one of his books described him, was becoming the "Most Distinguished Canadian." Taxi drivers need only be asked, "Take me to Dr. Penfield's house" for the reporter to be taken there and treated, en route, to an informed report of Dr. Penfield's many miracles. Border officials, if a reporter were driving across from the U.S., became instantly friendly when they heard that Penfield was to be interviewed.

As much as the publicity flattered Wilder, it made him strangely uneasy. He took the attention extremely seriously, though not in the way one might think. He or Helen would clip out the articles when they appeared and add them to the thickening file in his study, but although the articles gave him a warm surge of pride and pleasure, he was unlikely to dig them out again for a second look. He did not wonder whether or not he deserved the acclaim; he wondered what it *meant*. He took his work seriously and assumed journalists, editors and publishers did too. If they came to him it must be because what he was doing was important. What did they expect from him, and was it something he could, or ought to, provide?

Underlying the stream of theories and conclusions was his deep sense of the responsibility of science and scientists to society. Scientists should break new ground and follow where their data took them despite public criticism or ignorance, but scientists were also fundamentally servants, obliged to somehow see that the directions of their investigations serve society's best interests—or at least what the scientist judged to be society's best interests.

Although Wilder's faith in science as a "higher calling" to which men and women of high calibre were quite naturally drawn, was fundamental, he was not blind to the abuses. The making of an atomic bomb he thought an abuse of the scientist's responsibility, though at the time he was more relieved that the war had been brought to an end than outraged at the method. That came later. He admired Robert Oppenheimer for publicly regretting his role in co-ordinating the Manhattan Project, and was outraged by the persecution that subsequently fell on him for his unpatriotic heresy during the McCarthy witch hunts.

In his own field, the development of "psychosurgery" and the practice of lobotomizing criminals and maniacs appalled him. The American psychiatrist Walter Freeman who, like many psychiatrists in the early days of psychosurgery, felt that the results justified lobotomies in certain cases, recalls Penfield saying to him, "Walter, don't you realize that you're doing a very dangerous thing?" In the words of William Feindel, a long-time colleague, Wilder was also "outraged by the technique of chronic implantation of a massive series of electrodes in deep areas of the human brain in order to provide electrical recordings for some scientific project that had little or no relationship to the treatment of the patient." During the brief period when this practice was in vogue, Feindel recalled, Wilder would stand outside a conference room "with a tense pallid face... literally sickened by the accounts so callously delivered" inside, struggling with the urge to throw open the door and angrily denounce the speaker.

Bold and daring in his removal of damaged or diseased brain tissue, Wilder was fundamentally opposed to altering the functioning of a physically healthy brain, whether it was the brain of a child molester or mass murderer. Surgery of the brain was a means to relieve suffering and sickness, to help people, not to turn them into harmless and happy idiots. It was a cure, not a punishment.

If it was true that public attention to science and adulation of scientists brought the burden of responsibility, the phenomena also offered scientists great opportunities to make public statements. Along with others in the scientific community who were struggling to make philosophical sense of the growing data on the brain, Wilder discovered in these public forums that a strange reversal of roles was underway. Since the end of World War I, many philosophers had fallen under the spell of the behaviourist school of psychology, whose proponents held that since no objective study of man had turned up anything that could be called mind or consciousness or will, it would be better if these terms were dropped altogether from discussions about human activity. Meanwhile, a small but growing number of eminently respectable scientists began voicing their reservations about a strict, materialist approach. "It is not that easy," they said, "to dismiss the concept of mind, and it is getting *more* rather than *less* complicated the further we go."

Both sides met in battle in an illuminating series of programs for the BBC in 1950, later published as a book, under the title *The Physical Basis of Mind*. Among the ten contributors, Wilder Penfield was the only neurosurgeon, and in fact the only non-British contributor. The distinguished company included Sir Charles Sherrington and Edgar Adrian (later Lord Adrian, first Baron of Cambridge), who shared the Nobel Prize with Sherrington in 1932 for discoveries of the function of the neuron. The two physiologists were joined by two distinguished professors of anatomy, a psychiatrist, a neurologist, and three philosophers. In eight separate broadcasts the distinguished assembly discussed the physical basis of mind, occasionally taking shots at each other's views, but mostly just laying out their own. A quick summary is enlightening.

The task of introducing the discussion went appropriately to Sir

Charles Sherrington: now ninety-two, he had spent half a century grappling with the deceptively simple question, is there after all such a thing as mind? In 1906 he had written, "That our being should consist of *two* fundamental elements offers, I suppose, no greater inherent improbability than that it should rest on one only." And again, "We have to regard the relation of mind to brain as still not merely unsolved, but still devoid of a basis for its very beginning." Forty-four years later he saw no evidence to revise his opinion. He made a flattering reference in passing to Penfield's discovery of the "doubling of awareness," but concluded: "Aristotle, two thousand years ago, was asking how the mind is attached to the body. We are asking that question still."

Adrian, Sherrington's pupil and co-worker agreed. The real trouble with trying to understand what goes on in the brain, he said, is "the feeling that there may be an important part of the picture which can never be fitted in, however long we may work at it." The missing part is "the part which deals with the mind." Adrian suggested that the psychologists take over such speculations, since it seemed a fruitless and, he hinted, inappropriate preoccupation for neurophysiologists like himself.

Next in line was W. E. Le Gros Clark, professor of anatomy at Oxford. His workmanlike account of what was known of brain structure avoided altogether the larger issue, and implied that it was enough just trying to figure out how the bloody thing worked on the purely anatomical level, without straying into the ether.

S. Zukerman, an anatomist from Birmingham University, followed Le Gros Clark with a speech on "The Mechanism of Thought: The Mind and the Calculating Machine," proposing that the brain is no more than a sophisticated machine and that mind is better viewed as simply "a verbal cloak for such processes as perceiving, abstracting and reasoning." The mechanical devices from which he could draw metaphors for his thesis were dictaphones, cameras, tape recorders and the calculating machine of his title, and he spoke prophetically of the likelihood that in the future there would be such a thing as a machine capable of playing chess against a human player. Such a machine would prove his thesis, that for "all these things there is certainly a physical basis."

Next came a psychiatrist, E. T. O. Slater from Queen Square, whose conclusion was that, at least for the moment, "the relationship between body and mind is so intimate that they are best regarded as one."

Slater was followed by a neurologist, Russell Brain, from the London Hospital. For Brain, as for Sherrington and Adrian, the jury was still out on the question of the existence of a non-physical mind.

It was now Wilder's turn, but his argument is best saved for last. Before the philosophers entered the arena, the score so far on whether mind could be separated from brain was three wait-and-sees (Sherrington, Adrian and Brain), one probably-not (Slater), one avoid-the-question (Le Gros Clark), and one emphatically-not (Zukerman). The final program, called "Philosophers' Symposium" was added seemingly as an afterthought and compressed the views of three philosophers into one broadcast.

In the brief time allotted to him, Viscount Samuel, author of *Creative Man*, threw in his lot with Sherrington *et al*.: "Some meeting place there must be to account for the brain-mind relations." He regarded the whole argument as a species of monist heresy and warned: "The whole effort—to resolve mind into matter or else matter into mind—is the outcome of what T. H. Green called 'the philosophical craving for unity.'...But a craving is something irrational, and we had better beware of becoming addicts. What ground is there for requiring any such unification, either of the one kind or of the other? An essential duality in nature is the alternative that is left."

Viscount Samuel yielded to a very businesslike A. J. Ayer, Grote Professor of Philosophy of Mind and Logic at University College, London, who dispensed with "the whole muddle" in which the scientists found themselves by saying that if they were not lumbering about under the freight of antiquated and misplaced notions of 'mind' and 'thought' they would quickly see that the physical mechanisms accounted for everything. "Once the facts are fully described, there is no mystery left."

The third, and last, philosopher was scathing in his contempt. Gilbert Ryle, Waynflette Professor of Metaphysical Philosophy at Oxford, had only the year before (in *The Concept of Mind*) invented the phrase "the ghost in the machine" to dispose of so-called "mental events" altogether. The term—"deliberately abusive" he called it—pointed out the absurdity of confusing metaphor with reality, analogous to taking an expression like 'horsepower' literally. To illustrate, Ryle told a parable of peasants examining the steam engine of a train, the first they'd seen, peering into every crevice of it and saying, "Certainly we cannot see, feel, or hear a horse in there, so it must be a ghost-horse which, like the fairies, hides from mortal eyes."

Said Ryle, "Poor simple-minded peasants! Yet just such a story has been the official theory of the mind for the last three very scientific centuries." Like Ayer, his immediate predecessor, he treated the very question of whether there was such a thing as a mind as nonsense invented by insecure and unreasonable humanity seeking comfort in the dark and windy universe. "What prevented the peasants from finding the horse was not that it was a ghost-horse, but *that there was no horse.*" [author's italics.]

It is hardly possible to imagine two more contrary and antithetical views than those of Ryle and Penfield. As far as Wilder was concerned there was a horse all right, and he could point to its probable location amid the gears and pistons of the locomotive.

He began his address, titled "The Cerebral Cortex and the Mind of Man," by saying, "Some of you may raise eyebrows in surprise that a neurosurgeon should presume to consider so abstract a problem as the physical basis of the mind." Pointing to illustrious predecessors "whose addiction to the use of the scalpel did not exclude [them]...from such preoccupations," he proceeded to argue for the existence of the co-ordinating mechanism and its role as the doorway through which the mind entered the brain. In doing so he calmly walked into every trap Ryle, Ayer and the other disbelievers set, airily referring them to their Shakespeare to prove that what he was saying was "the commonest of common knowledge." Shakespeare, as he reminded them, referred to the "brain which some suppose the soul's frail dwelling house." He went on: "It is obvious that there must be a co-ordinating centre within the 'house,' a sort of telephone exchange or switchboard to which messages come, and from which messages depart after appropriate decisions are reached, decisions that are based upon memories of previous experience and influenced by present desires."

Wilder explained that this "master motor area" would be found in the upper brain stem. "Such a headquarters switchboard as that is so delicate, so complicated, as to stagger the imagination, but the evidence is overwhelming that it does exist.... The higher brain stem, together with that portion of the cortex which is being employed at the moment, is the seat of consciousness.

"It is the 'physical basis of the mind,' this hypothetical mechanism of nerve cell connections....

"What is the real relationship of this mechanism to the mind? Can we visualize a spiritual element of different essence capable of controlling this mechanism? When a patient is asked about the movement which he carries out as the result of cortical stimulation, he never is in any doubt about it. He knows he did not will the action. He knows there is a difference between automatic action and voluntary action. He would agree that something else finds its dwelling place between the sensory complex and the motor mechanism, that there is a switchboard operator as well as a switchboard."

No doubt he was regarded as an impossible adversary, this brain surgeon who conducted scientific investigations with conscious patients with one hand and waved poetry at his opponents with the other. But out they went over the airwaves, these conflicting views. Some of what Wilder was saying struck home, especially to people already familiar with his work as a surgeon and scientist, and among his admirers in those years were people in high places.

When the Queen's New Year's List was broadcast at the end of 1952, Wilder Penfield had been awarded the highest civilian honour in the empire, the Order of Merit. Only one other Canadian had ever been so honoured, Prime Minister Mackenzie King, and the O.M. was the only award Winston Churchill would accept from a grateful monarch at the end of the war.

There are only twenty-four holders of the Order of Merit at any one time: the one that was awarded to Wilder had been Sherrington's before he died, just months after the BBC broadcast. It was only fitting that it should go to Wilder. As a scientist he had tried to emulate Sherrington, and like Sir Charles he believed that scientists had a role to play in the world at large. No one could have been better suited to take up and bear into the future Sherrington's unusual scientific credo that the search for an explanation of Man's fundamental nature "will long offer to those who pursue it, the comfort that to journey is better than to arrive."

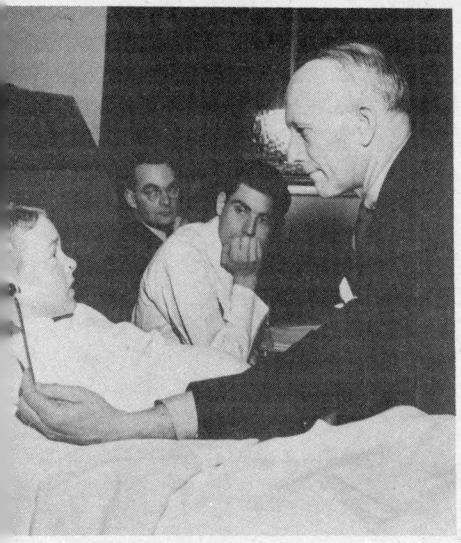
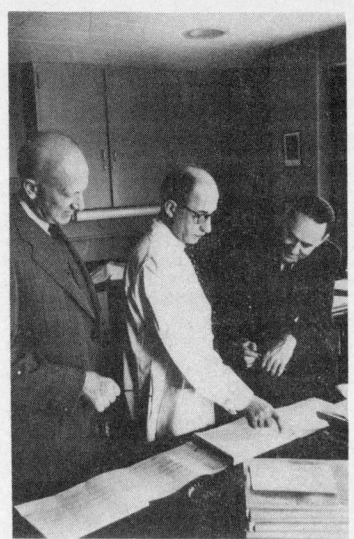
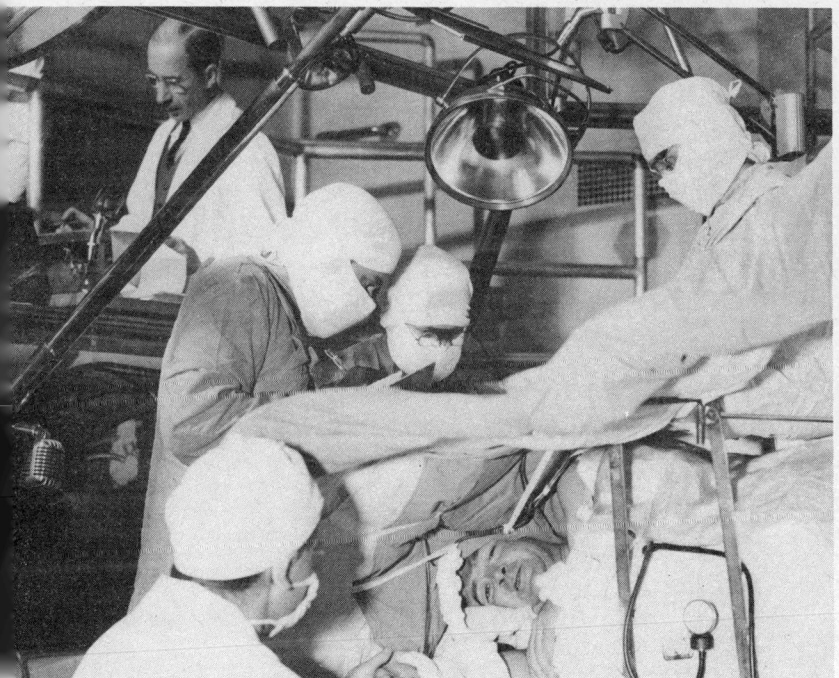

TOP LEFT: Wilder and patient circa 1945.   TOP RIGHT: Wilder (*left*), Herbert Jasper, Theodore Rasmussen.   ABOVE: An operation at the M.N.I. circa 1950. Herbert Jasper is in background.

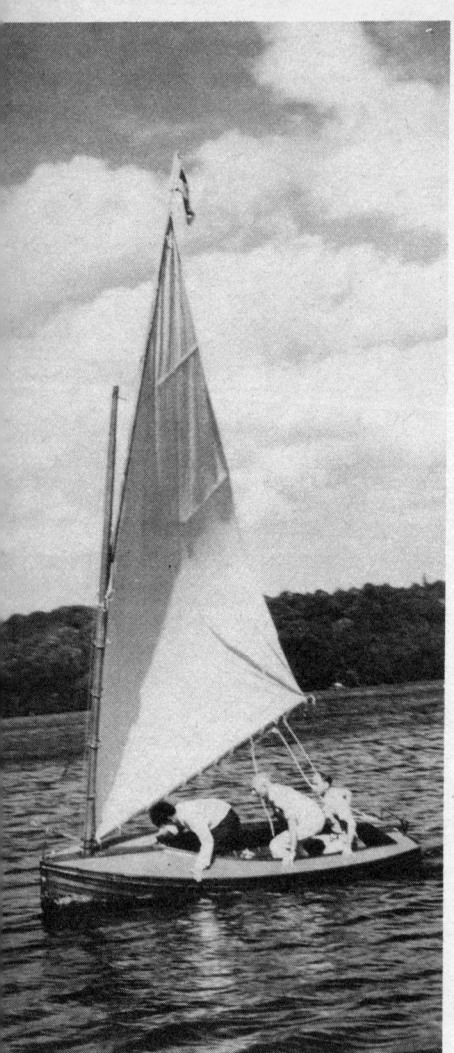
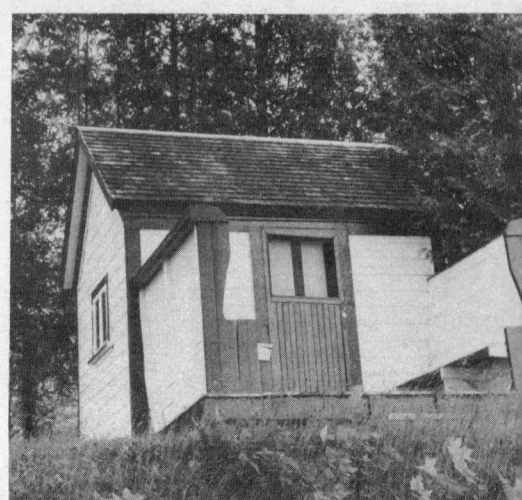
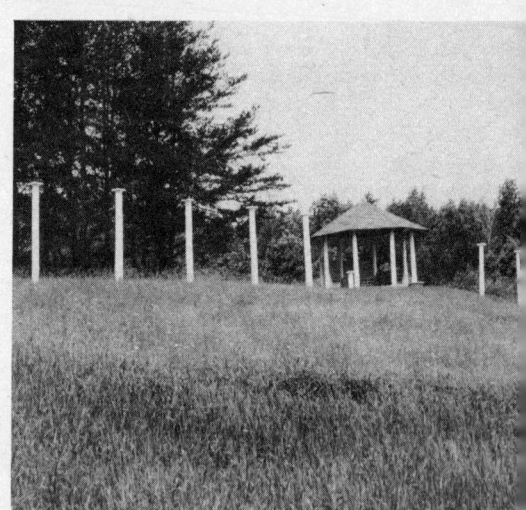

ABOVE LEFT: Wilder, Herbert Jasper and an unknown third sailing on Lake Memphremagog. (Gordon Matheson)   TOP: Wilder's writing house at Magog Meadows. (Sarah Chester)   ABOVE: The tholos and philosopher's walk. (Sarah Chester)   TOP OPPOSITE: Sussex House.   BOTTOM OPPOSITE: Wilder on lawn of Sussex House circa 1953. (Herbert Jasper)

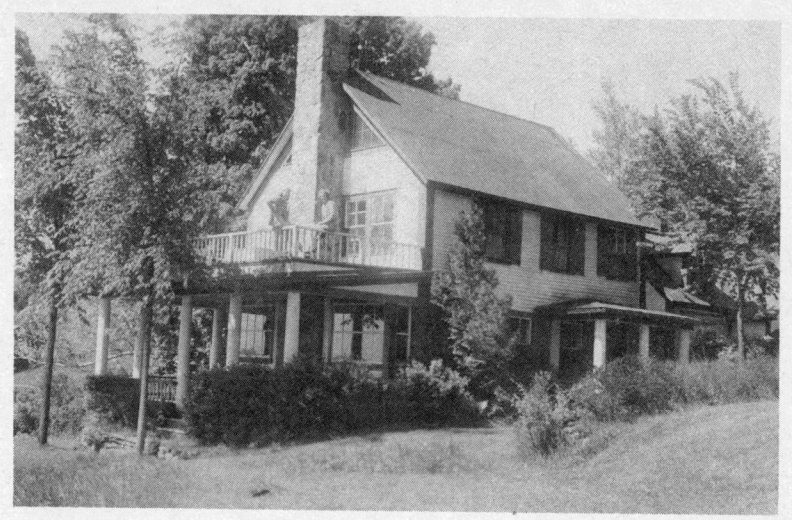

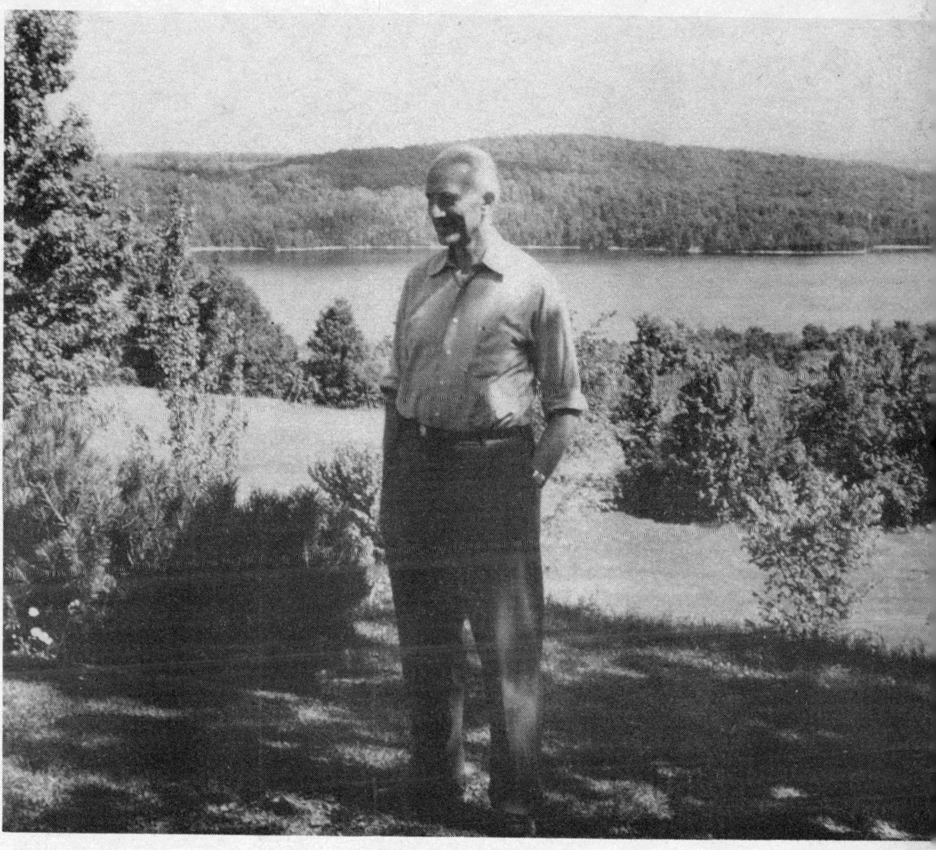

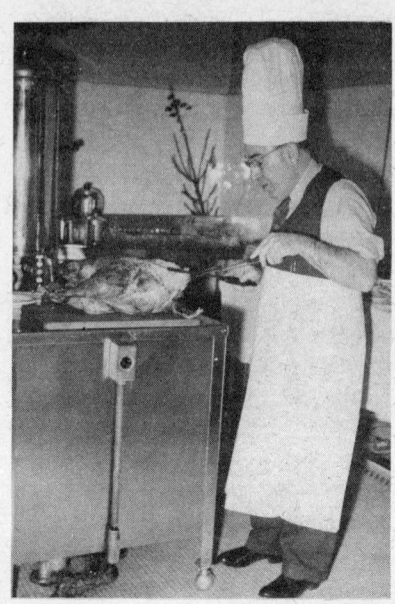

RIGHT: Bill Cone carving the turkey, Christmas 1952. BELOW: Wilder and Helen with their grandchildren about to depart for the Granby Zoo, 1956.

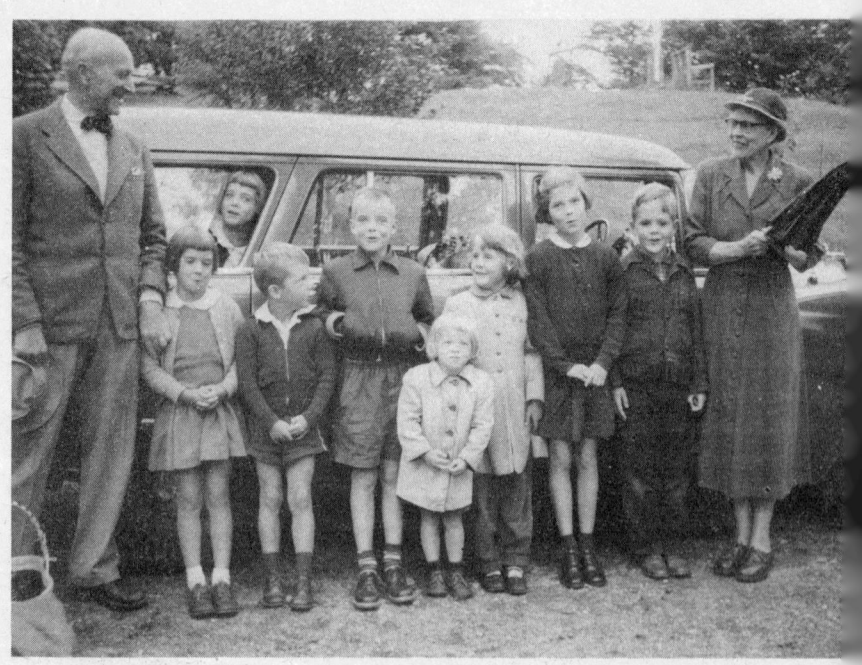

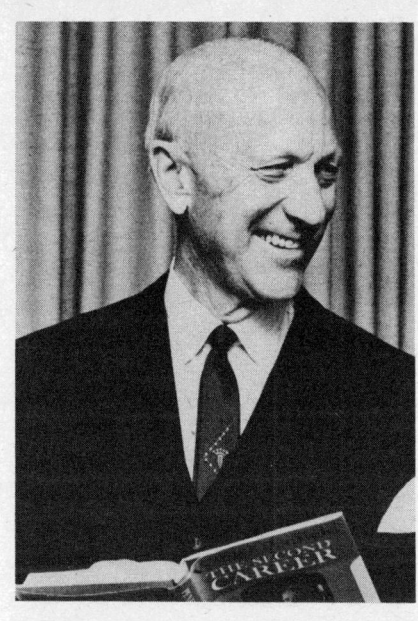

LEFT: Wilder at launching party for *The Second Career*, 1963.
BELOW: Wilder's study in the Gleneagles apartment.

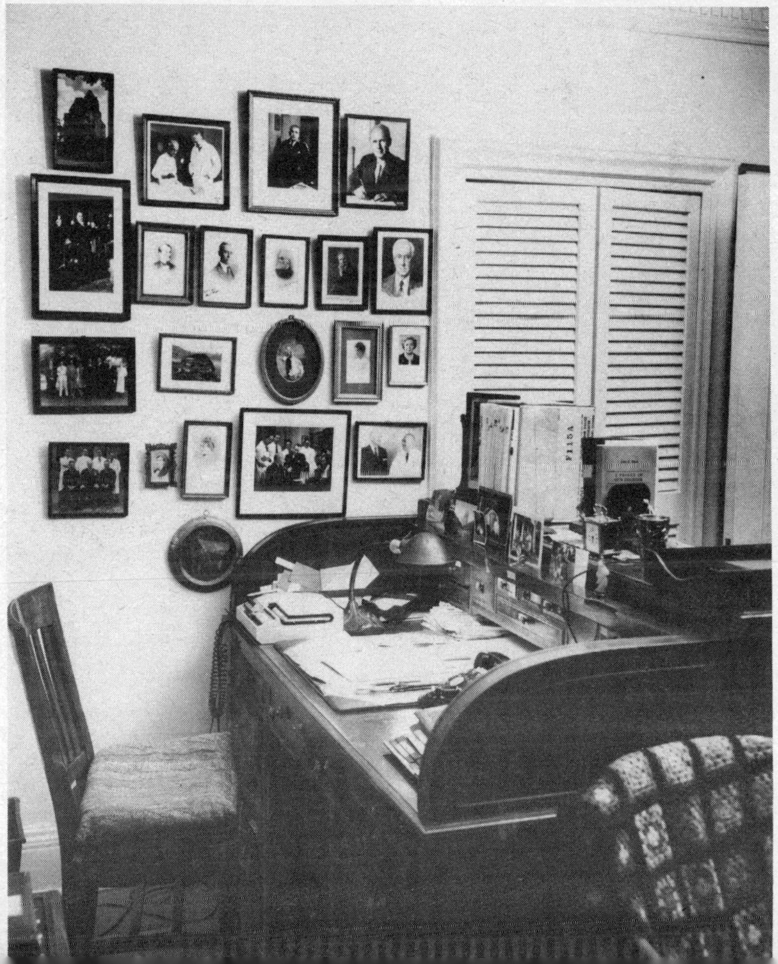

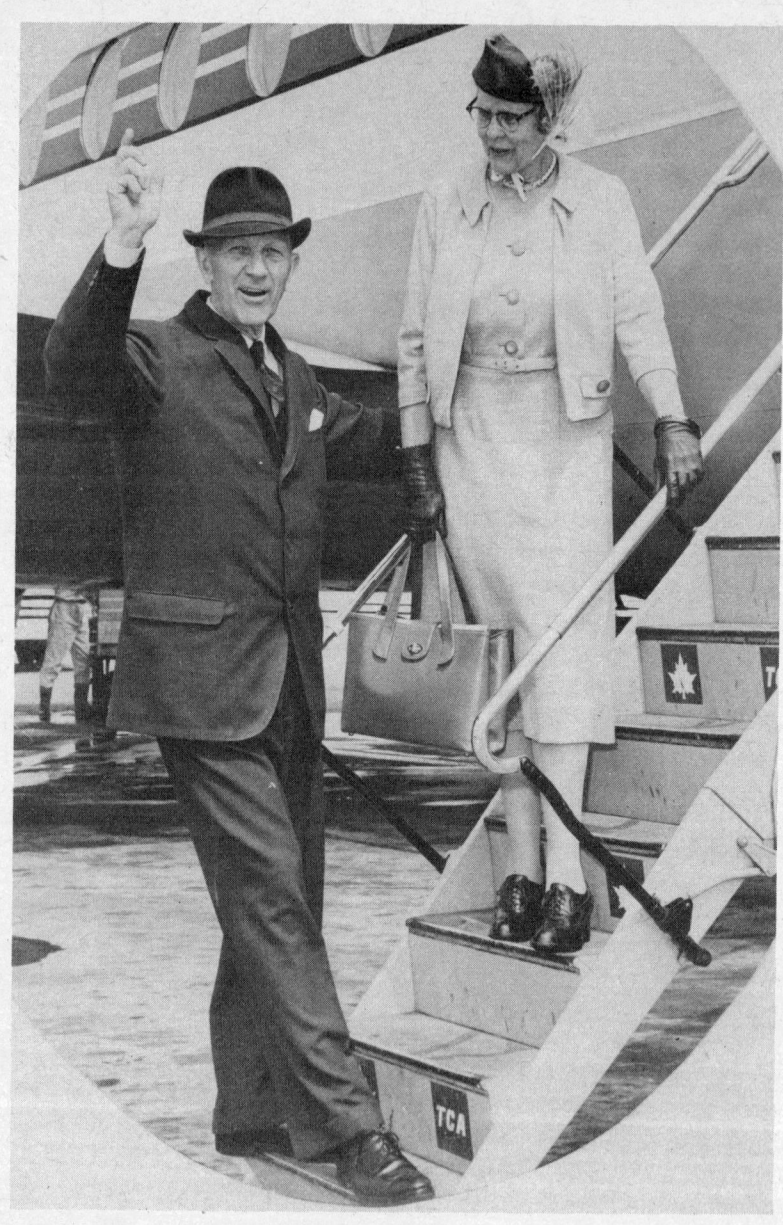
Wilder and Helen off to China in 1962.

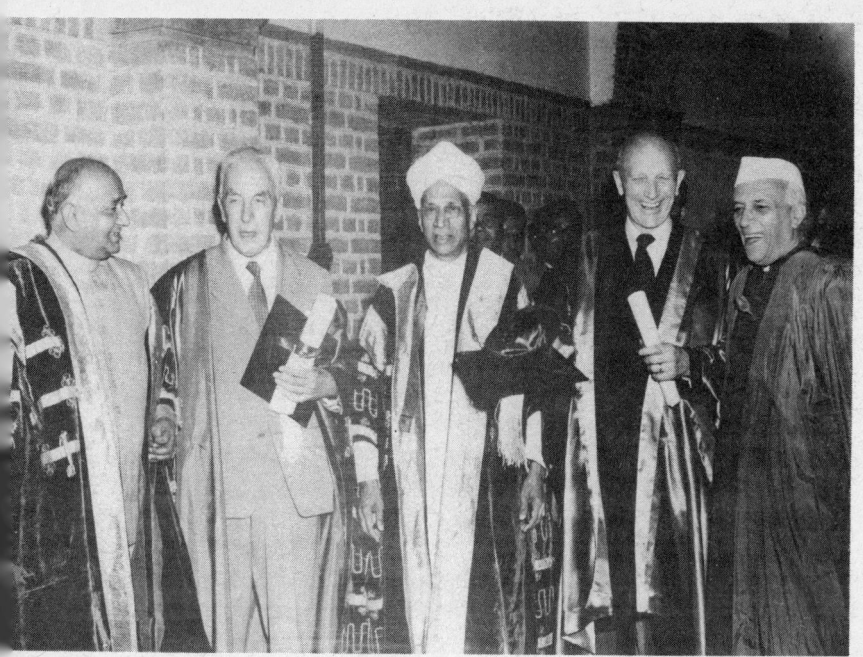

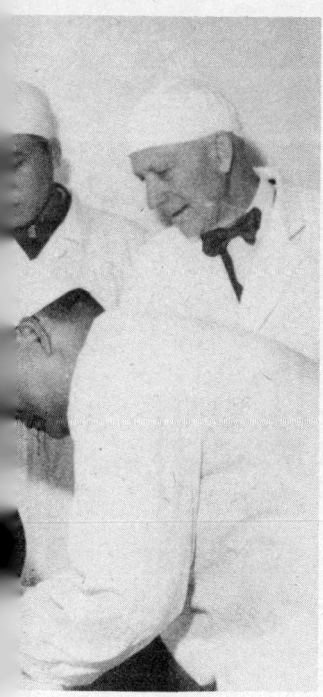

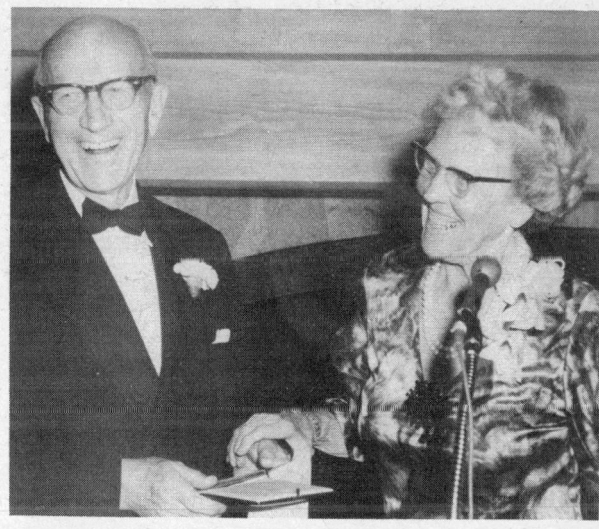

TOP: Degree ceremony at University of Delhi, 1957. Arnold Toynbee is third from left; Wilder and Nehru at far right. LEFT: In China in 1962. ABOVE: With $50,000 Royal Bank Award "for outstanding citizenship," 1967.

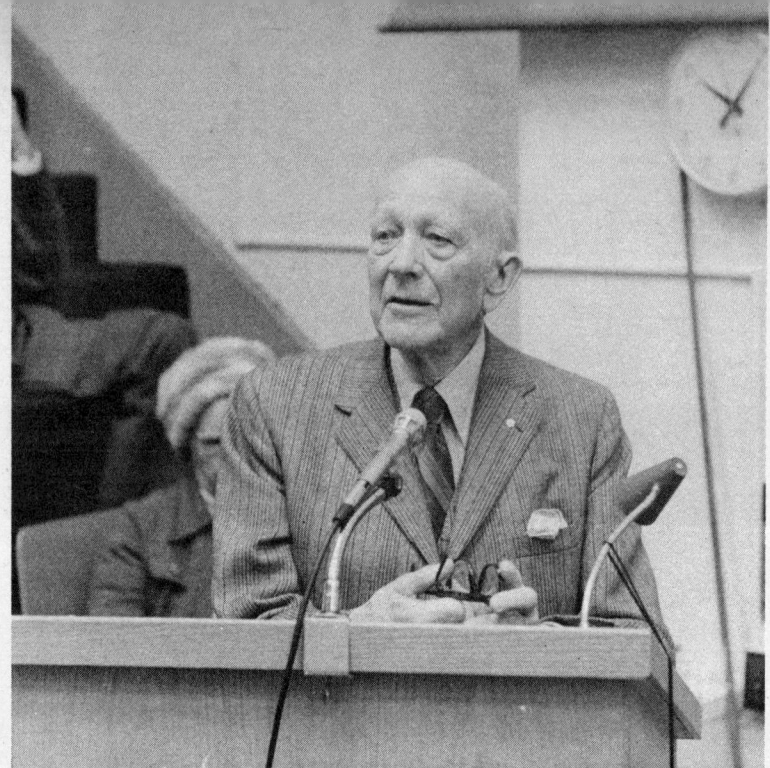

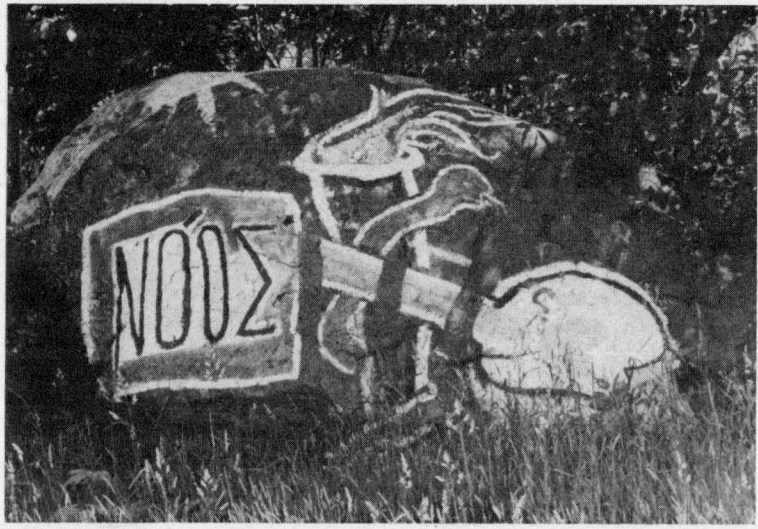

TOP: Wilder speaking at the M.N.I., 1973.   ABOVE: The painted rock at Magog Meadows. The Greek word for "spirit" is connected by a line to the Aesculapian torch, symbol of medicine. The line continues to a drawing of the human skull and inside it the outline of a brain and within this a question mark. On his last weekend there Wilder painted through the solid line in three places, making it an interrrupted line. (Sarah Chester)

PART THREE

*And indeed there will be time
To wonder, "Do I dare?" and, "Do I dare?"
Time to turn back and descend the stair,
With a bald spot in the middle of my hair...*

*Do I dare
Disturb the universe?*

— T. S. ELIOT

CHAPTER NINE

Other Doors Open

∞ A SECRET WRITER

Wilder was to be awarded his Order of Merit at a ceremony at Buckingham Palace on July 7, 1953. By mid-March he and Helen had already booked passage on a ship to arrive the week before, when a most unexpected invitation came in the mail to attend the Coronation of Queen Elizabeth II at the beginning of June. It came while Wilder was delivering lectures in Boston and Toronto, and when he arrived at the house he found Helen and a friend, Margery Mitchell, in a state of great excitement. Margery had come to stay and help Helen, who couldn't dress herself because her right hand was in a cast after a fall on the sidewalk a few weeks before. (The only servant in the house at the moment was a Chinese cook named Charlie, "who has certain male defects," as Wilder put it. Charlie's habit of punctuating his cooking with frequent nips from a bottle of scotch was, by this time, well established, and on more than one occasion Wilder had found himself in the kitchen plying Charlie with black coffee, leaving Helen to distract their hungry dinner guests. But he was a wonderful cook when sober.)

Helen and Margery had decided the Penfields must go to the Coronation, and Wilder gave in. The new plan was to go over at the end of May for that ceremony, following which Wilder would have the rest of the month of June to work on four addresses he had promised to give in July, after their return. The itinerary already included side trips to Oxford and Cardiff for honorary degrees, and it would end with the O.M. investiture, "All of which may call for some kind of preparation," Wilder wrote in his diary, "intellectual for me and sartorial and emotional for Helen!"

For the next four weeks the preparation kept them both busy, Helen packing, closing up the house, and tending to the long lists of household affairs, Wilder taking care of the urgent business at the Institute and compressing a two-month operating schedule into half the time. On a Friday afternoon, a week before they were to leave for England, they set off to the farm for a brief respite.

By this time Magog Meadows, as they had decided to call it, was greatly changed from the ramshackle farmhouse and outbuildings they had bought in 1928: their country neighbours shook their heads and lifted their shoulders in amazement at what "the doctor" and his wife had done with the old Manning place. Gone was the flat roof and the false front which had given the house such a peculiar appearance. The roof had been raised and porches now ran along two sides; the one facing the lake was deep and comfortably furnished with wicker couches and chairs with brightly patterned seats. Above the white clapboard walls and the green shutters, tin roofs painted a deep red now connected the main house by a long, covered walkway to the barn, transformed into a guesthouse at the other end.

Between the house and the barn, in the curve of the walkway, a spring flowed into pools (dubbed Liver and Kidney because of their shapes) through a fountain, and over the rim of a brass cymbal with a merry tinkle, then under a little bridge and down into the bushes at the bottom of the garden. The walkway itself was a delight: cool, mossy flagstones underfoot, vines curling up a lattice wall on the outside, and the garden stretching out below. Halfway along was a swinging loveseat and a small table, at which guests could pause and admire the view of the lake on their way to breakfast.

The transformation inside was no less striking: it was a house made for cool summer evenings and long, hospitable dinners with the family and good friends. No detail escaped Helen's keen eye: on the carved oak refectory table, brought from a monastery in Spain, candles were placed just so among the cut glass bowls, in which blossoms from the garden floated; the silver glowed, wine sparkled in crystal goblets, and Wilder and Helen would smile at each other over the bobbing heads of guests down the length of the table. The food was usually delicious, and Charlie's drinking could be forgiven for the moment.

After dinner, there would be cigars and coffee, their aromas swirling in the breeze from the screen doors opening onto the porches. Here, if you paused to listen, you could hear the delicate music of bells which had been hung about the porches—cow bells from Switzerland and Austria, temple bells from India and Japan, blending with the more distant patter of notes from the fountain's cymbal. Over the lake below the moon would rise, lighting a path across the water, and so bright on August nights you could almost read by it. There would be a fire in the red-tiled fireplace, and the light would flicker over the horse brasses, the buffalo rug, and the ancient, square Steinway in the corner.

It was this place and the life they led out here, as much as the Institute eighty miles away, that had bound the Penfields to Montreal. This was home. Among the flattering offers that had come to Wilder since the war was Osler's old job, Regius Professor of Medicine at Oxford. After brief consideration, he turned it down and when Sir George Pickering—who took it instead—came to visit at Magog Meadows, he walked around in silence, then came back and said, "I understand."

They had spent most of their lives living in big cities, and enjoyed the sophistication and amenities cities offer, but at heart the Penfields were both country people, people from a small town in western Wisconsin. In Montreal Wilder would work long hours at the Institute: administering, operating, supervising the work in the laboratories, seeing patients, teaching. He had never learned to pace himself properly, and he often needed to be dragged out of the thick of it by Helen, out to the peace of the farm.

That had always been true, yet, lately, Wilder had begun to rebel against the forces that drove him, and to wonder from time to time if he wasn't missing something important in life by running so hard. Even as his scientific work had grown more exciting, he had felt the urge to break away from it as well. And suddenly, with the O.M., the stream of invitations to speak to graduating classes, to be given yet another degree, to address scientific congresses and attend benefits for a variety of worthy causes, had accelerated dramatically. "The race I run is really against time," Wilder wrote in his diary, "to finish the analysis of the evidence that has come to me—memory, cortical function, epilepsy, man's thinking about life and religion. But I would not believe my work on these things to be of too great value. I would take time to laugh and play and be a companion [to Helen]."

It was only at the farm, or off on some trip, it seemed, that he could laugh and play. And out here was the intense pleasure of an endless number of small, manageable tasks necessary to maintain the property. There were trees to be planted, rowboats to be bailed, docks to be fixed, and always he or Helen had a new scheme for one more thing to make it better. Reshaping the house and the hillside was a perpetual task, and one he and Helen enjoyed doing together. A handyman named Andrew Marion from a village nearby would carry out the details for which Wilder hadn't time or skill.

It was at Magog Meadows that the Penfields did most of their entertaining, and staged events like the annual picnics for the Institute staff, which never seemed to stop growing. The summer before Wilder and Helen had held a party there for "the young people" at the Institute—eighty-four of them not counting babies, who seemed so numerous and to turn up in such strange places that Helen worried that some might be left behind. Helen, in one of her "round-robin" letters, which circulated still among the members of the Class of '13 at Milwaukee Downer College, described the ebb and flow of visitors and family for a typical July. Aside from the friends invited for most weekends and some sandwiched in between, another dozen guests were unexpected: from New York, a niece and her husband; from Brazil, a nephew and his family; from Milwaukee, Priscilla with husband, baby daughter and Great Dane in tow. (Priscilla had married the son of Bill Chester, Wilder's Princeton roommate.) In the hectic years since the war, the family had more and more often gathered out here in the summers. There were now ten grandchildren, and on weekends when everyone was there, the beach, Helen wrote, "looked like Coney Island."

Even though Herbert Jasper and his wife had bought a place down the lake, and Herbert and Wilder could spend an afternoon going over their work, they were more likely to meet in the fiercely competitive Sunday sailing races on the bay.

One of the first changes Wilder had made to the farm was to drag a little milk house along the brow of the hill to a spot with a view down the lake all the way to Vermont. It had been furnished as a writing house, simply, with a desk, a few shelves, and an iron cot. And though Wilder needed the time out here to write and to reflect on the directions of their research, since there never seemed to be enough time in town, the time spent on writing was instead set aside for another project. It was the novel, now called *No Other Gods*; Wilder had found a publisher eager to bring it out as soon as the final work was done.

The novel had taken nine years of stolen moments and summer holidays to write and the Penfields had to reorganize their lives; it was Wilder's hope and dream for the future; it was the source of greater anguish and frustration, and more pure delight, than anything he had ever tackled. His mother had handed over her original manuscript in 1935, and the few revisions he tried over the next few years "were burlap patches on a fragile silk garment." He gave up and the unfinished novel lay in a bottom drawer until he returned from Ur in 1943, his imagination fired by his trip to the desolate ruins and by Sir Leonard Wooley's book on the excavations there. That summer in the milk house he had begun to write his version of the story of Abraham.

Wilder did not discuss the project with his colleagues, imagining their amusement. The manuscript remained in a battered briefcase when he was in town, emerging only in the country, on weekends and during the summer. But all the while it percolated away in the back of his mind, a teasing counterpoint to the round of operations, the ceaseless effort to keep the M.N.I. on an even keel, the scientific papers and books and speeches. Half the time it struck him as lunacy, but then, "when I am suddenly alone, with empty hands, the romance of Abraham opens to my inward eye as though a curtain had gone up and I stepped on to the stage to direct the actors"—and he would return to it with renewed enthusiasm.

As great a challenge as learning to write fiction were the thorny questions the story presented. What made Abraham decide that one god was better than many? That making graven images of the gods was sinful? After all, Abraham's own father made his living from making and selling idols. And how was God revealed to Abraham?

The novel served a useful function through these years as a place where he could speculate freely about the issues of faith that underlay his life, keeping them out of the scientific papers, where he felt they had no place. He and Abraham had much in common, he decided. Both were seeking for an absolute truth which would put an end to restless speculation. Both were fighting against the tide of popular opinion: Abraham in the pantheistic world of Sumer with his idea of One God, Wilder in the world of twentieth century science with his notion of the central switchboard in the brain.

And yet in some strange unthought way Wilder's assumption of the similarity between Abraham and himself echoes his scientific theory that the mechanisms of consciousness lay in the 'old brain,' in evolutionary terms. Both argued that human nature was fundamentally unchanging—that Truth, whatever it was, was unchanging. Time could shift articles of faith around, could transfer functions from one part of the brain to another—Man could learn new tricks. But some part of him was unimaginably old, deeply rooted in the earth, in faith and in destiny.

And there were other puzzles for him to worry away at in the privacy of his writing shed, some finding their way into the pages of his diary: "For some time I have been thinking about the problem of the Jew. Why he walks alone, is driven out, disliked and yet contributes the work of inspiration to our civilization from time to time." The story of Abraham must somehow answer questions like this, for himself as much as for the readers of his novel. There had been no Jews in Hudson, Wisconsin, and he had grown up with the full complement of prejudices of his age. Since coming to Montreal he had made a few Jewish friends, but no one he could discuss such things with. "It would seem to me that the basis of the hatred which other people bear him [the Jew] lies in the fact that he does not become one of them. He will not stand shoulder to shoulder with them in adversity, will not face extinction with them. By carrying along his Hebrew religion and his conviction of superiority he erects a wall, or perhaps better a protective tent, that hides his thoughts and ambitions. This has preserved his race from being swallowed up.

"If they build again a Jewish state in Palestine, they may contribute again great things to religion and philosophy, but if these contributions are great enough they will reach the teaching of Christ and if they accept it they will come to the end of the philosophy that has led them back to Jerusalem.... They will be Christians."

Reading back through that he must have realized how silly it sounded, because he went on to add, "This is not expressed just as I would have it.... When one tries to apply this generality to individual Jews it breaks down. There are many who work hard and play the game, but they inherit the dislike that comes to their race, and many of them are Jews first and Americans or Canadians afterwards. They resent anti-semitism and we their friends deplore it," and so on.

From 1943 to 1948 Wilder plugged away at the novel when he could, turning to Shakespeare or the Bible for inspiration. The plot that emerged covered Abraham's rebellion from the priesthood of the Moon God in the city of Ur, the smashing of the idols in his father's store, the escape into the marshes, his vision and the final victorious descent into Canaan, where the Book of Genesis takes up the tale. In 1948 it was done, and he had a typed copy of the manuscript to show for his efforts. But alas, his love for the beauty and the thunder of the Old Testament had played him foul, and one reader after another suggested diplomatically that he had perhaps written something that sounded *too* biblical.

They didn't need to tell him: he could see it for himself. The writing was stilted and awkward and, without a doubt, more than a little reminiscent of the Old Testament. But there were passages, descriptions of the landscape of Ur for instance, that needed no apology. He refused to give up. Perhaps a trip back to Ur would inspire him.

So, in the summer of 1949, Wilder took two months off and set out for Mesopotamia, this time with Helen. She had been an honest critic and a stalwart believer throughout the writing, and she was as keen as he for an adventure.

It had to be more than just play, this struggle to learn how to write. And on board ship for London, the first stop on their journey, Wilder asked himself why he was doing it, especially now. "This is the most exciting period in my career from an intellectual point of view, and yet here I am starting on a two-month holiday.... Why all this when the physiology of the brain is calling for mature analysis? I'm not sure. Perhaps it is because the book has been undertaken since I was in Baghdad in 1943, and so lies on the desk of my conscience. Perhaps it is because of my promise to my mother. Perhaps it is to learn a new vehicle for creative work after I give up active surgery. If I can learn to write, I might then undertake biography in my twilight time before night closes in. Whatever the real reason may be it seems to me a new door is swinging open and I must enter it while I can."

And so off they went, he and Helen, into the desert. They rode on camels, crossed from Damascus to Baghdad in a bus in the heat of summer, wandered from shelf to shelf in the dim coolness of the Iraq Museum in Baghdad, making notes, drawing maps, arguing into the evening over details of dress, architecture, animal husbandry, cooking, in this volume or that. They loitered like a pair of dockhands on the waterfront of Basra, listening to conversations and making mental notes of how people walked and talked and crouched and ate. Following Abraham's path, they paddled through the reedy channels of the Great Marsh at the head of the Persian Gulf, and came back once more to Ur to climb the steps of the Ziggurat.

After two months they returned home, and Wilder set to rewriting his manuscript. On the first effort someone had said "Put in more sex," so he did, rewriting scenes between Abraham and the king's daughter Princess Shub, to liven them up:

"Spiral rings of gold trembled in her hair; jewelled necklace and earrings glowed against her smooth brown skin. A clinging cloak was thrown over one shoulder, but left the other lovely shoulder bare and revealed, rather than hid, a rounded breast.... He looked down into her face. Her soft eyes seemed to melt into his, and he realized that it would be so easy, yes, so pleasant to kiss those parted lips."

In early 1952, as he was approaching the end of the revisions, he and Helen decided to take a midwinter holiday (their first) in order to finish the book. They chose a lodge in the middle of the desert in Arizona, reasoning that it would be easier there to write about events that took place four thousand years earlier in another desert across the world. "It isn't," Wilder wrote two weeks after they arrived.

Nonetheless, at eight o'clock on the morning of their last day, Wilder finished the last chapter, ending, as he noted with satisfaction in his diary en route to Chicago, "with a column of smoke rising in the still air over the meadows of Drehem."

By the end of the summer there were no more excuses for postponing the inevitable. On his way through Baltimore to lecture in Washington, he stopped at a post office to mail the manuscript off to Little, Brown & Company in Boston. George Hall, the son of Wilder's fellow Johnson Club member, worked for Little, Brown, and on hearing of the project the summer before had asked him to send the novel along when it was finished. The size of the package and the care Wilder took to register it made the contents clear to a man in line behind him at the post office and as he turned to go, the man smiled and said "Good luck!" The remark turned out to be prophetic. Just three weeks and two days later, as Helen carefully noted on her calender, came a letter from George Hall saying that the book was accepted, and that one of the firm's editors would be in Montreal in November to discuss the publication details with Wilder.

It is easy to imagine the Penfields' excitement. When the editor arrived he said that Little, Brown would accept the manuscript as is, but that he preferred to see the first four chapters dropped, and the love affair run through to the last chapter. In spite of his delight at the prospect of getting the manuscript published, Wilder held his ground on retaining the first four chapters. With that concession won, he agreed readily to the other criticisms, and after the session, the editor took the Penfields to lunch at the Ritz with another Little, Brown author, the novelist Hugh MacLennan. Wilder was impressed by MacLennan and extremely flattered to feel himself somehow classified with him as a writer. In his diary account of the luncheon, Wilder observed that MacLennan "looked at me with surprise and what shall I say, suspicion that I should venture into the field of stories."

Four months after the meeting with Little, Brown, Wilder was still not finished revising the novel. The affairs of the Institute and planning for the trip to England to attend the Coronation had interrupted constantly. Finally, he put the manuscript away and closed his little writing house with the resolve to finish the rewriting task when he and Helen returned home.

∞∞ INTERLUDE IN ENGLAND

On the thirty-first of May, after a twelve-hour flight, the Penfields arrived in England to find it "cold, wet and cheerless," and there they stayed until the third week in July.

Wilder's diary of the period is filled with vivid sketches of the events that took place in bewildering succession, scribbled each night in an attempt to get all of his impressions down on paper. Of the Coronation Day, which came first, he recorded the picture of the two of them and Sir Henry and Lady Dale arriving at Westminster Abbey an hour and a half early, Helen resplendent in "a lovely blue net dress with a circlet of blue flowers holding a blue veil that fell to her shoulders," and he in a morning coat, his decorations sparkling on his chest. He described Vaughan Williams, who had composed some of the coronation music "a great, ponderous man with enormous head and face," straining to follow the ceremony through his hearing aid; Winston Churchill, sweeping in to the cathedral in the flowing robes of the Cinq Portes, stopping "to glower about him"; the maids who emerged with brooms to sweep off the gold carpet before the Queen herself arrived—even the toilets labelled LADIES, GENTLEMEN and PEERS, were duly noted in the diary.

Then the Queen made her entry and faced each of the four quarters of the Abbey while the Archbishop of Canterbury called out for their approval. He remembered the resounding shout of "Long Live Queen Elizabeth!" and the "curious tightness" that took hold of his throat at the sight of her standing "simply, but with calm dignity." Finally, he wrote of how the Queen and the Duke of Edinburgh took communion with the Archbishop of Canterbury "as though no one else were present—a family affair in the midst of her elevation to the throne."

The record continues, a succession of brief, poignant images: a rambling Sunday-morning walk with Edgar Adrian at Cambridge, which took them by Adrian's laboratory, where they paused and Adrian said, "Not much use going in" so they walked on; a visit to an ancient almshouse outside of Oxford, traditionally the responsibility of the Regius Professor of Medicine, where Wilder learned two new stories to add to the legend of Sir William Osler. One was told by an old woman who had worked for the Oslers when her grown son was a baby, a story of how Sir William would babysit while she did her housework—a picture Wilder found easy to accept. The other story came from the (apparently) level-headed nurse who ran the almshouse. She told Wilder solemnly that Osler haunted her cottage, knocking on the wall once a month and inquiring if all was well, to which she dutifully replied, "All is well!"

At Oxford Wilder went to St. Cross Cemetery to visit the grave of his old friend Cuthbert Bazett, with whom he had laboured in Sherrington's lab as a graduate student in 1919. "He lies under a simple headstone—'Fellow of Magdalen'. The sun shone, a breeze stirred the long grass and perfume came to us from flowers. In the silence an English robin in a nearby cedar sang delicately. That melody seemed all that there could be between our spirits and that of dear old Bazett."

After the ceremony at Oxford, from which he emerged with a D.C.L. (Doctorate of Civil Law) to add to his other degrees, he walked alone in the night through the grove by his old college. The sight of Merton tower floodlit against the dark sky, the silence, and the shadows on the lawn moved him to wish he could write poetry.

On the morning of the Order of Merit investiture, Wilder, "oppressed by a curious feeling of sadness and unreality," and Helen sat in a car by the side door to Buckingham Palace, waiting for his turn to come. Once inside there was another long wait. Then, as he was walking down the corridor to the royal chamber, he heard children's voices. "Princess Anne came jumping into our path, blond curls and a smile were my only impression. Behind her was Prince Charles.

"'Why are you wearing those?' he said, pointing to the ribbons on Campbell's breast. Campbell, a war hero, turned back smiling.

"'Because I have been helping your mother to give people medals.'

"'Why do you give people medals?'

"'Because they have been brave.' ('Some of them' in a lower tone.)

"'What did they do?'

"'I'm afraid we must go on now.'

"'Why?' The little fellow stood with feet apart, his face alight with keen, boyish interest. A woman took him by the hand and we went on."

Finally Wilder found himself in a large room with a desk in one corner and the door closing behind him. "I was startled when I realized that there was a woman standing quietly in the centre of the room. She was dressed in a yellow silk gown. She smiled slightly but did not move. I recognized the queen with a curious feeling—no royal coach, no trumpeters and the thought occurred to me—'could this be someone else.' I approached her. She was holding a brown leather case in her hand. She opened it and gave it to me. I looked down at it—a dark red cross and in the centre in gold—'For Merit.'

"'It gives me great pleasure to give you this. You deserve it.'

"I thanked her and said 'But I don't deserve it. You have been badly advised.' She smiled and said 'It has the new inscription.' "I looked at it puzzled and turned it over. She pointed to $E\ II\ R$.

"'It is one of the first to have it.'

"I said, 'Is it the first?' She hesitated & said 'One of the first.'"

Wilder and the Queen chatted for a while longer about the problems of trying to remember everything people said to her on a day like the one at hand, with three hundred investitures to get through. Wilder compared the Queen's problem to that of a physician trying to remember each patient's story, and then the two chatted about Wales and motoring. "I made a move as though to turn away and she held out her hand. I shook it (I have wished since that I had kissed it but it would not have been in character). I turned and walked to the door. Then I turned back. She was watching and bowed."

In his own words, "the award of the Order of Merit makes me feel that the Queen has recognized me as her subject." Where others must be satisfied with a simple declaration of citizenship, it was not until this moment that Wilder could say without regret, "I am no longer an American." Writing this, he noted that it was only that year that he was elected to the American Academy of Arts and Science—and then as a Foreign Associate. The Queen, and by association, Canada, had outbid the U.S. for Wilder's enduring loyalty and affections, and henceforth he would in his most unprotected thoughts consider himself a Canadian.

The pageantry of the Coronation had moved both Helen and Wilder deeply. When, on one of their forays through England, they passed a theatre in Hereford where *The Queen is Crowned* was showing, they promptly went in and sat through the film twice, missing their dinner altogether and emerging quite as touched as they had been at Westminster.

∞∞ TROUBLE AT THE INSTITUTE

Montreal was noisy, crowded and hot after eight days at sea. The

Penfields paused there barely long enough to unpack and take care of pressing business before fleeing to the country early in August.

With Charlie, the cook, in the back seat of the Buick, they motored out across the St. Lawrence, eastward through the rich, riverbottom farm country to Chambly on the Richelieu, through Marieville, St. Angèle de Monnoir, and Ste. Brigide to Farnham. There, as the road undulated through the foothills of the mountains, signs with French place names yielded to those of English villages and towns, where the Loyalists had pushed up across the Vermont border to scrabble a living from the thin, rocky soil: Sweetsburg, Cowansville, Iron Hill and Knowlton. Here the tarmac ran out and the dusty road twisted alongside a dry stream below the cliffs, through the Bolton Pass to South Bolton, the last village. From there, one final lunge over the mountain road and the lake was in sight, a long, narrow glimmer of sparkling blue. The Buick skidded down the gravel driveway to the house and grounds, "this green stillness to which we return."

Each morning through the month of August, when he was not called away to Montreal, Wilder went to his milk house to put the final touches to *No Other Gods*. His last stop in England had been to see Sir Leonard Wooley, the archaeologist whose book on Ur had provided much of the background for the novel. Wilder went over with him some of the puzzles he was trying to sort out in his own laboured manuscript, and then listened to Wooley explain that for his part he never went back to correct what he had written, and sometimes didn't even reread it—which promoted this outraged note in the diary: "I do not understand how a man can be a scientist and write that way."

By the end of the summer, with the editor's comments taken care of and Wooley's suggested corrections made, the manuscript of *No Other Gods* was sent back to Little, Brown, and was scheduled for publication the following spring. The publisher had asked for another novel, to Wilder's delight, and there was an idea forming at the back of his mind, but for the moment he was busy with something else: orchestrating his own retirement.

At his sixtieth birthday party two years earlier, a gala event held in a ski lodge in the Laurentians, he had looked out over the gathered staff of the M.N.I. and realized that he was, at last, the oldest. It made him feel queer, after a lifetime as the young challenger. Although he had originally planned to retire at sixty, he noted in his diary, "I know, or perhaps only think, that it is much better for me to continue till sixty-five instead."

It was more than simply vanity that made him feel indispensable in the affairs of the M.N.I. The staff had grown from fifteen in the early years of the war to well over a hundred. Reorganizing the

Institute and raising more money had taken more and more of his working hours, while the demands of the increased staff had placed even greater burdens on the Penfields' home life.

As Helen explained in a letter, it was a constant struggle "just to know everyone well enough to guide us to maximum happiness and efficiency which, of course, includes everything from housing problems, and care of first babies, opportunities for social contacts, library, music, etc., and just plain 'mothering' of the lonely ones, to getting to the bottom of why a brilliant man is not producing the work that was expected of him." These were questions for which Wilder relied heavily on Helen's "intuition." Every Sunday members of the staff were invited to dinner at 4302 Montrose, and after their guests departed Wilder would compare notes with her.

With the growing staff, the Institute was bulging at the seams. Room was needed for more labs, more beds, to house new equipment. And money was needed to pay for it all. Once again J. W. McConnell came to the rescue. He made the Institute a gift of $1,500,000 to pay for the cost of construction, and when word reached him that Penfield was having trouble raising the funds to endow the research—so the researchers wouldn't have to scrabble each year—he sent a message asking Wilder to come by his house the next morning.

Wilder found McConnell in bed, about to eat a boiled egg. When he had finished explaining the difficulty he was having persuading the city fathers to help in a permanent way with the deficit, McConnell wrote out a note that would ensure another million if the city came through. It did, and construction began on The McConnell Wing of the M.N.I.

The opening was scheduled for November, 1953. Wilder had come up with the term "Second Foundation," since the opening of the new modern wing was, in a sense, the second foundation of the Institute. But he had also picked the title with a private reference to his own retirement, having decided that if the right person could be found to take over, he would step down sooner than his sixty-fifth birthday, three years hence. Now that he could feel he was leaving the Institute with sufficient facilities and endowments for the next period of years, he was ready to step aside in favour of some younger man—though not without some regret and trepidation about his own future.

While the various senior members of the staff pitched in as the opening day ceremony grew closer, Wilder bore the brunt of the organization: arrangements with guests, patrons, donors, politicians, the details of dinners, exercises, speeches, the hanging of the

McConnell portraits, last-minute furnishing of rooms, labs and corridors, even the threatened resignation of the building superintendent in the midst of the preparations because of the head nurse's temper—"all seemed to fall about me as though I were inside a kaleidoscope."

As the day approached Wilder felt more and more isolated from them all, feeling "that we were approaching something important that only I could understand." He had, in secret, drawn up a nominating committee from outside the Institute, "men whose ideals are like my own," to choose a successor from a list that included several of the senior members of the staff, and candidates from elsewhere.

Friday the twentieth was a glorious autumn day. Governor-General Vincent Massey unveiled the plaque on the outside of the wing and all those who were gathered saw carved into the stone the words Wilder had chosen from Job: "Where shall wisdom be found and where is the place of understanding?"—words, he wrote, "that have returned to me so often."

As the day unfolded they listened to Alan Gregg, his hair and bushy eyebrows now turned white, describe the M.N.I. as the most successful project the Rockefeller Foundation had undertaken during his tenure. In the afternoon, Wilder delivered the Director's Lecture on the need for greater endowment for science "listening to it as though someone else read and I listened." Describing that evening's dinner party, he wrote, "I heard Geoffrey Jefferson chuckle and drawl through his graceful speech and I heard him call me 'saint' and attempt to place me with Osler." There followed several other salutes to Penfield, which pleased and embarrassed him, and then Phillips, the medical editor at Little, Brown, stood up and presented him with a leather-bound first copy of the first edition of Penfield and Jasper's *Epilepsy and the Functional Anatomy of the Human Brain*, their magnum opus, a brilliant and definitive treatise on the disease and the conclusions they had drawn together from their study of epilepsy. Like *No Other Gods*, it was scheduled for publication the next spring. The presentation gave Wilder an unexpected thrill, and brought a surge of affection for Jasper, who "had connived at it." For a moment Wilder basked in the praise and attention without regret.

Then, on Saturday morning, Bill Cone heard about the nominating committee and realized for the first time that Wilder actually meant to retire. Cone found Wilder drinking coffee in one of the reception rooms and immediately whisked him off to his office.

Bill was shocked. He admitted that Wilder had told him he was thinking of retiring, but he had never believed it. He wouldn't let him do it. He would go to the principal and the chancellor of McGill and get them to keep Wilder on. Wilder, it seems, explained that he was ready to retire, and Cone retorted (and the diary records), "[You] had no right to go back on the ideal we...built up together."

Oblivious to Wilder's words Cone did go to see both the Principal and the Chancellor and they said that the decision was up to Wilder; they weren't forcing him to retire. In desperation, Bill went around to the house while Wilder was elsewhere and pleaded with Helen to make Wilder reconsider. And Helen, though she was delighted that Wilder was at last ready to leave the Institute, said, like the others, that Wilder had made up his own mind to try his hand at a second career while he was still young enough to learn a new craft.

By Sunday evening the committee had come up with a list of the best candidates, beginning with the two they favoured most: Ray Adams from Boston, and Ted Rasmussen, who had been on the staff at the Institute for periods during the thirties and forties and who was now at the University of Chicago. That evening Wilder told Cone what the committee, (which Cone had refused to sit on) had concluded. "He stood looking at me and walking about my room—dazed and angry. He had asked to have my term extended to 70. I was 'selfish' to leave. I should 'die in harness.' But deepest no doubt was the wound that he was not to succeed to the job I have had....Unspoken in his mind was the question, didn't they even consider me? And my spoken reply was that he would be much happier with someone to run the administration and that he was recognized by them all as the most important asset of the M.N.I.

It was a terrible blow to Bill Cone. Wilder had handled the whole thing badly: not just Bill but almost everyone else at the Institute had assumed that Cone would take over when Penfield retired. Wilder had said as much in his diary when he first thought of retiring, and presumably said as much publicly when the matter was discussed.

He had thought to do Cone a favour, by handing over the Institute to someone else with more ability and tolerance for administration, fund-raising and maintaining the public image of the Institute. For all these things Bill had shown neither talent, nor inclination—and yet he had wanted the job, or at least wanted to be offered it.

It is a measure of the distance that had slowly grown between them that Wilder either didn't realize how hurt Bill Cone would be, or assumed he would get over it without any serious damage. To some extent, Wilder had come to think of Bill as a kind of eccentric, obsessed prodigy. Because they hadn't the same interests or ambitions, Wilder had been deluded into thinking that Bill had no ambitions at all. He was aware that Bill often considered the conferences

Wilder attended, the holidays he took, his many outside interests, as distractions from the time he should be spending at the Institute. And if that was a narrow view, then so was Wilder narrow to dismiss Bill because he wasn't interested in these things, and to assume that he would not be able to run the Institute after he (Wilder) left.

No one, admittedly, would be the director Wilder had been. His name was synonymous with the Montreal Neurological Institute by now; he had created it. Who could fill those shoes? There were few with his extraordinary ability as an administrator, fund-raiser and recruiter. Wilder's successor would have to be able to delegate some of the responsibilities he had made a part of the job, and the new man would have to substitute a degree of democracy for the iron will and occasional fireworks that were the mark of the Institute's founding director—not altogether a bad thing. But Wilder couldn't imagine Bill as the director.

As far as Wilder was concerned, Cone had become a first-rate surgeon, perhaps in some respects, a better surgeon than Wilder. But he was a surgeon who preferred to operate in the middle of the night, regardless of the inconvenience. He was a kind and compassionate doctor to his patients, without a doubt, but he spent an inordinate amount of time on the actual tending of patients, which Wilder preferred to leave to the staff in charge of that duty. Bill had a brilliant mind, but instead of turning it to the formulation of conclusions to his research, he preferred to tinker with a new apparatus to elevate beds. For all these reasons, Wilder had assumed that Bill would see the wisdom of his decision to hand over the running of the Institute to someone who would allow Bill to continue as he always had.

Instead, to Wilder's horror, Bill threatened to quit. If Wilder left and someone else was appointed director, Bill would go elsewhere. At first Wilder refused to believe the threat was serious. But Bill remained firm, and suddenly the prospect of losing the man who *was* the greatest asset of the Institute, next to Wilder himself, seemed a very real possibility.

Over the next few weeks, Wilder wrestled with his dilemma, while Bill silently went about his duties. Wilder talked to Ray Adams and Ted Rasmussen, the two candidates, and pleaded unsuccessfully with Bill to stay under a successor. Finally, Wilder realized he would have to change his plans. Much as he wanted to pull out of the Institute and spend the years ahead quietly writing and sifting through the data on the brain, he could not risk depriving the Institute of Cone. That, and the regret that he had hurt this friend and associate of thirty years, however unwittingly, finally tipped the scales.

The only alternative was a compromise. Wilder would stay on as director on a half-time basis, with Ted Rasmussen as assistant director handling the bulk of the administration. When Wilder proposed this solution to Bill, he accepted it and agreed to stay. Though the crisis had been averted, six months later Wilder noted ruefully in his diary that Bill had not forgiven, or forgotten. "It is a sorrow to me that he cannot accept my placing the M.N.I. on a basis that is above personal desires and even friendship. He accepts it all as a betrayal of our relationship."

Wilder was recording these thoughts while en route to Santa Fe for a meeting of the Harvey Cushing Society (after staying away for many years) "to demonstrate that I am remaining in neurosurgery, not retiring, and to read an analysis of the results of surgery as a treatment for epilepsy." To his remarks about Bill, he added: "Sometimes I am delighted at the prospect of carrying on with problems of memory and consciousness. Sometimes I wish I had arranged to clear out—looking at it selfishly."

Ahead of him now were, as he put it, "the perilous years between 65 and 70." "Confusing," or "disturbing" might have been more appropriate: half in, half out of the M.N.I., part-time surgeon, part-time scientist, part-time novelist—he would wish more than once that he had made a clean break, or stayed on full time. In science, the study of the brain was advancing so quickly that he was finding it impossible to keep up. Even as he and Jasper sent off the manuscript of the book on epilepsy he had observed with some distress that there was new information on the temporal lobe that was not in it.

A month before the opening ceremony for the McConnell Wing, Wilder had come away from a scientific conference troubled by a sense of foreboding of the pitfalls that lay ahead for him in science. The conference, organized by Herbert Jasper, was on Consciousness and the Reticular System of the Brain Stem. Distinguished speakers had come from around the world, and as he listened to the speeches and the discussion, Wilder's sense of isolation grew. He summed up in his diary: "I didn't follow them, and don't understand. But Bremer turned and told me that my paper on Memory [was] beautiful, etc. He had given a lecture on it to his students, etc. I went for a long walk over the golf course feeling discouraged in spite of what may have been an effort to cheer me up.

"The trouble is that all of the good physiological work of Magoun and his school, Lashley, Hess *et al.*, all deals with brain mechanisms, while my work with man works backward from the mind & consciousness toward the mechanism. I can see what has to be, but can demonstrate nothing, and surely an effort to relate the two will be wrong. I have to talk tomorrow and I feel suddenly that I can only speak like a prophet. I suppose prophets are always lonely men. They may be right in general outline, but they are doomed to be wrong in detail. If they are wrong in principle and detail too—they aren't prophets!"

Wilder knew it was illogical and unscientific to work backward, from his faith in the existence in the brain of a place where mind and brain interacted, to the hypothesis of the centrencephalic system. Still, he believed his conclusions were supported by all the available evidence of brain function—just as the evidence seemed to validate the "film clip" analogy for memory and his other theories about the cortex. "I really believe I'm right....I'd better try to formulate conclusions and then leave it."

Wilder's only comfort, for the moment, came from his budding career as a writer. With the extra time the new arrangement at the M.N.I. granted him, he began casting about for a suitable topic for his second novel, even as he waited anxiously for public reaction to *No Other Gods*.

The novel was published on schedule in the spring of 1954. It was 330 pages long, with eight pages of "Background Notes" and twenty-two bibliographic sources listed, including an article he had written for the *Bulletin of the History of Medicine* in 1946 called "Ur of the Chaldees and the Influence of Abraham on the History of Medicine."

In the preface of *No Other Gods* Wilder had written "This is a novel, not a history nor a treatise on religion," but his subsequent description of "certain facts...established by recent archeological excavations" and his longish account of his trips to Ur in 1943 and to various museums around the world had an unsettling effect on the critics. The book was clearly an anomaly—though no more anomalous than Penfield himself: was it a romantic novel written by a world-famous neurosurgeon or a thinly disguised treatise on the origins of monotheism by an amateur writer and archeologist?

The Montreal critics loyally heaped praise on the book, carefully avoiding any reference to literary merit beyond euphemisms like "the chaste precision of the prose," and made much of Penfield's other "protean" abilities and the strange story of how he came to inherit the manuscript from his mother. Reviewers elsewhere in Canada followed suit. In the U.S. the novel was generally ignored and sold poorly but within a year the book had sold close to twelve thousand copies in Canada—impressive figures even by today's standards—and it would continue to sell for more than a decade.

Trying to account for this success, Wilder observed shrewdly that "to know the author is more than to know the book." In places the labour of rewriting and rewriting had unquestionably borne fruit, and it was certainly no worse than many other first attempts at historical fiction. Wilder's own initial reaction to the news of the sales figures seems fairly just: that the novel did "perhaps better than it deserves in Canada and less, if possible, than it deserves in the U.S.A."

The publication of the novel was an anti-climax after so many years of effort, and in the depression that followed, Wilder resolved that in his next attempt at fiction he would move into an area where no one could challenge his authority, where he could do something other than "add to the flood of books." Gradually the notion of writing a novel about Hippocrates fixed itself in his mind. Who better than a doctor, he reasoned, could write about the father of them all? It was Hippocrates who had drawn up, in the fourth century, the Hippocratic Oath for all physicians to follow. His writings, copied and recopied over the centuries, were regarded as the first clear statement of the scientific method. His writings on epilepsy, in particular, had drawn Wilder to take a second look at the author and his life.

Beneath a plane tree on the Greek island of Cos, legend asserted and archeologists were inclined to agree, Hippocrates had taught the disciples who came to him, and had practised as a physician. Wilder decided he wanted to visit the spot. So in mid-July, the Institute running smoothly with Ted Rasmussen at the helm, the Penfields left for six weeks at the farm to prepare for a trip to Greece. A series of medical addresses had been added as afterthoughts, but as usual, the scientific writing took much of the time intended for reading Greek philosophy and history. And, as usual, Helen was kept busy with the family, all of whom came to visit at one time or another during the six weeks.

Wilder Jr. had recently moved from New York to Montreal with his wife and family, and there would now be two "constant clients" at Magog Meadows. Wilder and Helen were delighted. That summer they decided to give each of the children $10,000, rather than having them inherit it when they no longer needed it. That done, Wilder wrote, "we do not have to worry about passing on money on our death but can use what we may have for our own support."

With all of these outside interruptions, it was only after he and Helen had boarded ship at the end of August that Wilder could finally turn to the story of Hippocrates in earnest. "I am fumbling about for a basic plot," he wrote in his diary, mid-ocean, and resolved that it would be a "scaffold on which to hang or build the structure of the story of the birth of medicine."

Deciding that their travels and reading would be made much easier if he could at least sketch the outlines of the story, he turned to the historical accounts and, in a desultory fashion, began to embroider on the characters who emerged. Beginning with the family of the Governor of Cos, he listed each character and, next to each name, the adjectives that suggested themselves. Although the Governor was left blank and the Governor's son earned only "Olympic athlete and gymnast," the women, as usual, were clearer in his mind; the Governor's wife, he decided, was "brilliant, selfish, unprincipled," and her daughter "sweet-hysterical."

The family of the Governor caught his interest right from the start: "there is a mystery here" behind the historical record, he decided, and set about seeking for an explanation that seemed to fit. The explanation he came up with sounds like nothing so much as an historical soap opera:

"The wife is a brilliant woman, older than the Governor and with two of her own children—a daughter who has hysterical fits and a son who is a former Olympian athlete, handsome & a gymnast. The governor fancies his stepdaughter. The mother is jealous of her and the girl takes refuge in hysteria. Her own maid has temporal lobe seizures. The mother idolizes her handsome son and hopes that he can outshine Heracleides. He is engaged to the maid of Cnidos while her father Ctesias is away attending the king of Persia. Empedocles, in exile and suffering from incurable cancer & pain, comes seeking relief. He is a little mad, a dramatist who wants to die if need be to get relief, but he would like to be thought immortal. The woman of Athens had loved Hippocrates when he [was] a pupil of Socrates. She is now the mistress of a wealthy Athenian and comes to Cos seeking a safe abortion and hoping for other things. Finding abortions can not be bought from the Aesclepiads, she hides her condition and attempts to seduce Hippocrates so he will carry out the abortion for other reasons."

This was the stuff of racy and popular historical romances. At the end of this sketch he added a few scenes that he thought should be worked in somehow, and decided that "an exciting sea voyage" would help the story along.

London was the first stop on their itinerary. During their stay there, Wilder and Helen read in the London Library in the daytime, and in the evening went to the theatre. Feeling it would help put him in the right frame of mind for his writing, each day Wilder filled his diary with summaries of the play they had seen: Christopher Fry's *The Dark is Light Enough*, *A Day by the Sea* by N. C. Hunter, and *After the Ball*, Noel Coward's musical based on *Lady Windermere's Fan*.

From London, the Penfields flew to Rome and from there to Athens, where they settled into a room at the King George Hotel, planning to use it as a base for their preliminary explorations. Their daily schedule during this trip would have defeated a couple half their age. Each morning they were up early and out to some site they wished to see as the sun rose, and from then until sunset there was hardly a moment's pause.

This was the sort of thing Wilder and Helen did best together. In the evenings after the days explorations, they returned to the room to fill notebooks with drawings and diagrams of statues, instruments, clothing, vistas and anything else that might have a remote bearing on the story of Hippocrates. Often their discussions would go on for hours as each took a side and they tugged away at some issue, minor (how the Greeks tied their sandals or cooked their oat cakes) or major (the true nature of the Greek character).

For seven weeks they travelled about, to Rhodes from Athens, and from Rhodes to Cos; after two weeks there they returned to Athens and then they were off to Delphi and Boetra and eventually to Istanbul. There Wilder delivered his two lectures at the university medical school and wrangled a ride in a police boat out from Istanbul harbour into the Bosphorus.

Two days before they were to board the plane for London, on the streets of Athens, Wilder was mesmerized by a beautiful Greek woman, "the one I have watched for but never seen," Daphne of statue and legendary beauty. She was window-shopping with a friend, and Wilder followed her about from place to place discreetly, taking note of each feature: she walked with an "unexpected swing" with her head held high: dark eyes, black curls, narrow waist, broad hips, ankles that "curved back gracefully." He noted his surprise that she was wearing high heels, which struck him as absurd, so certain was he that he had found the original. Although he later regretted it, at the time he was too timid to approach her, certain she would be insulted, though, he wrote, "I suspect she was well aware of the fact she was conservative perfection from the topmost curl to the tip of her carefully rolled umbrella."

When the trip finally came to an end, Wilder left Greece with regret, "a lonely feeling" due to the parting from "Cos, Cnidus and Rhodes and...all the other doorways back to a past that I see through a haze. I wish I had this month for quiet in Greece instead of flying from place to place to lecture and dine and meet people and see new things, all so far from the Hippocratic landscape." Yet it puzzled him, as he returned to these duties of his busy life, the pull of writing: why, as he put it elsewhere, did he "let the writing of a romance that will have so little real value interfere with my real profession and responsibilities?"

Returning to Montreal he continued to wonder at what he suspected was a sign of some fundamental frivolity. Driving along Pine Avenue one morning "making my automatic journey to the Institute, I looked up. A bird was flying irregularly, up, up, and I exclaimed aloud, 'That's it!' Suddenly I knew it was the escape to freedom. When I write I see colour, light, distance, other people's thinking. When I was deciding what profession to enter at Princeton," he reflected, "and writing down a long list, I thought medicine had the virtue of being less disagreeable than the others, only that. Not that I wanted to continue playing football all my life. Certainly I was ambitious for achievement in many lines. But somehow any profession seemed an internship, a shutting away from freedom."

CHAPTER TEN

An Old Doctor

∞ "A HORRID RIVER"

In 1955 Wilder's sixty-fifth birthday was a year away, and he had earned the right to disengage, the right to a little freedom and the indulgence of writing. All the honours he could have wished for—all but the Nobel Prize, which every scientist covets—had come to him. His obstinate defence of radical surgery, such a challenge to the medical establishment in the twenties and thirties, was now old hat. The Montreal Procedure still had its critics, but patients continued to come in droves, and many went away cured of their epilepsy.

His honour and reputation had survived attacks on his "switchboard" hypothesis, the centrencephalic system, and he and Herbert were continually tinkering with it to account for new discoveries other scientists were making. His family was thriving, the four children and their families gathering each summer at Magog Meadows, "the sacred summer circle." He had enough surgical cases to support Helen and himself, and enough put away to live as he wished when he stopped operating. If his first novel was not a major success, he was convinced the second would be much better; anyway, it was a second career that would carry him through. And when he was not writing or at his desk at the Institute or operating, there was a seemingly endless number of clubs eager to hear him speak, universities anxious to confer yet another degree, medical societies keen to hear him talk about his scientific work. The future seemed assured—he could permit himself a time of indulgence.

And then, in 1955, there came a moment when he suddenly realized that in the world outside things were proceeding considerably less smoothly and predictably than they were in his own life.

On June 1 he and Helen were in New York for yet another honorary degree, this one to mark the opening of a new building at New York University's Bellevue Medical Centre. Wilder was to receive a Doctor of Science *honoris causa*, along with Edgar Adrian, the Oxford Nobelist; Salk, the discoverer of the polio vaccine, was there to be awarded a gold medal, and Adlai Stevenson was to receive a LL.D. (Doctor of Laws) and deliver the address. On the day before the ceremony Wilder and Helen decided to go see a performance of *Cat on a Hot Tin Roof*, then playing at the Morosco Theatre, which had earned Tennessee Williams a Pulitzer Prize and the New York Drama Critics Circle Award for 1955.

Helen was mildly offended by the play but Wilder emerged from the theatre outraged. Returning to their room at the Ambassador Hotel, he sat down at the desk and released a torrent of words:

"My sense of shock is that this, which men judge good, and which women crowd to see and hear, is admired. It seems to signify that degredation is rising like a horrid river to wash away good things in our civilization. Obscene language which men have used is now dished out to women, who laugh and applaud. Everything that is good is made of no account—The Church, family, children, affection, love, integrity: all laughed at.... If it is good drama and literature then I am all wrong. The writing of Shakespeare, the simple speeches of Lincoln are poor—feeble. They are pure water for which the pervert has no taste."

There, for the moment, he left it. But later that night, unable to sleep more than a few fitful hours because of "the cursed play," he got out of bed, pulled on his bathrobe and sat down again to write. "It is after 2 o'clock in the morning," he began, "and I have returned here to see if I can understand—what is happening to the modern mind, what may be wrong with my mind."

The play had shown him how the world looked through the eyes of a modern writer, and it was a far cry from the happy normality of his own family or the strictly ordered world inside the walls of his Institute. But the lines the actors spoke had a ring of authenticity that his own writing, he was forced to admit, lacked, and it made him wonder if his writing would ever become good enough to be convincing. He continued for several hours digging into his own life and examining his beliefs and achievements in the light of the success of Williams' play and what it implied about the world's standards of morality, covering page after page of hotel stationery. "What does it mean in regard to the story of Hippocrates? The plot has grown and looks quite impressive, 40 pages of it written out...Am I writing a fairytale?"

"*No Other Gods,*" he went on, "was naïve no doubt, spurned by the modern critic. So many have told me that it made them turn to read the Old Testament, that they have given it to their fathers or mothers or Sunday school teachers. That was what Mother hoped to do.

"The only characters people seemed to have liked, or at any rate refer to, are Princess Shub and Dudu—the naughty girl and boy. Some have understood the spiritual struggle of Abraham in the great marsh, those whose minds turn naturally to that sort of thinking. But the people I tried to make live—Sarai, Terah, Oni, even Abraham—came no more than half alive. Was this because my writing was so amateurish? It was, of course. Or was it because I don't see life true?

"I don't care whether a novel I may write is sold in large amount—I don't want to appeal to the public taste for family filth. But I want to understand the truth about men's motives and inner drives. Surely I do know them. Surely I can learn to make the truth into fiction, to animate characters that are real. But can I learn the art of writing today? Do I understand it? Does Tennessee Williams know anything I am blind to?"

If he could master the art of writing, Wilder reasoned, then he could use writing as a way to promote his own view of the world, "to help men to think right." Like Tennessee Williams, he knew men and women had evil in them, "levels...where thoughts do not belong." But life was struggling to rise above them and conquer them, not—as Tennessee Williams seemed inclined—to wallow in them.

But the reaction to *No Other Gods* made him wonder whether, even if his writing improved in his second novel about Hippocrates and the high calling of medicine, anyone would be willing to listen. Perhaps it would be wiser to stick to what he knew.

Detlev Bronk and Edgar Adrian, with whom Wilder and Helen had dined at the Cosmopolitan Club the night they arrived in the city, he continued, were satisfied with "a brilliant close" to their scientific careers. Why wasn't he? "Bronk is building a new University, the Rockefeller Institute, and hobnobbing with Rockefellers while he heads the American Academy of Sciences. Adrian is President of the Royal Society, Master of Trinity, the first Lord Adrian of Cambridge, and still justifies the awarding of the Nobel Prize to him by continuing to steal hours away to work on the mechanism of smell in a rabbit!

"Why," he wondered, "am I not satisfied to work on at my own carpenter's bench? The toys I've made are wonderful to behold, and many have come to life. They live in other men's clinics and in their minds. They don't know their own maker. Perhaps I'd better turn back to surgery and science. What can an impotent old man like me do to save the souls and spirits of mankind? Better stick to saving bodies from death and think nothing of the minds of men, nor worry about their ideals."

"But I want to turn away...I'm old in skin, hair, glands, joints. Others can work at my bench. They can take up the thinking about the mechanisms of the brain where I leave off. I want to write beautifully, be admired, much read. I suppose that is a silly bit of vanity. I want to be handsome, have thick curly hair, sparkling talents—all those things I wish I had. I'd like to run a mile in four minutes, to dance better than other men!"

If it was "sheer nonsense" for him to wish for such things, was it just as ridiculous for him to believe that he might, even at this late stage in his life, be able to make some contribution to the world outside of science? After all, the world had signalled its admiration for Wilder Penfield with all the honours it could give. Now when he spoke, people listened. He had taken the honours as his due, as permission to step down and become a writer. Suddenly he saw them as a mantle of responsibility he had unwittingly accepted, but accepted nonetheless.

It was more than his power as a public figure that made Wilder think he might be able to have an impact. He was a doctor, and doctors are by the nature of their work, infernal meddlers. He had spent much of his life being well-paid and highly praised for his inspired meddling in the lives and bodies of his patients. It was a habit by now hard to break. And if that is true of doctors, it is doubly, trebly true of surgeons—especially neurosurgeons. They play God every time they go into the operating room. It is not just the power over life and death, but the ever-present risks of brain surgery: one slip, one error on the surgeon's part, and the patient will live but never speak again, or live with all memory gone forever.

Some brain surgeons cope by denying the power and responsibility—the wiser ones, perhaps. "I don't think about saving lives, I think about performing that surgical procedure as best I can," they will say. But Wilder Penfield and those like him, because of their background, temperament, inclination and self-image, acknowledge and accept the role, and it becomes a part of them.

Should we blame them? Every brain surgery patient has come to the surgeon hoping for a miracle. There is no terror like knowing that something is growing in your brain, knowing that something is seriously wrong and understanding that it is not just your body that has been invaded, but *you*. A leg, an arm—you can separate yourself from these things, but not from your brain.

Those who inhabit neurosurgical wards, waiting for their turn in the operating room, are like people cut loose from normal society and everyday life. Everything not essential to the moment is stripped away: family, job, self-esteem. In their place, the only thing that matters is the sickness and the healing power of the surgeon, and the rest be damned. It takes a monumentally insensitive surgeon to ignore the patients' view of this relationship, and a profoundly humble one not to be affected by it.

As a surgeon, Wilder was neither humble nor insensitive to his patients. Before he operated he talked to them at length, about their lives, their expectations, their fears, their families. He could not separate himself as a surgeon from them as human beings who were putting their lives in his hands. He would see a patient dying slowly, draining the family's savings and leaving spouse and children destitute, and wonder if it was not more moral for him not to intervene. Or, as in the case of Ruth, the reverse: knowing how much she had to live for, he took terrible risks. In this era of malpractice suits he would have had to be much more careful.

But if patients wished to alienate him, they had only to suggest that they preferred a second opinion after Wilder had already made up *his* mind what was best. "You must trust me completely, and I will take you on and do everything in my power to save you," was his attitude, and he made no bones about it.

If not *Cat on a Hot Tin Roof*, something else no doubt would have awakened Wilder's concern at the changes afoot in the world. There were troubled times ahead; the impulse to intervene and the assumption that he had a duty to do so were too strong in him by now. But it would take a number of years for him to find a suitable platform, to shed his scientific disguise and emerge an unblushing social critic tilting at the threats to civilization and decency. For the moment he was uncertain about what to do, and would settle for the "enchanting occupation" of writing. There were scientific speeches, some that fell between science and social commentary, and a growing number that were more general and philosophical. And among the many people who listened there would be some who would have their uses for an old doctor with his wits about him and a famous name.

∞∞ THE WORLD OUTSIDE

In March of 1956, the Penfields returned to Greece for six weeks of research on Hippocrates, according to plan. Between the time of their departure and the shock of seeing *Cat on a Hot Tin Roof*, Wilder had done some travelling on his own. He had gone "a-lecturing" to Chicago, Los Angeles and Phoenix, Arizona, and had made a trip to the Soviet Union to address the Soviet Academy of Sciences. The Academy had elected him a member, and the vote, though supposedly secret, had been unanimous. A rare honour.

By now Wilder and Helen were seasoned explorers and amateur archaeologists. Off they would go, he in a light tweed jacket, a tie and deerstalker's cap, she in a silk dress and sun hat, the two of them poking about excavated ruins and wandering through tiny villages with their guide, busily making notes, drawing diagrams and taking snapshots. For three weeks they rambled over Cos and Cnidus, soaking up the countryside, exploring archaeological digs and looking for a village or stretch of coast or hillside to serve as the setting for this scene or that.

From there they went to Asia Minor and rattled about Turkey in a succession of decrepit taxis, staying in the worst hotels they had encountered in all their travels, and finally in Athens spending a few quiet days in libraries and museums before the return flight. It was, Wilder wrote, "a wonderful holiday, a remarkable honeymoon."

When they returned at the end of the summer there was an unwelcome surprise waiting in Montreal—a letter from federal Minister of Health and Welfare Paul Martin. The letter explained that the government of India had asked for medical teachers to come over and lecture for three months under the auspices of the Colombo Plan; would he be willing to go?

Unwilling to take the time away from Hippocrates, Wilder wrote back a refusal. A week later, Paul Martin was on the telephone from Ottawa: "Dr. Penfield, you can't refuse. The Indian government has asked for you. You could make the trip with stops in Pakistan and Ceylon, as short as you like." Then, the clincher: "The future of the world is to be settled in Asia and any little gesture we can make we must not overlook."

The appeal to his conscience worked, and on January 26, 1957, Wilder opened a new diary to announce that he and Helen were on board a B.O.A.C. Stratocruiser bound for "London, India and home around the world." In his customary stock-taking he wrote that he had agreed to the trip only on the condition that Helen could come with him. The itinerary had almost blossomed to include a visit to

Red China when he received an unexpected invitation from Peking, but at the last minute he realized he wouldn't have time to properly prepare, and so declined.

Both Wilder and Helen took the preparations for these trips seriously. In her "round robin" letter a few days before their departure, she wrote that they had read the Bhagavad-Gita and two novels "by a young Indian woman, Kamala Markandaya: *Nectar in a Sieve* and *Some Inner Fury*, which were "very readable and indicative of present conditions in India." They had also read a dozen other books, and had met with many Indians and others who had lived or travelled in that country. "One of our Indian visitors spent the whole evening expounding the philosophy which is the background of the Hindu religion," Helen wrote.

Although he was naturally flattered, Wilder was not entirely at ease with the role of goodwill ambassador. While Helen slept on the first leg of their flight, exhausted by the frantic race to pack and close up the house and farm in preparation for the trip, Wilder replayed his various conversations with Paul Martin. "His words— You can't escape, Dr. Penfield, you belong to the world,—keep coming back to me. Everyone does, of course. But is it my job to open lines of friendship & understanding? Why? I'm not much good at that sort of thing." Then, as though for a moment considering the role's potential as a retirement career, he added, "I can't retire and do it. I must be a doctor and speak as one. But I could retire and write."

Instead of a three-month long engagement, the Penfields agreed to thirty-five days, and their hosts responded by rushing them about without a moment's pause. Between February 2 and March 9 their whirlwind tour took them through Karachi and Rawalpindi in Pakistan, through the Khyber Pass and on to Delhi, Colombo, New Delhi, Madras, Vellore, and Calcutta, on to Rangoon in Burma, Bangkok, Hong Kong, and finally, Tokyo. "It was the most concentrated month I have ever experienced," Helen wrote to a friend after their return. "I thought how perfect it would be to be a queen—no packing and unpacking. But how Wide stood it, lecturing continually, I can't understand."

Judging from the diaries he filled as they went from place to place, he was delighted, more than a little flattered by the respectful recognition, slightly puzzled ("People have an extraordinary misconception of me. I suppose it is because of the O.M., which seems now a strange and forgotten accident of the past"), and endlessly fascinated by the sights and sounds of the passing spectacle. There was the dean of one of the many medical colleges they visited ("a little man with a black wart on the end of his nose that makes one long for scissors") and two students who had timidly approached after one talk he had given on the cerebral cortex. "In spite of the Principal's gestures and words of banishment, [they] stood their ground and asked how it could be that feeling was in the cortex? We talked for ten minutes while the Principal stood gloomily. When they had gone I congratulated him on having students like that, with great enthusiasm. I wonder what he will do later—nothing, I hope.

There is a long account of the tribesmen in the Khyber Pass, looking ferocious and all armed with long-barrelled rifles, many of them made from the stolen and bored-out railings of the bridges recently put up by the Pakistani government. "They live in walled villages made of clay and provided with one or more towers from which to spy enemies... [with] a rope ladder in each tower which can be pulled up so pursuers can't follow. They have a few goats but live chiefly on the tribute paid them by the British to keep them from making raids on the plains."

There were strange echoes of colonial empire. At the Mess of the famous Khyber Rifles, there was a wide, smooth patch of ground that looked like a lawn-bowling pitch, with no grass, just brown earth. Yes, they had bowls, but weren't sure how to play. At Wilder's mention of a game, "16 beautiful bowls appeared and the C.O. and I defeated the Major and Earl Drake" under the hot sun. At a luncheon in Karachi Wilder was seated next to the daughter of the Prime Minister of East and West Pakistan, who "said her father had gone to bed at one o'clock instead of 4 as usual, because I had told him it was wrong to go on 3 or 4 hours of sleep, which is his custom. He also told his daughter that I'd said it was too late for him to learn a new language!"

The Prime Minister was not the first, nor would he be the last, to misinterpret Wilder's theory on language learning, the topic of one of the speeches he had brought with him to deliver in various places on this trip. The theory, which had caused quite a stir when he first presented it in the early thirties, suggested that the brain of a young child can be more easily adapted to the learning of two, three or more languages than the brain of an older person. "The human brain has a plasticity at that time and a specialized capacity for acquiring speech, which is lost later," he had written.

Since the problem of language was one aspect of the work at the M.N.I. and elsewhere that interested him most during this time, he had brought the speech along, and had delivered it the day before in Karachi. He gave it again in Delhi a few weeks later and, in the enthusiastic discussion which followed, discovered that second language learning was a problem educators in India were grappling with in the wake of Independence. "Hindi is accepted as a compulsory secondary language," he noted in the diary later, "and they all seem to want to keep English. And yet since the English have gone, they speak a strange Indian English in many places, hard for us to understand."

In Delhi, there was a luncheon with Prime Minister Jawaharlal Nehru, "a quiet, quick man, muscular but rather small. His eyes smiled when his lips did, sometimes the eyes alone smiled when the lips were sad....He seemed to me a man who could be bored or angry but he was neither. Instead he was natural and friendly, with quick flashes of humour but no attempt to preach or make an impression."

Wilder found himself seated next to a tall, slender English woman whom he had observed acting as hostess, but to whom he and Helen had not been introduced. "I don't know your name," he said. "She looked startled and said 'It's Mountbatten.' I laughed a little and said, 'I had no way of knowing.'" Now that Lord Mountbatten's biographers have informed us that the relationship between Lady Mountbatten and Nehru was causing something of a scandal, we may wonder that her presence drew no more comment. Presumably the details were not for visiting dignitaries. Instead, there is the note that she was "charming and quick and completely unaffected. Helen was keen about her, which is high praise." So was Wilder. After lunch the Penfields and their hostess walked out to the verandah overlooking her old home, the Governor General's Palace, now the President's House. "Lady Mountbatten came and leaned on the verandah wall beside me. 'Were you happy there?' I asked her. 'Yes, I met my husband there when I came out to visit at 18. Then it came as a great surprise when we were asked to live there.' 'Where was your room? Did you have a room?' She smiled. 'Yes, it was at the back.'"

Back in the house there was another conversation with Nehru: "'I want to ask you,' he said, 'what you think of solitude and contemplation.' I was startled and said, 'You mean the way it is done here? I don't know India but I have seen the effect of solitude on men who had good minds and were put to bed for a year or two for tuberculosis. They had a deeper character afterward, more mellow, reflective.' "'Yes,' he smiled, 'prison is like that. I've spent years in prison, and then I've been in a single room with many men. There you have no privacy, no peace.'

"Escott Reid [Canadian Ambassador] told him my views of learning secondary language. He seemed interested and I asked him when he first began to speak English. I felt he was on his guard and he said 'Well, it was before the age of 10.' "I thought to myself it might be his best language and he would not want that said of him."

The next time the two men met it was a very different Nehru indeed. This time the man "who could be angry" *was*. At a degree ceremony in Delhi Wilder found himself walking down the aisle beside Arnold Toynbee, when a photographer leapt out in front of them to snap a picture. Nehru suddenly appeared, grabbed the photographer by the arm and shoved him off into the waiting arms of security guards. "As we passed the front entrance I saw the photographer being hustled down the steps as though he were being consigned to utter darkness. We reached a sunny courtyard where Nehru called out like a man who regrets his temper. 'Go get the photographer.' So in time the fellow appeared and photographed us all."

The trip and the diary entries continue, ending at last, on March 9, in Tokyo with a geisha party organized by one of their hostesses and a happy meeting with Dr. Leslie Kilbourn, the Canadian medical missionary to China. Since their last meeting in Chungking in 1943, Kilbourn had been expelled. Now he was dean of the medical school at Hong Kong University, but still "the servant and lover of China... counsellor and leader of all who escape" to Hong Kong. Like those of all the others Wilder had spoken with, Kilbourn's reports of the medical work in Red China were disappointing. They were turning out doctors on a two-year program as well as regular five-year doctors, and including acupuncture, of which most of these Western doctors disapproved. "I begin to fear my visit would serve no useful purpose....I'd so much like to stay home now."

It was time to go home, and Wilder's final entry, written in Hong Kong, is curt: "I lectured. A dignified audience, applause good, but discussion nil."

At the beginning of April, 1957, having had a month to recover from their Asian trip, Wilder and Helen left for a reunion of the Johnson Club at a lakeside resort in North Carolina. According to Helen's cryptic calendar note, the Penfields travelled by "plane to New York, helicopter to Newark, N.J. and train to Spartanburg, N.C." There, ten hours after leaving Montreal, they were met by their host and taken to the Chalet Club, set on a beautiful mountainside above a man-made lake in the Blue Ridge Mountains. Wilder, awakening early in the Honeymoon Cottage in which he and Helen were staying, could step out onto the porch and listen to the birds as they whistled and seemed "to wait for their own echo" in the stillness of the pine forest.

There were other guests of "late middle age, old age, wrinkled, with automobiles and agreeable smiles, and so like ourselves," Wilder wrote, "that I turn away from them disgusted. It is like looking in an unwelcome mirror." This rather crotchety mood eventually wore off during the four days that the Penfields spent discussing politics, world affairs and their own affairs with their old friends the Halls, the Myers and the Chesters. Wilder noted with some satisfaction, "the whole octet make good companions and are growing still in stature as well as age."

After this brief respite, Wilder and Helen returned to Montreal on April 12, and for the next eight weeks Wilder attended conferences in Philadelphia, Detroit, New York, Ottawa, St. Louis, Kingston, Winnipeg, Saskatoon, Atlantic City and again in New York, with barely time to unpack between trips. Helen was growing more selective as the years passed, and managed to avoid at least three of the trips, which were to specific conferences or meetings she particularly detested from past experience. Wilder accepted invitations to speak at these conferences because they offered him the chance to reconsider his own work in science and neurosurgery, and to hear the reports of new developments, but more and more he was aware that he was simply watching from the sidelines.

By July Wilder was in Belgium for the International Congress of the Medical Sciences where he delivered an address and was startled to find young men he had never met "waiting to speak to me in the corridors, as I did once." Perhaps, for this reason, the congress gave him a strange sense of déjà-vû. Or perhaps it was because he could remember the very first meeting to include neurologists, which had been chaired by Gordon Holmes and Sir Charles Sherrington back in 1933. Now, in 1957, the study of the brain had expanded from neurology, and present at the conference were specialists in neurosurgery, electroencephalography, neuroradiology, neuropathology and a number of other specialties. As he delivered his address, he later wrote in his diary, "I was vaguely aware of an altered point of view—I was a figure to look back at, not a man to help solve the future problems."

On occasions like this, Wilder sometimes found himself regretting the distance which grew year by year between his own work and the work being done by a new generation of scientists, and he missed the thrill of being the author of a discovery that challenged old ideas. He still had the fascinating responses from the temporal lobe, which no one else had been able to duplicate with anything like the same degree of success, and each time he was invited to talk about them, he tried to use the occasion for a progression of ideas, rather than simply a restatement of earlier conclusions. As for the centrencephalic system, he now tried to avoid the term. Privately he admitted that he had fallen into a trap by insisting that the brain's co-ordinating mechanism had a specific location. The trouble was that more recent discoveries about how the brain worked were making it more and more evident that any such mechanism must be just part of a complex process of interconnections within the brain. There was no doubt in the minds of most neuro-scientists that the upper brain stem, where he had insisted the "switchboard" would be found, played an important role in integrating incoming data and formulating an appropriate response. In fact the evidence in the years ahead would continue to reinforce the importance of this so-called old brain.

Though criticism of the theories he and Jasper had formulated could still arouse his ire, more and more Wilder was likely to shrug his shoulders and say of the revisionists—as he did of one at the symposium on the history of brain function—"He was only trying to establish the importance of their own work. We all have some of that in us." And walking about the exhibit rooms with a young researcher, the pupil of one of *his* pupils, noticing how little of the new work he was up on compared to his young companion, prompted the remark, "It's all a relay race. You may run well and be in good stride, but the time comes to hand on the stick to a fresh runner."

Wilder made notes on some of the more intriguing reports: "Eccles with his ideas of function in individual nerve cells...Gastaut with a theory of conditioned reflexes that is different from Pavlov... Herbert Jasper with fastidious records of single nerve cell responses in motor area...Malcolm recording neighbourhood electrographic records of cortical cells in permanently installed electrodes in free cats—changes of sexual behaviour in cats...." But at the end of the symposium he found himself asking what all of this work had to do with the more fundamental questions that increasingly interested him. "All these things hardly touch the question of the frontier between brain and mind. Perhaps we must approach the inter-relationship before we can know very much about behaviour." It was an interesting thought, but for the moment, with the scientific conferences over for a while, he had more important things to think about. "Now for two months I can turn back to Hippocrates. It is not a less difficult problem. Perhaps it calls for more—more of the sort of skill I have not learned, more of the vision of the past and of men's minds and emotions than I can comprehend easily."

Back in Montreal at the end of July, the Penfields began packing to leave for the farm. While he waited for Helen to take care of the final details, Wilder found that a book for schoolchildren entitled *Famous*

Doctors had just come out in Canada, with profiles of Osler, Banting and Penfield. Protesting that he didn't belong with them and vowing that he would "never write an autobiography," he admitted, "I've had a varied enough career. There have been 'close shaves' for life and for character too. The latter are covered over and hidden, the former to be boasted about."

These thoughts led inevitably to musings on the relation between fiction and autobiography. He confided to his diary that the task of the next few months, "to find the thought and character of Hippocrates," was fraught with perils, an observation based partly on a candid and somewhat cutting criticism he had received on this very point: "Someone who had read *No Other Gods* told me that I had drawn myself in Abraham's clothing. If I can do no better than that with Hippocrates it will be a poor counterfeit of the true man. Time is running out and I may yet turn back to my task of writing the book with the failing capacity of a senile pen. To draw a picture of an old man's fantasy is hardly worth the effort. The figure I draw will be a much better one than my own self."

Despite the gloomy tone of these diary entries, Wilder had little to fear from senility, and he knew it. His unhappiness was no more—or less—than the symptoms of artistic growing pains. With grim determination Wilder struggled with the novel about Hippocrates off and on throughout the summer, fall and early winter of 1957. Helen, meanwhile, struggled off and on with Charlie's drinking problem, which seemed to be getting worse or, at any rate, more visible. Two years earlier the Penfields had fired him but Charlie had refused to leave, and they were so fond of him between his drinking bouts that they let him stay. Helen noted the growing frequency of these episodes with ever greater exasperation in her monthly calendar, and reported that the crisis came finally New Year's Day. "Blow up over C's drinking" was followed two weeks later by "Chas. leaves for Good!"

Before Christmas Wilder and Helen had decided to drive down to Princeton in early spring so Wilder could use the library there, and Wilder had sent off a letter to the head of the history department, to make arrangements. Then came a letter from Robert Oppenheimer, now director of the Institute for Advanced Study at Princeton, inviting Wilder to become a member of the institute and stay in their facilities on the edge of campus. So on March 4, in the middle of another snow storm that had already left five-foot drifts in front of 4302 Montrose, they packed up their Humber station wagon and headed for New Jersey. They arrived the following day to find the lawns of Princeton turning green, the air balmy, and the birds singing. "Spring!" Helen noted with relief.

The Institute for Advanced Study had been set up in the early thirties to provide scientists who were fleeing Nazi Germany, like Albert Einstein, with a place to live and work. It existed now to provide visiting scholars from around the world with a place to spend a year on their studies in the stimulating company of other distinguished visitors, free from the pressures of earning a living.

Accordingly, the Penfields were given a modern apartment on the second floor of one of the buildings at 55 Einstein Drive with a thirty-foot window in the living and dining rooms looking out across the lawn and over rooftops to the woods beyond. "Wilder," Helen wrote in the round robin several days later, "is purring over his spacious bookshelves and enormous desk in the little study here, and he has also an office at the institute where he can get his manuscripts copied."

Helen's brief notes on the interlude in Princeton also make reference to the "strange and interesting personalities" occupying the institute apartments. Below them lived Sir Llewellyn and Lady Woodward; he was working on "British Army secret material" and moved "with a properly furtive air" through the corridors. And among the most interesting of the Princeton residents were a number of the archaeologists, including Benjamin Meritt (who had arranged for the Penfields to be welcomed at the institute) and the Wade Garrys, a husband and wife team. Wade Garry and Benjamin Meritt had recently written a four-volume report on the Athenian decrees at the time of the Delian League, when the cities of Greece paid a tribute to Athens in return for protection in case of war. These decrees were carved in marble and set up in the market places of the various cities. Each inscription indicated the date, the location and population of the city, and the amount of tax due. This period was just before the Peleponnesian War, during the lifetime of Hippocrates, and the research and general knowledge Meritt and Wade had gathered was invaluable to Wilder. During the two months the Penfields spent at the institute there were many long argumentative dinners in their respective apartments revolving around obscure details of life in Greece in the fifth century B.C.

"Thirty days in the life of Hippocrates," Wilder noted at the end of their stay in Princeton, "has gradually formed itself into a romance and an evolution of medical thought," entitled, temporarily, "Shadows on Cos." Winter had returned to Princeton almost overnight and during "an amazing blizzard" that broke trees and brought down electric wires, leaving them with only the fireplace for heat, and no light or phone, "Helen and I sat inside our big window and read the first chapters of the book while the miracle of snow drifted and blew past." Although some of the characters now stood out clearly in his thinking, others (such as Daphne, Hippocrates' romantic interest) were still shadowy. When a temporary membership was offered for the following spring, the Penfields leapt at the chance to return once again.

And so, after a busy ten months in Montreal and at the farm, in March of the following year Wilder and Helen were back in an apartment similar to the one they'd been in the year before, sticking to a rigid schedule that had Wilder working eight to ten hours a day with an hour off at noon for a walk, six days a week. On their way down to Princeton they had stopped in Boston to discuss the manuscript (now called "The Torch," a reference to the Aesculapian torch, the symbol of medicine) with the editor at Little, Brown. He and Wilder agreed on a number of changes and the outline of the final scenes, and Wilder was determined to finish the novel quickly. Back in Montreal, at the beginning of May, 1959, the round robin left on its circuitous flight with the following note from Helen:

"Well! 'The Torch' is finished (except for some work on glossary and appendix) and has been accepted by Little, Brown and will be published early in 1960—*d.v.*—such a relief! And yet, we shall probably go through it all again, I mean, writing another novel or something. A scientific book on 'Speech' comes out this month, but I don't believe Wide is half so excited or pleased about it. And now he has dropped what he calls his 'secret sin' and is a doctor full time again!"

What pleasure there was in at last having the novel off to the publishers vanished a few days later with a call at 5 A.M. from the M.N.I. It was the Night Supervisor. Seeing a light on in Bill Cone's office he knocked on the door. When there was no answer, he pushed the door open and found Cone dead. He was lying on the floor with his head on a pillow, and potassium cyanide powder on his lips and spilled on his coat.

Wilder dressed quickly and hurried to the Institute where Ted Rasmussen had taken charge. After the coroner left, they drew up a statement for the public, which said simply, "Dr. Cone was in the hospital at midnight checking the conditions of his patients and seemed in excellent spirits. He was found in his office at 5 A.M." That, and the announcement that he "died suddenly" was what the newspapers printed, followed by lengthy tributes from his colleagues.

Bill Cone's death was a terrible blow to everyone. He had been the lurking spirit of the Institute, always there, it seemed, walking the hallways in the early hours of the morning to check on his patients, sleeping on a cot in the cloakroom, always available, always with a kind word or a smile. He was a healer, quite simply, loved and trusted by his patients, the staff and his friends.

Although in the next few days Wilder went through the motions of issuing statements and arranging the funeral, inside he was stunned. He had gone to see Bill's wife, Avis, to break the news to her that morning. He did not say the word "suicide," but from her comments he knew that she had guessed. He had talked of suicide before, she said, and had mentioned cyanide. Was it unhappiness at home? Unhappiness at work? Wilder wondered, and yet just the night before, they had gone together to the Fellows' Dinner, and Bill had seemed his normal self: it made no sense. "What was wrong?" Over and over again in the months and years ahead Wilder searched for an answer. "Somehow I should have helped...I should have understood," he wrote some months later. In the interim he filled a diary with thoughts about Bill Cone and their years together, trying to make sense of the suicide, but that diary he had lost on a train, and it seemed to have resolved nothing for its author. "Bill was neurosurgeon-in-chief...at the height of his capacity as surgeon. Yet when his face was at rest he seemed sad. He was happier when he and I worked alone, doing all things together. As the Institute grew and new men came, he seemed less contented. When I started to resign in 1954 he was furious and never quite forgave my separate action in having my successor chosen by outside advisors. He told me often that I must not resign but should die in harness. But what was wrong? Why he was so unhappy within himself I cannot fathom."

Wilder could not understand and no one, it seemed, was close enough to Bill to provide the answers; perhaps that itself was one of the causes. He had had a hand and a kind word for everyone, and none of his colleagues, not even Wilder, had known that Bill Cone was terribly unhappy. All of them would carry that burden of guilt, but Wilder most of all.

For the moment, Bill Cone's death threw his own life into sharp relief: all the things that Bill had disapproved of, the long holidays to travel and write, the many outside interests, pulled at Wilder more strongly than ever. Without Bill Cone the Institute was not the same, and an era was coming to an end. Wilder decided he should delay no longer and pull out himself, at long last.

Accordingly, he began the withdrawal. In the fall, after a summer spent travelling and lecturing and making final changes to *The Torch* he threw himself into the organization of the quarter-century celebrations at the Institute, which were to be his swan song as director. With the approach of his sixty-ninth birthday, he decided it was time to stop operating. Though surgeons in other specialties will go on operating into their seventies, brain operations are too risky for the patient and too gruelling for the surgeon. In October Wilder operated on his last patient, a difficult tumour case that, like a warning of what would have been in store if he insisted on continuing to operate, gave him a few bad moments. After the operation, the patient's right arm was paralyzed, and though Wilder fully expected—and assured the patient—that movement would return before long, "I go about with a weight in the pit of my stomach because of him and his accusing eyes. I think I did as expert a job as I ever did....He would soon have been paralyzed by its growth, but he doesn't know that. His chance of final recovery would have been nil....It is fair now."

Even after thousands of operations, so little changed. For each patient it was the first time, and the risks as great. Shortly after the operation Wilder wrote, "It seems harder than ever to take such things. I wonder, too, whether my skill is really all I think it is, and all that others seem to think."

Two weeks later, the patient moved the finger and thumb of his right hand just slightly. He wouldn't believe it, and still refused to smile, and then several days later, the diary records jubilantly, "he closed the hand very weakly and he grinned at me." Wilder went on, "Today when we went around, the resident said 'We have a pleasant surprise waiting for you on the third floor.' All the residents were smiling....'Howard?' I asked, 'his arm?' 'Yes, he moved it at the elbow both ways.' He is content to stay here the six weeks for his X-ray treatments before he goes back to Utah."

"Patients," Wilder added, "are never twice the same. One must take time to know them and talk to them and look out at their lives through their eyes. How different life looks then from the world the Doctor lives in, the world he may continue to live in if he treats the sick as bed occupants not people. It's easy to be preoccupied and not to see the dreadful spectres that crowded about Howard's bed and made him choke and the tears come when he spoke, after much prodding, of wife & two children and the chainstore he manages."

At last there were no more patients, and at the annual meeting in May, 1960, Wilder made his last report as director of the Institute and announced he was retiring: "Just pipe me over the side of the ship and I'll go ashore in the pilot boat," he told those who had been his friends and colleagues for so many years. He wanted no fuss, no formal ceremony, but it was nonetheless gratifying that the Canadian newspapers treated the event as newsworthy, and he noted later in his diary with some satisfaction that it had been reported in the U.S. papers too, "even in *Time*."

All took their cue from him: "Famous Surgeon Puts Down Scalpel, Takes Up Pen," went a typical headline. Knowing how difficult it must be for him to sever the connection altogether, and unwilling to lose the benefit of his counsel and experience, Ted Rasmussen persuaded him to accept the honorary title of "Fellow of the Institute," along with an office and a secretary there for as long as he wished.

"That is just as I would have it," Wilder wrote happily. He had a place to work away at his second career in earnest. *The Torch* was scheduled to come out in the fall, and it was "the best I can do at this stage & it thrills me." And he had another book project ready and waiting. He was free at last.

CHAPTER ELEVEN

Champion of the Old Order

~~~ SECOND CAREERS

For the moment, the writing of *The Torch* had exhausted his imagination, and he had no urge to start on another novel. In the preparations for his retirement, as he cast about for some new writing project, one dropped into his lap.

In May, 1959, a letter arrived from Alan Gregg's widow. Alan had died in 1957, and now she wrote to ask: "Have you thought sometimes, during the past almost two years now...that writing a biography of Alan might interest you? The idea is not new to me. In fact I've had it on my mind for some time to write you on the subject. Alan's biography could be a fine, interesting, delightful, worthwhile undertaking for someone who knew and admired and loved him, someone who, as a scientist, understood his work, someone who, as a friend, thought of him in terms far broader than his career with the Rockefeller Foundation, someone with the light touch.... Nothing would make me happier than to learn that 'someone' might be you."

"As Alan would say," she added, "don't answer until you pass through the negative stage." Her timing could hardly have been better. Wilder passed through the "negative stage" while he was preparing to leave the Institute and realizing just what a big step he was taking. It was one thing to write romantic novels when it was just "playing hooky," as he put it, from his professional life. It was quite another to write that sort of thing full time. Now that he was to be a full time writer, it occurred to him that he should perhaps be looking for a more dignified subject, one more suited to an eminent doctor of advancing years.

A biography of his old friend Alan Gregg, who had persuaded the Rockefeller Foundation to back the proposal for a neurological institute so many years ago, would be a way of repaying Gregg while giving Wilder a subject that was unquestionably respectable. What's more, he could use Gregg's life as a vehicle to write about medical education and philanthropy, the "difficult art of giving," to use the modest phrase coined by John D. Rockefeller.

In November he wrote to the Guggenheim Foundation to apply for a grant to write about Gregg, medical education and philanthropy, and in February of 1960 while in New York he made a detour to the Rockefeller Foundation to talk to the president, Dean Rusk. Rusk explained that the Rockefeller Foundation doesn't go in for memorials to former employees. They had once made a grant to a writer for a history of the Foundation's General Education Board, and the writer returned the favour by calling it *Escaping From the Baptists* (John D. Rockefeller was a Baptist and much of his original philanthropy was through the Baptist Church). Besides, Rusk pointed out, biography was difficult—he did not add "more so than writing romances," but the implication was there—and what made Penfield think he could write a good biography?

Rusk could hardly have given Wilder a better reason to say yes to Mrs. Gregg. They talked on, and Rusk eventually agreed that the foundation would open the files, subject to whatever censorship the board decided was necessary after viewing the contents.

In March, though still not committed to the project, the Penfields went to see Mrs. Gregg at her house at Big Sur, California. She showed him into Gregg's study and wisely left him alone to explore. He found an unfinished autobiography, a charming children's story and Gregg's private writings: book after book filled with notes to himself, aphorisms, witty observations on his colleagues at the foundation and people he met, and much more. It was a goldmine, and Wilder was sold. He left for Montreal with the lot—over a hundred pounds of paper, neatly packed into trunks.

Soon after he returned, the Guggenheim Foundation awarded him $30,000 over three years to write the book. Wilder sorted the material out in his office at the M.N.I., shut the door, and began working.

He took his second career as a writer as seriously as he had his first, and his expectations were just as high. The only justification for being a writer, was to be a good writer. He wanted to master the craft, and have his ability recognized by literary awards, critical praise and book sales. Only a wide and admiring audience would satisfy him.

In September the advance copies of *The Torch* arrived at Magog Meadows while he was out sailing with one of his grandsons in the annual Labour Day Regatta. He and Helen went off by themselves to her dressing room in the boathouse and opened the package. It was the first time she'd seen the dedication: "To H.K.P.—wise critic and good companion." The cover was fine, they decided, and the words inside were his all right, but leafing through it later in his study, it seemed as though the characters spoke their own lines and all he'd done was "described the setting and polished their thoughts and rang the curtain up and down." The reaction to the book was now the important thing: "What this book seems to critic and public may determine my plan for the next ten years."

If he had been willing to settle for more modest success with *The Torch* he would have had every reason to be delighted with its reception. It was published three weeks later in Canada and the U.S., and was followed by a British and a Dutch edition. It was reviewed just about everywhere in Canada and abroad in such august journals as *The New Yorker*, *The New Statesman*, *The New York Times* and *The London Times*. Some of the reviewers were a trifle condescending, but the majority were quite enthusiastic about the book. The worst criticisms were that his touch was a little heavy in places ("The stilted romance is only a slight imperfection in a work that is based on careful research and written by an eminent physician") and that some of his assumptions were questionable ("Perhaps Hippocrates has been too much assimilated to Mr. Penfield's scholarly temperament, perhaps he made his discoveries with less equanimity than Mr. Penfield shows.")

The reviewer in *The New York Times*, on the other hand, spoke for a fair number of the others in his review: "It is not because Dr. Penfield understands medical practices and the process of the medical mind that he has written an excellent book," he wrote. "It is not because he understands the zest of contest. The book is excellent because of its human story—a story that is both moving and suspenseful."

There followed translations into half a dozen languages in the Soviet Union, and even an option from a Hollywood producer. It was, as one reader remarked, "as good a picture of Victorian Greece as any." In *The Torch* he had, in fact, drawn rather heavily on his own life—to the point of writing about Hippocrates and his courtship of Daphne in phrases remarkably like his own diary account of his courtship of Helen Kermott by the Saint Croix River fifty years earlier.

And though the book went into paperback and would continue to sell for years, the sales were disappointing to Wilder, who had hoped for much more. It sold around 15,000 copies in Canada, and perhaps half that many in the U.S.—substantial for a book written by an old doctor, but certainly not enough, in his view, for a professional writer. Besides, for all the praise *The Torch* received, he wrote, "not a single prize in the U.S.A. or Canada. It lacks something I can almost understand....If I could understand it clearly and fully I could rid myself of the deficiencies." And again, later, "Probably there is a more fundamental failing that I shall never understand."

For a while he kept a copy by his bed and read a few pages before he went to sleep, trying to figure out what was wrong with it, but that only led to nightmares in which he struggled to write better. It was dispiriting, but eventually he resigned himself to not being a novelist. He would continue to write, though, and by now Gregg's biography was taking up more and more of his time and effort.

Wilder spent six years puzzling through the life of Alan Gregg, working at it off and on in binges whenever he wasn't away giving a lecture or accepting one more degree or consulting on a patient or advising on some problem at the Institute. Hoping to make the book a major statement on the things that occupied Gregg, as well as on Gregg himself, Wilder dug into the history of the Rockefeller Foundation, travelled around the U.S. and Europe interviewing former employees of the foundation who had known Gregg, sifting through the mountain of material that accumulated in his files. Alan Gregg was full of surprises, he discovered.

Growing up in Colorado Springs during a period of bitter union struggles, he had listened eagerly to fiery union orators as they cursed John D. Rockefeller and the other capitalists—and later he had become Rockefeller's representative. Gregg had gone into medicine but discovered he didn't want to be a doctor, and became instead, a man, to quote from Wilder's introduction to the biography, "inevitably set apart from his fellows. Thirty years ago, his arrival in any medical school sent a ripple of excitement through the faculty, from the dean down to the hopeful experimenter and teacher. He brought with him the possibility of a grant from the greatest of all philanthropic foundations. His very name when heard in academic conversation had the warm overtones of hoped-for favours. He liked to compare himself with the banker's daughter who wondered whether suitors loved her for herself alone."

Gregg voted socialist; son of a Congregational minister he stopped believing in God; he wrote a sweet children's story about a kingdom called "Trobania" populated by little creatures six inches high, and filled his diaries with biting portraits of the high and mighty in whose company his work obliged him to spend many weary hours.

During the six long years of the writing, Wilder's interest in Gregg and the book waxed and waned over and over; and he doubted he could do it, doubted its worth and wondered if he would ever, ever finish it. In May, 1962, on a train to Rome he wrote, "Sometimes I am tempted to realize I am an old man, but I don't do it. It's like looking over a bridge to discover the stream is now far below in a gorge and the railing is rotten, and you grow dizzy. No. I'll keep on...continue the romance. It is fun. It may look like comedy to others perhaps." In September, 1963, he wrote in the same vein, "I refuse to accept what may be evidence of slow, stupid performance. I will not take No for an answer, but will go on and will finish, *Deo Volente*. This could be a wonderful book." Only four chapters were written, and a month later, when Hugh MacLennan called to say with infuriating confidence that he was off to France and Greece to write a novel in seven months, Wilder issued himself a challenge: "Can I finish the Gregg biography in that length of time? I think I can." And then more interruptions, and instead of finishing, a year later this weary note: "Back to the Gregg grind until the damned thing is finished."

As the years passed, the rumblings of the world outside grew more and more insistent, distracting him from Gregg's biography to put this thought or that theory into a paper and then stand in front of an audience and speak. From each foray he returned with greater impatience to the book and its demands. And yet, curiously, it was probably the best writing he would ever do. It was not the sort of verbal brilliance from which you can pluck a phrase and say "there, that's what I mean," but a fine and exuberant portrait of a very interesting man. Its strength was a certain consistency—he had learned to write—and an eye for scenes that make Alan Gregg's story come alive.

Here is his description of Gregg's arrival, a sandy-haired and freckled freshman, at Harvard in 1907:

"From Boston over the Harvard Bridge to Cambridge, the electric streetcars were clanging along, full to their doors. In front of the college gates, Harvard Square—which was triangular and not square at all—was crowded. Cabdrivers shouted and cracked their whips, and there was a general din of greetings and laughter. An automobile of the steam variety came puffing through the throng; a horn was squawked and a cabbie shouted as his frightened horse reared. But Alan Gregg, crossing the square with his loose-swinging stride, entered the gates oblivious of everything except the importance of the moment. Here he was at last in his own right."

The book has the ring of authority and familiarity: Gregg's life and Wilder's own had crossed and crisscrossed so many times, not just in connection with the grant to build the Montreal Neurological Institute. They had in common their age and the important fact that both came from the outside—one from the West, one from the Midwest—in the first decade of the century, to big Eastern colleges and the fast and heady life where rich young princes from old East Coast families held sway. They had friends in common, ideals in common, a shared humour and the same odd innocence. In writing about Gregg and the medical world in which he had been so important, Wilder often found he was writing about himself. The fundamental difference between Wilder and Alan Gregg was Gregg's detachment: he had more faith in human nature and less in himself than had his biographer. Whereas with age Gregg's detachment grew, Wilder's concern and his compulsion to involve himself in the world increased as he grew older. Society in the sixties was to a certain extent a product of science in the fifties. Technological advances had helped create an increasingly affluent society—and all of its problems. What disturbed Wilder even more was that science, by seeming to hold out the promise of an answer to every question, a solution to every problem, had pushed religion into the background. As a scientist, he felt responsible for science's part, and felt that he must do something, somehow, to help restore lost faith, traditional values.

When the anti-Establishment protests began, he took them personally too—it was his world and his values that they were challenging. Politically, he was no hard-headed Jeffersonian democrat, determined to evoke an intelligent, open discussion of ideas. Rather, he was a prairie fundamentalist—passionate, certain, closed-minded and conservative.

On the subject of morals and manners he grew more and more disturbed as the years passed. They mattered a great deal to him, not as social conveniences, but as representing an entire set of values he held to, strictly and utterly. And in the 1960s, morals and manners were the first casualties of change. His reaction was, in short, like that of many other seventy-year-olds viewing the 1960s with alarm and dismay. The difference was that he had an audience, and the vanity to think that he could, as he would write, "change the course of civilization."

This attitude set the patterns for the years ahead, as he struggled with one threat after another to his view of the world. As he worked on the biography of Alan Gregg, a strange reversal gradually took place. The book became his official occupation and took on the role the Institute and its affairs had formerly played. Travelling, making speeches, and writing essays about the modern world and what was wrong with it became his escape from routine—now the routine of biography writing. The public speeches grew into something quite new and exciting. The invitations began to pour in to his office at the Institute. In a country that pays inordinate respect to doctors, a famous retired surgeon and scientist who could actually *talk* was a real catch.

And he could talk. He prepared for each address as carefully as if he were preparing for a delicate and complicated operation, spending days and sometimes weeks on his research, writing out the text carefully on cards, keeping a few with jokes or amusing anecdotes to one side in case the audience's attention wavered. He obstinately refused to talk down to his listeners when the topic had some reference to scientific theories, and he had nothing but contempt for 'high-falutin' jargon, scientific or other. Instead he said what he had to say in the simplest plain English, trusting to the audience's intelligence and his own oratorical skill. As he spoke, in his soft, clear voice with just a trace, still, of a midwestern drawl, in the back of his mind he was constantly taking the audience's pulse: "How am I doing? Did they like that?" Helen usually sat near the front and on the way home they would go over the speech and the audience's reaction, making notes for the next time.

And though the fat manilla file in his desk in which he collected material for his talks was labelled "NONSENSE MATERIAL," the label was more in the nature of a warning to himself not to let the success go to his head than an accurate reflection of his attitude to public speaking. If anything, these speeches gradually become more important to Wilder than the biography or the steady flow of scientific lectures.

His career as a public speaker began fairly predictably with talks on "A Doctor's Philosophy"; they progressed to "The Second Career" and "The Uses of Idleness," reflecting his thoughts about his own life and retirement, and they took on a more urgent note as his sense of foreboding about the state of the world grew during the 1960s: "The Changing Purposes of Youth," "Mankind in the Atomic Age," "The Family and the Moral Fibre of a Nation," "Canada at the Crossroads—Alliance or Civil War?"

But long before the name Penfield became attached to such controversial subjects, he had made a speech that more than any other catapulted him into the public consciousness in his new role as a public speaker. The title was "Pseudo-Senility: Osler's Dictum Reconsidered," and it was delivered as a challenge to the whole prevailing notion of old age and retirement barely a few months before he himself publicly retired from the Institute.

Fifty-five years before, Osler had made his final address at Johns Hopkins Medical School before stepping down as director, taking as the title for his parting words "The Fixed Period," from Trollope's fanciful novel about a college of men who agreed that each of them would be chloroformed on reaching the age of sixty.

"I have two fixed ideas," Osler said at the farewell dinner. "The first is the comparative uselessness of men above forty years of age....My second fixed idea is the uselessness of men above sixty years of age, and the incalculable benefit it would be in commercial, political and in professional life if, as a matter of course, men stopped work at this age." Then, tongue in cheek, he went on: "As it can be maintained that all the great advances have come from men under forty, so the history of the world shows that a very large proportion of the evils may be traced to sexagenarians...all of the worst poems, most of the bad pictures, a majority of the bad novels, not a few of the bad sermons and, I hesitate to add, speeches."

All of this Wilder quoted in his speech, and then went on to describe how the papers had picked it up and run headlines saying "MEN USELESS AFTER FORTY," and "SHOULD BE CHLOROFORMED AT SIXTY." The phrase "Oslerizing the aged" entered the language, and in St. Louis a man of sixty killed himself, leaving an empty chloroform bottle and newspaper clippings referring to Osler's speech on the bed beside him. Osler apologized publicly, but maintained his conviction that by the age of forty a person's most productive days were done, and that after sixty it would be better for everyone if they "rested from their labours."

All this was the launching pad for Wilder's own vehemently different views on the subject: "Let me describe to you the evolution of a little-recognized disease. It is a psychological malady which we might name *pseudo-senility* or *false senility*.

"A worthy citizen employed in business, for example, or in industry or education or government, reaches his time of statutory retirement. Some colleague, who happens to have a larger bank account of unspent years, comes to him and gives him a gold watch and tells him to take a well-earned rest. That man, who yesterday was busy and capable of contributing something that was of value, now stays home. He mows the lawn and carries out the garbage for his wife while he thinks about his future. When he is well-behaved she lets him wash the dishes. He notices that his recent memory is not as good as it was when he was younger, although distant memory is good enough. He doesn't know that this is caused by the fact that the hippocampal gyrus in the temporal lobe of each side of the brain often suffers interference in its circulation, while the rest of the brain is as good as ever for many years to come.

"Perhaps, then," Wilder went on, "some friend who is well-meaning but devoid of a sense of humour comes to comfort him. 'Enjoy yourself,' he says; 'that is all there remains for you to do. Just have a good time.' Then, in a little while, people begin to say, behind his back of course: 'He is going to pieces, poor fellow.' And so he is, fast.

"The whole trouble," Wilder concluded, "was that what he needed when he was given the gold watch was a new job, a difficult job—not a rest. Beyond the normal rhythm of work and sleep, rest was not what he needed. Rest, with nothing else, results in rust. It corrodes the mechanisms of the brain. The rhubarb that no one picks goes to seed."

Citing the examples of soldiers-turned-statesmen like Eisenhower and De Gaulle, of Verdi composing his greatest operas between seventy-four and eighty, and Michelangelo painting the Last Judgment at sixty, Wilder ended with the example of Winston Churchill, who when he reached seventy-nine was too busy with his second career to go to Stockholm to accept the Nobel Prize for work in the field of his second career as a writer. "His wife had to pick up the Prize for him as though it were a notice from the post office!"

"To most men," Wilder concluded, "there should come a time for shifting harness, for lightening the load one way and adjusting it for greater effort in another. This is the time for the second career, time for the old dog to perform new tricks. The new career may bring in little or no money; it may be concerned only with good works. It may, on the other hand, bring in support that is much needed. It can be a delight to a man, who comes at last to a well-earned job instead of a well-earned rest. It can be, too, what society needs most from him.

"The problem to set before the wise men of today is simply this: How can each individual be given the chance to work? Sometimes the race is not to the swift nor the battle to the strong. It may be that the last work of the old man's hands will serve society best—and him as well."

This speech hit a nerve. A reporter from The Canadian Press news service wrote a story about it that was picked up across Canada and the U.S. In the next few years Wilder was invited to give the same speech half a dozen more times. The reprints were in great demand, and it became the title of his first published collection of addresses in 1963.

The speech was successful not so much because he was saying

something startlingly new, but because of the scientific edge he added—that and the fact that he himself was a living example of what he preached. It was in character for him not to be satisfied with quietly going about his second career, but instead to formulate a theory about second careers, drawing rather arbitrarily on his understanding of how the brain worked—knowing that what he said at this point would be taken as gospel. While no neurologist would dispute that the brain, like any organ, benefits from continued normal use and atrophies if unused, it was a purely personal interpretation that made Wilder regard quiet reading, pottering around the house and contemplation as insufficient use of the brain. Similarly, while it is true that the acquisition of new skills calls on previously unused areas of the brain, it was stretching things a bit to conclude that "the 'old dog' will increase his previous capacity by taking on a challenging new job," as he put it.

But to the public he was speaking as a scientist who had devoted his life to the study of the brain. He could coin phrases like "pseudo-senility," and "retirement neurosis" with easy assurance. He was a scientist, what's more, who spoke in comfortable homilies: "The rhubarb that no one picks goes to seed"; "Rest, with nothing else, results in rust." The prescription made such good, common *sense*, and it spoke directly to a large proportion of the population in North America during those years, those who were, in the words of the head of the United Auto Workers Walter Reuther, "too old to work, too young to die." By mid-decade in North America, those over the age of fifty numbered over fifty million, and in an era that adored youth and all its fashions and ideas, its music and its politics, the over-fifties were a disenfranchised, puzzled and resentful group who took Wilder Penfield very seriously. He was one of their own, after all, for all his elevated status as a scientist, and he spoke about the things that concerned them: the problems of growing old, the immorality of youth, the importance of religion and faith, the increasing lack of respect for authority and tradition. They were the people who crowded into meetings of The Canadian Club, the Empire Club or the Rotary Club to listen eagerly to what Penfield had to say, and it was they who bought his novels, and his collections of essays on the modern world and what was wrong with it.

While for some of us even the phrase "The Sixties" has the ring of reckless energy, the bursting excitement of new ideas and grand schemes, and a deep and abiding nostalgia for lost innocence, those were not years from which a seventy-year-old man with strong conservative views of morality and social intercourse would derive either much pleasure or much reassurance.

At the beginning of May, 1960, a crowd of students at the

University of Texas in Galveston moved into the Jack Tar Hotel and spent the night splashing in the pool, drinking beer, and shrieking with laughter. Tomorrow was "Splash Day" and they were getting an early start. The ruckus kept the Visiting Professor from Montreal awake until 4 A.M., "worrying about young people who go in for body exhibitionism, alcohol and casual sexual encounters. They didn't even sing."

Two months later he was in Paris doing some interviews for the biography; he was "shocked at the bearded, sandalled, strange young men and the young girls who walked about the streets and let crude youths maul them continuously in public, and stop for long, slobbering kisses....Such actions are an offence that would make ancient Greek and modern communist, Indian and caveman no doubt, blush." It offended his midwestern prudery, but more than that this behaviour seemed a dangerous portent of a general breakdown. "Ancient Rome must have been like this in its last years."

Those were the unrestrained notations in his diary, but two months after that, in September 1960, he spoke from a podium in a crowded auditorium and pointed a finger at the culprit: "We all know that the minds of men can be influenced by teaching and preaching, by conversation and suggestion. Communist countries use propaganda to create a conscience in their citizens that will make them loyal to the state's own ideology. There's no advertising there....That is a capitalistic phenomenon. Our advertising propaganda, with a little assistance from TV and with publishers' overtones, includes a bombardment of invitations to strong drink, the misuse of sex, the thrill of crime."

He was in fact at a medical conference, a rather unusual one. It was called "Great Issues of Conscience in Modern Medicine," and to address the subject Dartmouth College had assembled a group that included people like the geneticist Hermann Müller; scientist-authors like C. P. Snow and René Dubos; Aldous Huxley; an ambassador; several psychologists and psychiatrists; politicians and professors; and powerful men from the government agencies and foundations that direct and finance scientific research of all kinds. Each had been chosen because he had somewhere, in some public forum, expressed a concern with the moral and ethical questions facing science. And if the fifties had been a decade of great scientific advances, the sixties were beginning as a decade of grave doubts about the Pandora's Box that had been opened.

It was a concern that ranged from Huxley's frightening portrayal of the future in *Brave New World* to the crusades of Hermann Müller, who had won the Nobel Prize for his classical experiments demonstrating the effects of X-rays in 1946 and had gone on to become a campaigner against the dangers his discoveries held for the human race.

As for Penfield, he had long since, in forums like the BBC symposium on "The Physical Basis of Mind," established his credentials for such a gathering. In recent years his interest in the broader aspects of his work had taken on an edge of anxiety as he witnessed the assimilation of his discoveries about the brain into psychology to rationalize a view of humanity that dismissed out of hand the belief—so dear to him—that beyond the physical matter there was an intangible, spiritual essence as well. To a degree his research is still used that way, as Richard Restak pointed out in 1979 in his book *The Brain: The Last Frontier*. Restak, knowing how this view of Wilder's work contradicted his intent, wrote: "Ironically, Wilder Penfield is still erroneously cited as an exponent of the view that the mind can be reduced to some sort of clockwork mechanism within the brain."

The Dartmouth Conference was divided into three separate areas of discussion: "Man and His Environment," "Man's Biological Future" and "The Issues Involved in Influencing the Mind." Wilder had been invited to speak on the last topic. The various addresses generated considerable heat and only a little light on an array of extremely complex topics. The first panel discussion debated issues that have a very familiar ring twenty-odd years later: smog, industrial waste, nuclear waste, nuclear fallout; short-term advantages versus long-term effects; who makes the decisions and on what basis; who is to control the levers of the machines that make modern industrial societies work, and on and on. Likewise, the second panel in which the ethical questions were malnutrition and its effects; population control; the touchy issue of mass sterilization in poor, developing countries.

In the third area of discussion, "Influencing the Mind," there was, if possible, even less agreement than there had been in the others—not surprising when the vagueness of the subject is considered. Rather than force the speakers to address directly one aspect of the issue, the idea behind the conference seems to have been to simply provide a rough framework and allow the distinguished speakers to go where they wished. Thus, one speaker proposed that World War Three might be prevented by obliging heads of state to prove that they were speaking the truth, in moments of international crisis, by submitting themselves to lie-detector tests. Another, a psychiatrist, took as his subject "Rage, Violence and Conscience," and the premise that the greatest problem in the modern world, where individual heads of state had the power to obliterate life on the planet, was to control the fit of rage that might bring on the end.

Wilder began his speech by dismissing the possibility that science could, or ever would, be able to control the mind, summarizing briefly his own experiments with conscious patients and concluding that if the electric probe could not convince someone to believe anything, than brain-washing and mind-control were so much nonsense. From there he passed to a matter he considered more important, the responsibility of medical scientists in the modern world, harkening back to Hippocrates and the standards he had set for those who followed:

"Now the essence of the Hippocratic Oath is this: *'I will keep pure and holy both my life and my art.'* What an extraordinary thing that was and in the fifth century before Christ. There were rules for behaviour, too, but the kernal of it was this: 'I will keep pure and holy both my life and my art.' Hippocrates meant this to serve physicians as an ethical guide during the practice of medicine and at other times. He did not attempt to derive his ethics from the little he knew of science. Teachers of other arts in Greece called upon their disciples to sign an indenture as apprentices—the sculptors, the poets, the Sophists, the philosophers—but none, as far as I can discover, added an ethical resolution to the indenture. But it could not be otherwise. Medicine dealt with life and with men and women and children, not with marble, and rhythms or abstract concepts. Physicians looked into the heart and minds of patients and of those close to the bedside, at a time when they are most vulnerable, most in need of counsel. To influence them for the good of society is part of the art of medicine. But the code of medical ethics and the conscience thus created is not enough to guide the race of man, now moving so swiftly in the stream of social evolution. The meanings we read in the study of nature are not clear enough to guide us. The study of the brain has not explained the mind and science can neither prove, or disprove the existence of the spirit of man and of God. Therefore, we must act in the light we have.

"It was said at the opening meeting of this symposium, 'Science cannot be immoral and science cannot create morality.' This is true, but philosophical and religious thought has been retarded by the general impression that science had proven something in this sphere. Physician and scientist must make reasoned conclusions each for himself.

Let us take, then, the best conclusions of the past and create a working religion—a faith that will seem reasonable to all men—one they will welcome. How? I do not know. The world has need of great religious leaders, men who, like Gandhi, will discard no good thing in the faith of Christian, Mohammedan or Hindu, men who will show us how to live by our beliefs.

"As Hippocrates turned from the practice of a profession to a code of ethics, so must all men turn from the rush of life to discover a reasonable faith. Only an interpretation of religion suited to these times can create in the hearts of men of every nation a better conscience. Make them see that they must love their fellow man everywhere or be destroyed. Only this, I say, can save this unbridled generation rushing on—confused—to self-destruction."

Wilder's speech was a hit with the audience—professors and their spouses, students, and members of the public—and a bit of a puzzle to the other scientists among the speakers. As the chairman of the discussion, Ralph Gerard, a professor of psychiatry and physiology remarked dryly when the applause died down, "Thank you, Dr. Penfield, you have obviously struck a receptive chord in the audience. You have said some of the things that many people here, I think, have been hoping someone would say, and I'm not sure all the rest of us would say them." Sir Charles Snow commented at the end of the conference that Penfield was the only one who turned to religion, while "the rest of us have not the help of this but should be called, I suppose, humanists."

His religious faith did indeed give Wilder at least the comfort of a clear starting point for discussions like this one at the Dartmouth Conference. But over the next few weeks he turned back to his diary several times with questions his speech had raised in his own mind. Although he was an elder of the Presbyterian Church, his criticism of organized religion in general was growing less restrained: "The Unitarians offer a very exciting approach to truth and the personal worship of God without symbols and mysticism, but see what small progress they have made in a century. I would join that church if it were not for the apparent insult to the Presbyterians. Perhaps we shall anyway."

And then, later: "No! The movement that might spread and succeed with all men of all nations must be extra-church—devoted to the fellowship of man as an ideal, the love of man—to thinking like the thought of Christ. His philosophy and message is walled about by ecclesiastical forms and choked up there, available only to those who belong to the self-chosen. He should be born again outside the wall of churches. Then he might speak again to all men as Gandhi began to do."

Wilder was in full swing by now. If his willingness to leap across chasms separating science from philosophy, philosophy from religion, religion from politics—as much by dismissing the chasms as illusory, as by any particular skill as a dialectician—tended to isolate him more and more from his scientific colleagues, it delighted what he referred to more than once as "the most conservative elements." It brought a host of other invitations to speak, and encouraged him to speak in ever larger and more sweeping terms.

In January of 1961 he was one of the keynote speakers in a symposium called "Man and Civilizations: Control of the Mind" held at the University of California School of Medicine, San Francisco. His speech there was an update of the 1950 BBC address on "The Physical Basis of the Mind," ending with the same stubborn insistence that science had not yet answered the fundamental questions, and restating his conviction that the ultimate answer would be an affirmation of God's existence rather than the reverse: "In attempting to describe the physiological basis of the mind here in San Francisco before this great symposium...my predicament is like that of a certain astronomer who was invited to inaugurate the proceedings of a religious gathering by describing God's handiwork in outer space. There is a relationship. But it is difficult to define!"

Some months later Wilder was invited to speak at a symposium in Montreal under the heading "Mankind in the Atomic Age." He had to choose between the symposium and a meeting of the International Neurological Congress in Washington, D.C. He cancelled his plans to go to Washington and set to work. He called his address "Let Us Wage an Offensive of Human Understanding and Friendship," and argued that such an offensive was the only way of "winning this cold war."

His solution to the Cold War with the U.S.S.R. was "an uprising of people who have no desire to proselytize and who are willing to discover that the philosophy and social system and religion on the other side suits their needs there as ours suit us." Specifically, he proposed that Canada and the U.S. recognize Red China, that Russian and Chinese courses be widespread in towns and universities across the continent and that a large-scale program of exchange visits be instituted so that doctors, lawyers, engineers, teachers, businessmen, farmers, artists, religious leaders and athletes could meet and get to know their counterparts in the rest of the world. He was doing it, why couldn't the rest of them? The long-awaited return to China was now scheduled for July, 1962, and as Helen noted in her round-robin letter a few weeks later, the "offensive of human understanding and friendship" was the purpose of the trip, "little as it may accomplish." As it turned out, Wilder wouldn't have to wait more than a couple of months to put his words into action with a great deal of drama and publicity.

Near the end of February, just weeks after his seventy-first birthday, he and Helen had planned to go skiing in the Laurentians with Wilder Jr. and his family. But a great blizzard began in the night and by morning the roads out of the city were closed off; they were forced to wait at home, listening to the weather reports. While they were waiting an urgent phone call came from the Soviet Embassy. Professor Lev Landau, a distinguished Soviet theoretical physicist and one of the key scientists in the Soviet space program, had been badly hurt in a car accident. Would he fly over immediately for a consulation? Never mind visas, all he needed was his passport. Off he went. The press got wind of it, and at the airport television cameras and reporters waited to record "Penfield's Mission of Mercy." Seven hours to London, then a three-hour delay by a blizzard there as well, then four hours to Moscow. A delegation from the Soviet Academy met him at the airport and whisked him directly to the hospital. Landau's pupils and colleagues had descended with nurses and technicians and equipment on the small Moscow hospital where he had been brought, and Penfield found several dozen of them waiting anxiously when he arrived.

It was by now after four in the morning, Montreal time, and he had not slept on the plane, but the consultation began immediately. It was the physicists who had insisted on bringing in Penfield, as well as a distinguised neurologist and a neurosurgeon from Paris—not trusting their own surgeons, Wilder guessed. Here is his account of what followed:

"They gave me the history. I examined Landau with the room packed. We returned for consultation. Prof. Garcin with typical scholarly exactness outlined the location of the lesions deep in the R. & L. hemisphere....I sensed a good deal of tension.

"Finally I could only say that the anatomy described by Garcin must be correct but since there might be a round clot still making some pressure near midbrain and since physicians could be wrong and since the outlook of the patient was hopeless unless something was done, I would transfer him to the Neurosurgical Institute and carry out a ventriculogram at once. Every sentence was translated into Russian by Lifschitz (the physicist in charge and Landau's closest friend and colleague). Finally I said risks were of no importance. If the patient were my father I would do that and probably only learn that there was nothing to do but possibly a slight chance of better life."

His verdict was received sombrely, and he left them to digest it while he went to the Ukraine Hotel for a bit of supper and to get some sleep. The phone rang the next morning at ten. It was one of the Russian neurologists calling to say that they had summoned a neurosurgeon from Prague, Professor Koontz, and would Wilder be able to go immediately to talk to Professor Kapitza, another physicist, who was anxious to have a word with him. Giving up any hope of breakfast, he agreed. An hour later he was being driven with Lifschitz into a compound on the outskirts of Moscow, through remote-controlled gates and up to a large stone house:

"Lifschitz rang, and a shrill barking resulted. Finally a man opened the door and stood waiting with a little Pekinese dog. Lifschitz left us and Kapitza led me through a bare hall into an enormous study and library. Enormous windows looked out on a river on one side, and an orchard on the other. An enormous desk was heaped with books and papers. There were two of the largest overstuffed chairs I have ever seen in front of a stone fireplace. He motioned me to one and he collapsed in the other.

"'These chairs were brought from England. They don't make comfortable chairs anywhere else.'

"Peering over the top of the arm of my chair I could see only his face, a rugged, smiling face with a rounded nose and chin and long brown hair that fell over his eyes and was often brushed away. He laughed and we recalled friends in Cambridge....

"He jumped up and opened a drawer filled with photographs in great disorder. He found pictures of Landau, a tall, thin alert man with strong aquiline features and a reflective smile. 'If an operation is necessary, who will do it? Will you? You have authority. They will do what you say. They are afraid to touch him. If they did and Landau should die...Egorov, well, young men are sometimes better.' I realized that although I had said the night before that there was nothing to lose, there were some there who were worried about such a decision..."

The decision had been left to Wilder. After lunch they returned to the hospital, where he found Landau's wife waiting. "She entered the room with me, and the nurse stood aside. The patient's left arm was making slow, sinuous movements, the right hand was clutched against his side. He breathed through a tracheotomy tube, another small tube, for feeding probably, emerged from his nose. His face was turned away and the chin moved slightly, rhythmically.

"She took his left hand and bent over him and I leaned close over her shoulder. Landau's eyes turned slowly toward her, and focused on her. She spoke in Russian. He nodded slightly and looked then at me, focusing. I moved my head and the eyes followed. Then his head turned away out of contact again.

"Outside the room another woman, a friend, joined us. The wife took my hand and held it and spoke. The friend said in English, 'She says she believes in you as though you were God. She knows you will help him.'

"I have taken time to describe that. So many times those about a seriously ill patient say things like that. I suppose they do to all doctors. We pass it off and forget it. But now when I am at the end of a medical career I have set it down this time. How often people look into your eyes searching, pleading for strength and ability to do something for one they love. Sometimes the impossible. But always I have been sure I could comfort, point to a ray of hope that seems to fall into the darkness of every desperate struggle for life.

"How long since she saw her husband?

'This is the first time in more than a month.' No more explanation. Lifschitz coming up said, 'She has been ill'; something unexplained in the situation, curious...

"Back in conference, Prof. Koontz from Prague now added to the medical chorus. I thought Graschenko [the head neurologist] would talk. No one did. I looked around at the silent people and finally at Graschenko.

"'You speak,' he said.

"'The man is better. He knew his wife and understood something. Since he seems better, I withdraw my suggestion of ventriculography.' Egorov [the neurosurgeon who would have been the likely candidate for such an operation] nodded violently, his face all smiles.

"'I would transfer him at once to the Neurosurgical Institute, use physiotherapy, and increase activity. I think he will steadily improve. I believe he is not aphasic [speechless]....'

I wonder what they thought. They would have carried out the radical steps they feared if I had insisted. The physicists were, I suspect, disappointed.

If this were Montreal, Wilder concluded, and the facilities of the Montreal Neurological Institute were available, he would have gone ahead with the ventriculogram. But here there were too many elements beyond his control.

(Landau would never really recover. A year and a half later Wilder was passing through Moscow on the way back from China and paid Landau a visit. Struck by the tragic change in the brilliant mind of a man compared to Einstein in his broad grasp of mathematics, Wilder recorded the return visit as well. He found him "sitting up in bed in a fresh white shirt looking at me anxiously.... He had an air of understanding, he was stubborn in his confusion and I could appreciate why he asked Lifschitz to bring him poison several months ago.... When I asked Landau if he had received the Lenin Prize he said yes but could not tell me when. When I asked him if someone had shared it with him he looked around and, finding Lifschitz standing with the others, smiled and pointed to him. 'I think he and I shared it.'" Lifschitz had been Landau's disciple and co-worker, and seeing the grief in this man "who feels he has lost his closest friend and his leader" reminded Wilder of his own recent tragedy. "Their relationship seems a little like what Bill Cone and I once knew, and lost, alas.")

For three days his Russian hosts took him sightseeing and to look over the facilities in their hospitals and laboratories, and to long dinners in their homes. Finally, just as he was boarding the plane, a man and woman from the Soviet Academy rushed up, and pressed a package into his hands. He opened it up after takeoff and found a watch inside. "It was a gold wrist watch, a present from the Academy, no doubt the watch I don't want in lieu of the fee. But I am content to do what I can toward more mutual understanding. I want no fees for it." Which was just as well since none was offered, and after one or two times on his wrist, the watch stopped.

Wilder came back from the U.S.S.R. on the first of March, and set off again ten days later for Italy with Helen. They had been invited to spend two months in the Rockefeller Foundation's retreat for visiting scholars and writers, Villa Serbelloni, on Lake Como, to work on the Gregg biography. At the beginning of May, they headed back to Montreal, stopping for three or four days in London, where Wilder sat for a portrait commissioned by McGill University from the artist John Gilroy. That done, he and Helen returned to Montreal and spent the next two months preparing for the trip to China.

They prepared as they always did, reading books about the country, talking to people who had been there, going over Wilder's notes from the last trip in 1943. They were to be the guests of the Chinese Medical Association; obviously the Chinese hoped that he would return favourably impressed and one more influential ally in China's struggle for formal recognition by Canada and the U.S. "You will see what they want you to see, believe what they want you to believe," they were told by one of the China experts they consulted. Wilder dismissed that sort of cynicism out of hand, convinced that he would not be duped. "What he [the unidentified China expert] had forgotten," Wilder wrote on his return in an article 'A Doctor In Red China' for *Atlantic Monthly*, "is that the way to the truth about men and women is through friendly contact at first hand, rather than through analysis of data derived at a distance from spies and expatriates."

The plan was to go via Hawaii, New Zealand, Australia, Manila and Hong Kong, giving speeches and accepting more honorary degrees along the way. In China, the Penfields were to visit hospitals and colleges, lecture at various medical centres, and see the sights. It had been twenty-two years since they had seen Y. C. Chao, a Chinese neurosurgeon who had graduated from Peking Union Medical College and come to Montreal for two years, in 1937, to study at the Institute. Chao had become a friend, and they had kept in touch; it was he who had originally proposed this visit.

On September 12, with a film about Norman Bethune under his arm and reporters and photographers there to record the moment ("for going into China seems to be an event"), the Penfields left Hong Kong, walked across the short iron bridge over the Shumchun River and into China. They stayed for a month—a month, as usual, crowded with lectures and hospital tours, celebratory dinners and evenings at the theatre, exploring each new city on their itinerary, making several new friends, going on shopping expeditions, and stealing a moment now and then for Helen to send a few postcards and Wilder to scribble in his diary.

Their hosts commented frequently, Helen wrote with amusement, on such great energy for people "of such extreme age." As for the Penfields, the trip left them overwhelmed, puzzled, irritated, enchanted: "so much that is admirable mixed with such a profound misstatement of the intent of the U.S.," according to Wilder.

He had reacted with considerable skepticism to the arrangement that had been made to translate his lectures. The night before each lecture he would hand over the text and the accompanying slides. One of the young Chinese doctors appointed to the task would first translate and then memorize an hour or two-hour speech, which he delivered the next day without notes. These performances Wilder watched from a seat in the audience, sipping tea, marvelling at this demonstration of "superior brain power" while Chao, sitting beside him, compared the translation to the original. There were no mistakes.

The highlight of the visit came near the end, when the Penfields were invited to a formal dinner celebrating the thirteenth anniversary of the founding of the People's Republic of China, and met and spoke with Mao Tse-tung. They had shaken hands and exchanged greetings early in the evening. And though the only words Wilder could make out when an official presented him to the Chairman were "Norman Bethune"; the connection was enough to make Mao's face light up in a friendly smile. After a few polite questions, the officials moved the Penfields along, but a while later Mao came over alone to talk to them. As he approached, Helen caught Wilder's sleeve and whispered, "Tell him you have read his poetry." They shook hands again, Mao spoke; eventually Wilder's translator recovered sufficiently from his excitement to make a conversation possible, and Wilder did as his wife had suggested. Mao looked surprised, according to Wilder, and said, "I don't write anything very good." He did not speak again but looked off into the distance, then turned away slowly and walked off while people made way for him as he passed through the crowd and out of the room.

Something of Mao Tse-tung's presence, the combination of great power and quiet reflectiveness, impressed Wilder so strongly that, nine years later, he would leap to the Chairman's defence when news of his cancellation of the twenty-second anniversary parade came out of China, accompanied by wild rumours of Mao's death. In an article in the Montreal *Gazette*, Wilder would recount his meeting with Mao and write: "He is a man quite capable of calling a halt to the Peking parade...provided he thought it best for his people." There was no reason to conclude that he was "either mad or dead....He is to China what George Washington was to the United States." And though, nine years later, Wilder would have nothing but contempt for the resurgence of traditional Chinese medicine and the use of techniques like acupuncture, he would write: "There are more important things than scientific medicine. There is much that we in the West might sacrifice if we could only see our way to check the present moral and social trend toward decadence." But by that time China had passed through the Cultural Revolution. In the West the "horrid river" of immorality had burst its banks and Wilder Penfield had, at last, found a cause.

The next few years were to constitute a rare lull in the Penfields' busy lives—the lull before the storm. Although the travels continued, the trips were shorter and the itineraries less ambitious. They spent more and more time at the farm, and by half-past six each morning Wilder set to work in the refurbished writing house—now working away at the biography, pausing to write another article or a speech he had agreed to give, finishing the corrections to the galley proofs of *The Second Career*, his first collection of speeches, or polishing up a monograph on the brain. Helen was slowing down a bit, tiring more easily and plagued by the small ailments that come with advancing years, but keen as ever. Wilder, on the other hand, felt as fit at seventy as he had at sixty. For a time after the war he had developed a stiffness and soreness in his joints, and had started taking injections of testosterone. The male hormone drug not only kept the joint trouble at bay, he believed, but "also gives me drive in the rough and tumble of daily life, as well as in those matters which Aphrodite dwelt upon." So he had confided to his diary, and had added wryly, "Synthetic youth! I may break my neck skiing."

Whereas Wilder's diary erupted from time to time into angry tirades, Helen was a more phlegmatic observer, and her contributions to her college class's "round-robin" are a nice skipping summary of where their attention alighted. At the end of March, 1963, she wrote: "Since November 21st life has been interesting but more prosaic for us, with a steady background of writing for Wide; lectures, radio and T.V. broadcasts on everything from bilingualism—second careers—Science—Red China and euthenasia!" Wilder was President of the Association of Canadian Clubs, with chapters across the country which met regularly to hear speakers on various subjects, she reported, and he was the only speaker in the history of the Montreal branch to be invited back four times. He had accepted invitations from Yale, Bishop's University, Syracuse University and New York University for brief periods as Visiting Professor. In New York they had gone to the Museum of Modern Art to see slides of Le Corbusier's extraordinary buildings, and to half a dozen plays: *Photo Finish, Beyond the Fringe, A Man for All Seasons,* ("a *great* play,") *Threepenny Opera,* (which they walked out of in disgust during the intermission).

Lester Pearson had just been elected Prime Minister, she wrote in April: "We are very hopeful of the new regime.... But we are aghast at the growth of crime, from petty to bombing, which accompanies the accelerated growth of Montreal. We have every hope that the Separatist Movement will gradually settle down with Pearson at the helm.... Much fanfare in Montreal newspapers because a twenty-two-month old child won 1st prize at an Art Exhibition! Her father (also an artist) pasted a sheet of paper on the refrigerator, gave her some paints, and let her loose!"

In October they were off to spend a week with Paul Myers (from the Johnson Club days) in Pennsylvania, where they alternated between riding around the fields on the back of a tractor and having "heated argument of world affairs—revolution, civil rights, segregation, relationships between countries (ie. U.S.—Canada), Red China, Formosa, Korea, Indonesia, Malaysia. How much broader is our comprehension of the geography of the world than it was when Roosevelt urged us to get out our atlases as he gave his 'fireside talks' during the war! The others still think we were 'duped' in China. 'That is as may be!'"

They had gone to the spring meeting in Philadelphia, of the American Philosophical Society founded by Benjamin Franklin, who had hoped that the Society's meetings would help "promote useful knowledge." There were talks on everything from "The Origins of Chinese Law," "Symmetry and Finite Simple Groups," "Mesopotamian Historiography," to "Cuneiform Law and the History of Civilization" and "Molecular Relaxation Times." "One of the

Chairmen," Helen wrote, "expressed my feelings: 'I have never been so interested in so many things of which I have understood so little!'"

And so on: "Beatlemania has hit us hard but we count it more or less a blessing in disguise," with no further explanation, in April of 1964. And a note shortly after about the Chinese couple from Hong Kong who had come to work for them, neither of whom spoke much English. Despite the daily English lessons from Helen, there were still many puzzling conversations: "One night this week, Wide enquired of Yui Peng, 'Are you carving tonight or shall I?' He replied, 'I took the bus both ways.' But he is improving, and she is a dear and most intelligent. So we are hoping..." The rise of Barry Goldwater was noted with apprehension, and a dismissive column by Walter Lippmann syndicated to the Montreal *Gazette* was reported with relief.

In October of 1964, Helen's letter was full of news of a trip to Rome where they spent ten days. Wilder had been invited to join twenty-three scientists from around the world in a symposium organized by the newly formed Pontifical Academy of Sciences in Vatican City. The subject was "Brain and Consciousness," and at the end of the symposium, Helen wrote, the Pope "granted us all an audience and read a three-page address of his own on the changing attitude of the Church to Science."

A year later, a more sombre note: "In spite of strikes—of which we have had many in the last few months—gas-truckers, postal, etc., we build up an assurance that we are above warring. But when we were in Halifax in mid-June, on hearing booming cannons, we looked out our hotel windows at 6 o'clock one morning on a grim, grey, almost endless procession of USN battleships with sailors standing at attention from stem to stern. They were returning from NATO exercises." And an apology for the delay in writing, explaining that she had been interrupted "umpteen times. The last one was the arrival of Their Excellencies, the Governor-General and Madame Vanier for a 'quiet tea.' We heard a roar of motorcycles and opened the door with alarm—thinking there must be a fire nearby. No, just guardians! They were persuaded to leave the Vaniers in our care except for an extra car of plainclothesmen. But the two cars remained 'at the ready' for 1½ hours."

These were years of small victories and setbacks for Wilder. *The Second Career* was hardly a great publishing victory and certainly no financial success, but people read it and wrote to tell him how much it meant to them, which was something. The book, he noted, "carries my struggle to contribute to culture and civilization." He had turned back to Gregg's biography and the end was in sight, but "it is always what lies ahead that thrills me and challenges me and makes me feel unhappy when I am failing, happy and exultant when I surge ahead."

"What is driving me so restlessly at seventy-two? Some kind of devil I suppose. Helen says sometimes I see only my objectives—I see more and yet I drive on. But we stop and have more fun than anyone I know." *Time* Magazine had asked for an article on Red China, and had then rejected what he sent them: "Something wrong with my technique. What?" he wrote dejectedly. And then, when the weather was fine at the farm, and all the family was out, he wrote, "Our good fortune frightens me." There were fifteen grandchildren now, from infants to teenagers, gathered for at least a part of the summer at Magog Meadows. There were four houses apart from their own, plus a guesthouse and a log cabin that Jeff, their younger son, had built on a point of land jutting into the bay. Naming the houses was necessary, if only to spare their various visitors a great deal of confusion, and their own house at the top of the hill had been christened "Sussex House," after the ship. In these years, Wilder's grandchildren began to play an ever larger part in his life. In the days when they were younger—and fewer—he and Helen had each summer packed them all up in the station wagon and headed off with a picnic lunch to the Granby Zoo, several hours drive away, making up songs as they went. Now the grandchildren appeared at Sussex House on Sunday mornings with shorter skirts and longer hair, full of their own ideas and restless with his. The crowd at Sunday morning "Prayers" (a ritual he and Helen began when their own children were young as a substitute for Sunday church during summer holidays) now filled the living room and spilled over into the dining room. What formality there was—Wilder would read from the Bible, usually the Old Testament, and talk about whatever was on his mind for a few minutes, then they would all say a prayer and sing a hymn—had become more of a preamble to spirited conversations over coffee and doughnuts. And while he was not an easy man to talk to on touchy subjects like politics and morals, the grandchildren would come away each time puzzled by how *seriously* he took their arguments, and how vehemently he rebutted them when he disagreed. At summer's end when they scattered, there were letters of kindly advice, small sums of money as "stirrup cups" as one or another set off to college, letters of praise for a job won, a career chosen. Occasionally there were unhappy letters, often written late at night (sometimes sent only after the third or fourth draft)—letters to a granddaughter leaving home to live in rather too close proximity to a young man, or a grandson who left college to wander through North Africa with a sleeping bag and a knapsack.

All of this added an edge to Wilder's uneasiness about the world and rumblings from nearby and far away. The talk of something called The New Morality, the Cold War blowing hot, the Quiet Revolution in Quebec erupting noisily—all made it harder and harder for Wilder to return to the biography. And yet, as he wrote in his last diary entry for 1964, "HKP and I work on happily, if a little forgetful, and with just enough to live on to the end and the Hwangs caring for us and the house. I must finish the biography quickly. Perhaps there is still something more important to do. What? And then after that—what?"

∞∞ A CALL

The answer was not long in coming. Among the other engagements that year were several days in Ottawa at the first Canadian Conference on the Family, initiated by the Governor-General, Georges Vanier and his wife, Pauline. Deeply concerned by changing morals and the decline of the influence of the church on family life, the Vaniers had begun organizing the conference two years earlier. The idea was to draw together professionals working in areas that affected the family (social workers, ministers, priests, lawyers etc.) and concerned citizens to discuss the future of the family and what might be done to protect it in the turbulent years ahead. In June, 1964, fifteen hundred people gathered at Rideau Hall, the Governor-General's official residence in Ottawa.

Wilder Penfield was one of the concerned citizens invited. He had met the Vaniers ten years earlier at a party, soon after the Vaniers returned from France, where Georges had been posted as Canadian Ambassador. It was Madame Vanier who approached him first. Before saying "How do you do?" she blurted out, "Dr. Penfield, can you tell me where the soul is?" Madame Vanier recalls that he looked at her, blinked his eyes and then fixed her with that disarmingly bright stare and said, "We can't answer that quite yet." The conversation ended like that, and she turned away embarrassed, but the connection had been made.

At the conference, Vanier made the opening address to the crowd gathered on the lawn of Rideau Hall. He was an impressive figure with a military bearing—he had been a general in the army—a bushy moustache and the air of a man accustomed to command. It was an inspiring address and in tune with Wilder's own thinking on the subject. Vanier said, in part: "The transition from the religious and metaphysical ages to the age of science has unfortunately been effected so far not by addition but by replacement. In many ways science has been used not to emphasize but to weaken the essential truths of faith and metaphysics.... Creativeness, science, technology—without moral reason, without justice, without friendship, above all without religion and loving faith in God—will tend to make of man a heartless, automated thing. In its application for man's uses, science should be inspired by human and divine justice."

The outcome of the conference was a decision to create an organization "to promote the well-being of the family," to be called The Vanier Institute of the Family. When the Governor-General, his wife and their advisors considered who should be asked to lead it, someone whose ideas were in line with theirs and who was known to the public, they decided to approach Wilder.

At first he declined, but when he turned to his diary a year after the conference, it was to write that, although the biography was still far from finished, "in spite of everything I am to be president of The Vanier Institute of the Family. It will take much time and call for so many talents that are not mine. But the election, they say, was unanimous, and the Vaniers have asked me to do it repeatedly. Why? What am I? When did I become a public figure? I want to write quietly and well. This will mean organization, speeches perhaps.

"And after all, the family is the citadel of an affluent society that is becoming decadent. Oh dear! But I will do what I can. Perhaps Gregg is not really important. My pride is to finish & do a good job. But that is no more than pride, vanity perhaps—the other is a call."

With the decision made, he threw himself into the Vanier Institute with a vigour and determination that astounded everyone. As far as he was concerned, he had put together one institute and he could do it again. First, a strong leader was needed to be administrative head of the Vanier Institute. For his part, as president, he would raise money and publicize the cause.

Rather than begging from governments and private sources year after year to support the institute, they would need a massive amount of money to start with, the interest from which would be a permanent endowment. They would need a headquarters in Ottawa, with offices, libraries and conference rooms. From there they would make scientific approaches to the problems of the modern family, and establish the institute as *the* authority on the family, able to answer any (and all) questions. The Vanier Institute, and he as its spokesman, would defend the family from the undermining influences in the modern world, would re-establish the importance of discipline and lead people back to the old-fashioned values he himself had been raised by. He agreed whole-heartedly with the Vaniers' aim to make the church and religion important aspects of everyday life again. And the Vaniers, for their part, were delighted with the strength of his conviction and his grand schemes. The active head of the institute, Wilder decided, should be called "Secretary-General," like the head of the United Nations. As he explained to Stewart Sutton, who accepted the position after a lifetime of experience in social agencies, including work for the UN, the Vanier Institute was "more important than the United Nations."

Wilder's self-appointed task of raising money and making the public aware of the institute began immediately and took up much of his time for the next four years. As a fund-raiser he was brilliant—and ruthless. He went to Prime Minister Lester Pearson and convinced him to pledge $2 million outright and a dollar-for-dollar matching grant for all funds raised elsewhere. And while much of the fund-raising was done by members of a finance committee, no one could equal Wilder. He went to provincial premiers, to private foundations, he wrote letters to organizations like the Catholic Women's League. Not only had Pearson committed the federal government to contribute, but Pearson himself wrote letters to be sent to the provincial premiers, encouraging them to throw their support behind the institute. Canada's Centennial was coming up, and the Vanier Institute of the Family was to be one of the government's centennial projects, as well as a tribute to the Governor-General and his wife for their long service to Canada.

And when he was not raising money, he was talking about the family and modern society. For four years he stumped the country, talking to anyone who would listen. Wilder Penfield, long famous as a Canadian doctor, scientist and author, became even more famous as president of the Vanier Institute of the Family. He spoke in the style of the great reforming moralists of the Christian tradition, and he was just as difficult to argue with. He had not taken on this job to learn about the family and its different ways of adjusting to and coping with a world that was changing, but to seize the family by the scruff of the neck and shake it back to its senses. Here, ten years after *Cat on a Hot Tin Roof* opened his eyes, was the platform from which he could give vent to his outrage at what he saw as the decline of public morality and social responsibility. He had been called "the greatest living Canadian," in newspapers and magazines, and he'd damned well *tell* people how to behave, if need be. "You teach your children by what you think is right," he told one television interviewer, "that's a man's right. And he closes the door against what he wants to keep out. He's got to learn to do that with TV and radio and newspaper and movie and all the other influences he thinks are bad for his family. We need to do what the communists have done for their countries, in each family—and you may find you go back to reading, and writing and even talking."

Did he think that was likely, the interviewer asked? He paused, and then added sombrely, "It *must* happen. Or we're going to be lost."

At the suggestion of Stewart Sutton and others, Wilder tried to moderate his views when he spoke in public. But for each statement like, "The task before us is not to restore the family of the past but to adapt family life to the world of today and tomorrow," there were in any one speech or interview half a dozen like these: "Young men and women are in need of definite, unhesitating statements on moral issues," and, "The job society must face is to establish moral codes or suffer the consequences."

One of the most revealing of Wilder's interviews was with Charles Templeton, a Canadian television personality, for *Star Weekly* magazine in Toronto. It was published in October of 1966, a year and a half after Wilder accepted the presidency of the Vanier Institute. On the cover of the magazine was a picture of the actress Jane Fonda and the headline, "The Shocking Ideas of Henry's Little Girl." On the first page of the magazine, in a contrast that must have delighted the editors' hearts, "BEHIND EVERY SPOILED CHILD THERE IS A WEAK, A SILLY, OR A SELFISH WOMAN"—a quote from Dr. Wilder Penfield, whose interview followed and whose stern face stared out from a full-page photo opposite. The two stories make a nice contrast: Jane Fonda in a long filmy red dress showing plenty of thigh, posing for the camera and saying things like, "Wives should accept the need of husbands to be unfaithful," and, "If a woman has a beautiful body, I don't think it's immodest of her to show it to advantage in a nude scene. Sex is more than the size of your breasts, though I admit I wear sweaters a lot. Tight ones. The kind you can see through a little bit. And I don't wear anything underneath." Meanwhile, back on page two, Dr. Wilder Penfield (who, according to Templeton, "reminds [one] of Gary Cooper, because [he] conveys an impression of enormous quiet competence and does it with an economy of words") was saying, "Sex before marriage and outside of marriage is always wrong and harmful...anything that militates against the old-fashioned family relationship is a step in the wrong direction."

Templeton's comments at the conclusion of the interview are a good representation of the impression Wilder Penfield left, not just with journalists but with the audiences who heard him speak: "You are struck with a sense of the paradoxical as you talk with Dr. Penfield. He could not be regarded as other than a giant standing on the frontiers of the science in which he specializes, yet his views on the social attitudes and behaviour patterns of our time have an odd old-fashioned quality. His language, when he discusses the problem, is the language of a generation gone. The complex natures of the great social problems seem reduced to simple matters of cause and effect, subject to easy diagnosis and simple solutions. Are his conclusions the result of extensive research? 'No,' he replies, 'I'm just speaking as an old doctor.'" As they left the Institute where the interview had taken place, Templeton asked his wife (who had come along) how Penfield struck her. "He seemed like a kindly, old-fashioned family doctor," she said. "But I wonder if in our kind of world, anybody will listen to him."

Some did, and they wrote letters enclosing money, asking for advice, asking if they could help, thanking him for standing up and saying what was on their minds. But he was fighting a losing battle in a field in which he was ill-equipped to fight. In the second half of the 1960s in Canada, most people seemed to welcome, to some degree, the changes in their lives: the freedom to discuss new ideas, to explore alternatives and make up their own minds. People were less interested in listening to the warnings and reproaches of an Old Testament figure like Wilder. Fifteen years later he might have been a hit, when the young people who worried him so much had done their experimenting and subsided into marriages and mortgages and jobs. But in the years he spent as president of the Vanier Institute, his appeal was mostly to older people who shared his emotional reactions and, because they agreed, didn't question the basis for his remarks.

The first signs of trouble came from inside the institute. In fact, from the very first meeting with Penfield, Stewart Sutton began to have second thoughts about the job he had taken on. At that meeting Sutton recalls suggesting that the first order of business was to figure out what the institute was actually going to do, what its program would be. Wilder's immediate response was, according to Sutton, "Well, Sutton, if you don't know what we're going to do, I'll tell you. I'll tell you right now." He then went on to propose that he (Wilder) would write statements advising parents what books their children should and shouldn't read, what magazines and movies they should be exposed to, what television programs (if any) should be allowed in the house; and Sutton was to negotiate with the federal Department of Health and Welfare to have these recommendations sent out with family-allowance cheques "so the Vanier Institute would soon have the families of this country in good shape," Sutton remembers. "It was that simple, I think, in his mind at that time."

Stewart Sutton was not the only person involved in the Vanier Institute who had doubts about the wisdom of the Vaniers' choice of a president, but Sutton, as Secretary-General, bore the brunt. "I used to feel in his presence sometimes that it must have been a bit like this talking to Moses."

Sutton also found himself from time to time caught in the middle between Vanier and Penfield. "Well, they were very close in many ways, but I remember once when something came up and there was a slight difference of opinion between the two. I was telling Governor-General Vanier what Penfield's view on this subject was, and he said, 'Well, Stewart, you've got to remember Dr. Penfield's getting on and his judgment's a little different than when he was younger.' Some time later, when I was talking to Penfield on a different subject and relating Vanier's view, he said, 'Well, Sutton, you have to remember, General Vanier is getting on and he's not in very good health, and his judgment may not be quite what it used to be.'"

There were fundamental disagreements between Wilder and the more conservative, older members of the institute's board on the one hand, and Stewart Sutton and the professionals on the board and staff on the other. The professionals felt that the institute should be studying the family as it evolved and adapted, and helping people to understand and cope with changing circumstances and attitudes. Wilder and his supporters, including the Vaniers themselves, saw the institute as the last line of defence against The New Morality and all that ubiquitous phrase implied. There was another problem. Wilder's autocratic style of leadership was more appropriate to a bygone era and to the strict discipline that still distinguishes hospitals from most other institutions. In addition, many members of the staff and board of directors felt misgivings about his grandiose scheme for a headquarters building. They had not his fondness for symbols and monuments: such an expenditure of money struck them as immodest and likely to suggest to critics a certain implacability, a fixity of perspective more in keeping with his attitude toward the family than theirs.

By the beginning of 1967, Wilder's enthusiasm was beginning to wane. The battles within the Vanier Institute were growing repetitive and tiresome, and he was growing tired of the role in which he had cast himself: the lone champion of the old order trumpeting from the ramparts. The social-philosopher role had cast a shadow over his reputation as a scientist, he observed with regret. Just when he would have welcomed a serious and dignified lectureship to summarize his conclusions about brain mechanisms, he noted in his diary, "People think I can do nothing but entertain after-dinner, well-fed mixed audiences. Perhaps 'people' are right, and I am passé."

Each time Wilder went to Ottawa, he found Governor-General Vanier's health worse. On March 4, Wilder paid him a final visit, and the following morning, Sunday, he returned from church with Helen to a telephone call from Government House saying that Vanier was dead. With him went some of the spirit from their enterprise, and Wilder slowly began preparing to hand over his presidency of the Vanier Institute to someone else. He would stay on another year to finish the fund-raising campaign—they were now aiming for $6 million as a permanent endowment, and it seemed within sight—and the publicizing of the institute and its purpose. Throughout 1967, Wilder crisscrossed the country giving speeches (thirty-six in all), from Vancouver to St. John's. The strenuous schedule, he admitted privately, was "almost more than I am capable of." In fact, the whole business was more and more of a chore, and he was even starting to doubt some of his own, oft-repeated words. He had put his thoughts on the family together in a slim paperback published under the title *Man and His Family*, and reading back through it that summer, he judged it "as far as I can go in writing about social problems—perhaps too far." He had shown the draft to a number of people, including his daughter Ruthmary. She had responded with a spirited letter criticizing his remarks about a woman's role being in the home, looking after a husband and raising children.

There were other disturbing events that spring, including a horrible 3 A.M. telephone call from a woman whose voice, so he wrote later, was full "of the most heartfelt hate."

"Dr. Penfield?" "Yes." "Himself?" "Yes." "Dr. Penfield, thirty years ago you refused to come to save my sister—you rat! You're still alive. You're *still* alive? You rat, you *dirty* rat."

After that there was silence, and then the line went dead. Wilder returned to bed dazed and lay there for hours trying to remember a patient he had refused to see thirty years ago.

There were pleasant surprises, too, among them the Royal Bank Award "for outstanding citizenship" with a purse of $50,000. Two public-relations people from the bank arrived at the house and marched Wilder off to Ottawa for a presentation. That night when he returned, they turned on the radio expecting to hear news of "the great event in the Penfield family." Instead, he wrote, "The farmers had invaded Ottawa and mobbed Parliament Hill at the same time as our planned press conference, drawing attention away. Next morning, Helen quoted to me from the Bible—'what we need,' she said, is to remember 'not to think more highly of ourselves than we ought to.' We laughed. A very good watchword and I've said it to myself several times in the past two days when praise was fulsome." They promptly decided to keep part of the prize money for a new oriental rug and having the house painted, and to give the rest away to the children and the M.N.I.

That summer Wilder and Helen were scheduled to go to Government House for a dinner in honour of General de Gaulle, who was among the visiting dignitaries for Expo '67. However, the same afternoon De Gaulle made his famous "Quebec Libre" speech from a balcony in Quebec City, which so outraged Wilder that he sent a stiff telegram instead:

> THE AIDE DE CAMP IN WAITING
> GOVERNMENT HOUSE OTTAWA ONT
>
> DOCTOR AND MRS WILDER PENFIELD REGRET DEEPLY THAT IT WILL NOT BE POSSIBLE FOR THEM TO ATTEND THE DINNER THIS EVENING IN HONOUR OF THE PRESIDENT OF FRANCE. MAY I ASK YOU TO EXPLAIN TO HIS EXCELLENCY THE GOVERNOR-GENERAL IN ALL FRANKNESS HOW DISAPPOINTED WE ARE TO FOREGO THIS PLEASURE AND THE HONOUR OF HIS HOSPITALITY AND THAT OF MRS MICHENER IN ENTERTAINING THE PRESIDENT OF FRANCE WHOM WE ADMIRE AND WOULD DELIGHT TO HONOUR BUT ALAS DE GAULLE THE MAN HAS MADE HIMSELF A LEADER OF THE FRENCH CANADIAN SEPARATISM MOVEMENT. AS A CANADIAN CITIZEN AND A WORKER FOR QUEBEC'S MATURING STRENGTH, CULTURAL, ECONOMIC, AND INTELLECTUAL, WITHIN THE CONFEDERATION, I WOULD FIND IT DIFFICULT TO MEET HIM AT THIS MOMENT.

Then in November, he was invited to give a speech to *L'Institut Canadien du Québec*, in French. At first he refused, feeling that his awkward French would be more of an insult than a compliment. But the president of the association telephoned him and said, "Dr. Penfield, with the climate in Quebec what it is today, it is important that you should say yes to this invitation, important that you should speak of Canada and Quebec in Quebec in French." They were talking in

French, and then Wilder heard "You know, you are accepted today by French Canadians *'comme un de leurs'* (as one of theirs)."

"Those were the words," he wrote, "that I had hoped to hear since we came to live in this province thirty-nine years ago." He agreed to make the speech, hung up the phone, then realized with horror what he had taken on. Immediately he made arrangements with a former Berlitz teacher for lessons every day he was free. He had barely two weeks to prepare, and though some days the lessons were extremely depressing, by the end his instructor approved of his accent. Meanwhile, Wilder and a Jesuit priest, Father d'Apollonia, had been busy translating the speech, to be called "Canada at the Crossroads—Alliance or Civil War." With his teacher and his son Wilder, who spoke French with a very convincing accent, he began to rehearse.

Finally on November 27, Wilder and Helen took the train to Quebec City, and after a gay dinner, Wilder walked up to the podium. "I heard my voice and it seemed the old awkward sound of the English learner had disappeared....As I watched the audience and saw every face intent during the hour I knew I was hitting the mark. At the close there was that explosive quality of applause which I recognize occasionally and know it means a response from the heart."

The capacity audience in the auditorium gave him a standing ovation, and continued to clap while the others on the platform, including former prime minister Louis St. Laurent, shook his hand and congratulated him. Those in the crowd were touched, not just by the content of the speech, which was a predictable if heartfelt approach to the problems facing Confederation and the need for "charity and mutual understanding," but by the fact that this man of seventy-six had clearly put a tremendous effort into this gracious gesture. Wilder was delighted.

∞ THE MYSTERY OF THE MIND

In April of 1968, with his involvement in the Vanier Institute winding down, the biography of Alan Gregg published at last, and the Centennial activities and speeches over, Wilder and Helen left for a holiday in Greece.

On the island of Rhodes they sat on the beach in the warm sunlight, and while Helen read aloud from Dorothy Sayers' *Busman's*

Holiday Wilder marvelled at the smooth stones, the sea, the sky, and, in the distance, the low line of the distant coast. A subtle but insistent change was coming over their lives. So many of the things that had occupied the last few years were coming to an end and, almost puzzled, Wilder realized how old they were. It had happened so gradually, and so often in the past he had rejected the thought. In some vague way he had hoped that this trip away from the demands of Montreal and the Vanier Institute might clear his mind and help him plan for the future. Instead, as he was waking from a nap one afternoon in their hotel room he heard a voice saying, "You have no plan for the future—the first time in your life."

It was a voice he had heard in his head before, he wrote, months ago. Waking from a nap in his office at the M.N.I., he had stood up, pulled back the curtain at the window and looked out to see Montreal's towering buildings coloured gold by the setting sun, and heard himself saying aloud, "I don't want to leave it."

Now, in Greece, he turned to his diary to wonder how "to use my present talent and training and the place and influence that have come to me, for good. I can speak, if I work hard on the text. I could write, I suppose, as well as ever or better. I can study new material, though slowly (when wasn't I slow?). I can reason more maturely and, I think, soundly. At 77 I could labour hard at something for 3 or 6 or even 10 years."

It would be easier to plan if he knew how much time he had left. He had seen too many of his friends and contemporaries die suddenly, from a coronary or a stroke, to have many illusions about making elaborate plans at seventy-seven, and yet he couldn't resist. Despite recurring trouble with his knee, he felt well enough. He limped more and used a cane much of the time, he was more wrinkled, almost completely bald, a bit stooped, a bit forgetful. The most bothersome sign of age was that after three hours at his desk he found himself dozing off, but he had learned to take short naps and return to work refreshed. Helen was faring worse, becoming unsteady on her feet, and her memory faltered more and more frequently; it was terribly frustrating for her. Still, Wilder wrote, "I have never been happier than right now, on this month with her. I think she would honestly say the same, although I know well I'm hard to put up with very often. Our lives as lovers is just as rewarding in every way as it ever was, which is saying quite a lot." And yet, he acknowledged, "She will not be happy unless I settle the problem of what to do with one W.P."

The stay in Greece had produced no answers, but a few weeks later in Berlin, he turned to his diary to note that he had been wondering if it was preposterous for him to undertake one last, sweeping work of writing that would tie together his whole life, interests and beliefs, "a book entitled *Man*, perhaps." He listed the various things he had covered in his life: medicine—that could be a section on "Man & his body...Brain-Mind relationship." The writing of *No Other Gods* could be called "Man and God," *The Torch*, "Man and Profession," and the Vanier Institute, "Society and Family." There would have to be another section, dealing with the impact of "Experimental Science and Mass Communication on Man."

The idea excited him. "It would matter little," he wrote, "whether such a book were ever finished or when. If it constituted an honest and critical study I would be content to give it all the strength I have. It would be a new form of biographical writing, free of any concern for the appearance the author might make in the eyes of others. Thus the vanity that spoils autobiographical writing would not be a factor."

The idea stuck in his mind and he returned to the diary once or twice to consider some aspect of it, but by the beginning of May he had decided that such a book was beyond his skill. "The books I have written have brought me no prize for literary excellence. One hardly expects that for the scientific and medical efforts. But if the novels, the biography, the essays and the little book on Man and His Family were really excellent they would have received awards. So it is nonsense to consider a monograph on Man that would be read or that would have an impact on social evolution. For this the final stage in my life, the best I can do is to choose the projects that present themselves, wisely, whether scientific or social or scholarly....I can at least seek the truth in little ways and do each job as well as I possibly can."

Even though he concluded that he was not a good enough writer for such a mammoth undertaking, there was still something beyond little projects that tugged at him from time to time like a guilty conscience. From the first published results of his operations on conscious patients in the nineteen-forties, he had insisted, quietly at first but with more determination each time, that his discoveries proved nothing either way about the possibility of a separate element—the mind, or the spirit.

Many of his colleagues and contemporaries had been puzzled by his insistence. It was true, they agreed, but why insist on it over and over? Given time, improved methods and more sophisticated equipment, no doubt the study of the brain would be able to explain the intangible things—thoughts, dreams, hopes, emotions—in terms of the physical workings of the brain. For a fellow scientist, and a distinguished one at that, to keep insisting on how *little* they had accomplished struck most as inappropriate, and some as downright treasonous.

The simple fact is that for all his insistence that he was only trying to understand the true nature of the brain, Wilder didn't want to find out that the physical mechanism was all there was, that all the mysteries of faith and God and sense of mission and destiny could be explained away in brain cells, chemical reactions and hormones. The closer science came with each new discovery, the more strident became his insistence on what had not been discovered, at least in the study of brain function. On the subject of the search to understand the nature of the mind, Wilder's view echoed, as it always had, Sir Charles Sherrington's famous words: "It will long offer, to those who pursue it, the comfort that to journey is better than to arrive." Like Sherrington, Wilder believed that some day science would find the answer, but he had his own views of what that answer would be, and they were distinctly unscientific.

Wilder Penfield had come a long way from the basic scientific conclusions that had made him famous. In the years after his career as an active scientist and surgeon ended, he had watched science contributing to an increasingly materialistic world. He felt that scientists had allowed people to believe that science would ultimately provide all the answers, and in doing so had undermined their faith in God. If humans were no more than sophisticated animals then talk of the soul and God must be rubbish; love was no more than an excess of hormones, a sense of destiny no more than self delusion. He refused to believe it was so. Perhaps the time had come for him to speak as a scientist, to go back to his basic data and at least reiterate his point about the limits of scientific understanding. Perhaps in reconsidering the evidence, he would find that it justified a more positive statement.

"The die is cast," he wrote in his diary at the beginning of summer, 1968. He would take the invitations to make scientific speeches as they came to him, using them as opportunities to reconsider the conclusions he had reached in the past. "All my studies of the brain of man...were worked at with the secret hope that I would see more clearly in the end. But each study called for so much exact writing with care for patients and the team of workers...[that] I often did not get to the deductions that may have been there to draw. Will this late return to the brain detail give greater understanding of mind and spirit? I wonder....All my life I've expected to emerge somehow from brain to mind, and yet I tell people that science has proven nothing about the spirit. Why assume I shall succeed now?"

Even as he began the sifting and rethinking that would culminate, five years later, in a manuscript titled "The Mystery of the Mind," Wilder found himself embarked on the one book he had said repeatedly he would never write—"my pseudo-autobiography" he would call it in a moment of weariness.

It was Ted Rasmussen, Wilder's successor as director of the Institute, who suggested the following year that perhaps it was time for Wilder to put down on paper the events and decisions that had led to the building of M.N.I. It was now possible to talk about all the various aspects of the scientific study of the brain as "neuroscience," and he was considered one of the pioneers. His instinct that the various specialties could work together effectively, which had raised so many hackles in the early days, had been vindicated in Montreal and in research centres around the world.

At first Wilder rejected the idea, not just because he feared it might turn into an autobiography but because of his renewed interest in the studies of the brain. But Rasmussen persisted and others, including his children, added their voices, hoping that he *would* make the book autobiographical. By the end of 1969, they had prevailed, though as far as he was concerned it was going to be a straightforward account of the evolution of an idea that had resulted in the M.N.I. He had his letters to his mother, which she had typed and assembled in four, thick looseleaf binders and given to him before her death in 1935. From those he could draw for contemporary detail in his accounts.

But the building of the Institute and the idea behind it were inextricably connected to his own life, and at each point in the writing he found he was waxing autobiographical. Looking back over his life, he found that what he had accomplished by dogged determination, luck, and inspiration led so often to his mother and *her* ideas. Though he railed at the project periodically, it became a fascinating task—reviewing his own life as though it were someone else's, watching from the safe remove of his eighty years as the boy grew into manhood, went off to Princeton and then to Oxford, became a doctor, got married, grew more ambitious for a place to work out his ideas about the surgery and study of the brain, came to Montreal, and persuaded the Rockefeller Foundation and wealthy Montrealers to make his dream come true. It also turned into a chance, at last, to bury the skeleton of his father, which had been rattling around in his closet for so long. The first draft that he showed to friends and family members caused one of his colleagues, more blunt that the rest, to say, "What's the matter, didn't you have a father?" At that point he wanted to quit, but didn't. Reluctantly he rewrote the first section of the book dealing with his early years, struggling with the anger that still boiled up at the thought of his father's betrayals: "Others had fathers to advise them.... Not I."

"In a sense," he wrote in *No Man Alone*, as the book would finally be called, "this is, for me, a project in real research analysis." But in the end, he made no mention of the basic incompatibility he knew was the cause for the break-up of his parents' marriage. He chose instead to accept his father as an amiable, irresponsible man who could not resist "the call of the wild."

The book was far from being finished in April of 1971, a few months after his eightieth birthday, when he and Helen sold the house at last and moved into an apartment overlooking Montreal. The Chinese couple, the Hwangs, had left and Helen was simply not up to the task of training anyone to replace them. Her memory had begun to behave like a worn-out sprocket; now it worked smoothly, now it slipped a few notches, and sometimes it whirled around furiously, never connecting. She had always been so organized, so meticulous a housekeeper and planner; now as it all slipped through her fingers she tried harder and harder. She would write everything down, recopy a letter before she sent it off so she would have a record, draw up careful lists for the new maid in her shaky hand, but there were still bad moments. In May, 1972, a note in Wilder's diary: "Helen came into my study after breakfast to ask me to look at the schedule for the next two days for Mary. It was accurate after much work at her desk, except she had written Mrs. Feindel when she meant Mrs. Robb. 'I would be so afraid if I had to live alone,' she said. Sometimes when she realizes how difficult it is to remember and plan, she weeps. This morning she is reflective and quiet. Just now she came in again and sat on my lap briefly: 'Thank you, thank you for a lovely life.' Then she went out again after giving me a hug."

Five years earlier, in case he should die first, he had started a letter to her full of love and careful instructions and advice, and now and then he took it out of his drawer and added to it. But despite the occasional warnings of the end, and added difficulties, he continued to accept the invitations to give lectures and Helen would travel with him: "She is still my ablest critic." And Wilder was still connected with the Vanier Institute, as a "Patron," attending annual meetings and giving advice, welcome or not.

More and more now, since Helen needed his help, he worked at home in his study. When he had to go out he left tender little notes and funny drawings where she would find them. The Institute was a half-hour's walk away, and when his knee would let him, he went on foot. Behind the apartment building was a path which a neighbour had christened "Penfield Parade," because of the hours they spent walking there. Throughout 1972 Wilder worked steadily, if more slowly on *No Man Alone*, and by the end of January, 1973, a second draft was complete, and only the revisions left, he wrote triumphantly. With perhaps two or three months work, the book would be ready to go off to a publisher for consideration.

But eight months later the manuscript was still sitting on his desk, untouched, and Wilder was in a deep depression. The trouble began with a speech he had promised to give in April, to the spring meeting of the American Philosophical Society. As he had planned on their return from Greece five years ago, he had returned to his conclusions about the brain in a number of different papers, and in the pages of his diary. Each return had reinforced his conviction that the evidence of a separate element was there, if only he could see it, but each time he had been obliged to admit that he was still proceeding on faith. Partly this had been the exercise of native caution, and partly the advice of scientific colleagues like Ted Rasmussen and Herbert Jasper, whom he had asked at one point to tell him when he was in danger of "spinning nonsense."

The version of his argument for the American Philosophical Society was the boldest statement he had dared to make so far, and he had worked on it steadily since January with high hopes. But the speech had been a disaster. As though from far away he had listened to himself stumble through it, making pointless asides, forgetting his place and missing the most important points. The friends and colleagues he had known for so many years listened to his confused rambling with embarrassment and sadness. Later, he wondered wryly if they thought they had stumbled into a bad performance of *King Lear* instead of a scientific address.

But it was only the presentation that had betrayed him, he was convinced, not the content. When he returned to Montreal he ignored the manuscript of *No Man Alone* to work some more on the paper, and he delivered it to a symposium at the M.N.I. This time he did better with it, and the good response had been heart-warming. When summer came and he and Helen went out to Magog Meadows, he kept finding himself returning to it rather than the unfinished manuscript, wondering if the speech might not contain the germ "of a little book." He decided to take a month or two and work on it, and then try out the results on a couple of readers. He would listen to their comments, then decide whether it was worth trying to have it published or if he should put it away and turn back to the revision of *No Man Alone*. All through the summer Wilder worked at assembling the various pieces of evidence and trying to fit them together to form a coherent picture. In September he sent the draft to friends and family members who agreed to read and comment on his work.

The first reaction came from Ted Rasmussen, a long letter with many criticisms, both specific and general. As he read through it, Wilder realized that Ted was worried by the way Wilder had skipped from the scientific data, obviously written for scientists, to conclusions that were not scientific but philosophical. Rasmussen's criticisms struck home and Wilder wearily decided to put it away and go back to *No Man Alone*. Perhaps when that was done he would come back and try again. There was still a statement in all that data that he wanted to make— had wanted to make, in fact, for years. Perhaps he realized that, after all, it would have to be a philosophical statement, and perhaps his own words—"When a scientist turns to philosophy we know he's over the hill"—came back to him.

For a week or two he tried to concentrate on *No Man Alone*, but the other kept returning to plague him. "All my life I expected to emerge somehow from brain to mind." He had written that note in his diary in 1968, and had added, "Why should I believe I will succeed...?" Now he argued with himself that surely he had earned the right to make public the conclusions that he himself had drawn—for his *own* life—after a career studying the brain. And if he didn't do it, who would? Who would give ordinary people some reasons to believe that there could be such a thing as the mind, and the spirit, and God?

It was at the lowest ebb in this depression that a letter came from Charles Hendel. Hendel and Wilder had been classmates at Princeton, but they had only become friends in the nineteen-thirties when they both found themselves in Montreal, Wilder as the neurosurgeon at the Royal Victoria Hospital, Hendel as Professor of Moral Philosophy at McGill. Hendel had published an article in the mid-thirties in *The Journal of Philosophy* called "The Status of Mind in Reality," and he and Wilder had had a number of intriguing discussions on the subject of the mind before Hendel returned to the U.S. to become chairman of the Department of Philosophy at Yale. Now Hendel, retired, was living in Vermont, where he was working on a book of his own.

He had read through the manuscript and was excited by what Wilder was trying to do. "As I finish a second reading...I find the last pages are an eloquent, convincing justification of your hypothesis and belief that mind has a being distinct from body. The final statement is you *yourself*, speaking to the reader. The careful, modest, thoughtful assertion of belief and questions alike are the marks of a philosopher. And I salute you as a master."

The problem in the earlier parts of the manuscript, Hendel suggested, was that there Wilder was pushing the argument rather than letting the strongest element in the book speak for itself, "...the testimony of living, conscious patients. This is an *objective item* in your scientific evidence...[the] discoveries...which made you wonder about something that does not fit into the scientific picture, and you wonder again and again."

Charles Hendel had not only understood what he was trying to say, Wilder discovered with delight, he had found an eloquent way of describing the evolution: "How Wilder Penfield, operating on patients in order to cure them if possible, found out things about the cerebral cortex and the mechanisms of the higher brain stem that turned a suspicion or mere notion into a vital hypothesis, and this further led to practical results in the lives of patients.

"You became more and more convinced that the mind is something in its own right, that it did things with the mechanisms at hand in its own way, that it had an 'energy' of its own. You offer only suggestions.... You end aligning yourself with the prophets, the poets, and the philosophers who have emphasized the spiritual element in man."

Hendel concluded the letter: "For myself, reading this has been far more than instructive: it is something of an inspiration to find reasons for believing, what I have always held from the beginning of my own life and work as a philosopher: reasons for 'a persistent view in modern thought that mind is a very distinctive reality.'"

In order to make the book fit together, Hendel suggested that Wilder "make it plainer to the reader that this piece of writing gives the autobiographical sequence of your development. Yours is a story of 'how I came to take seriously, even to believe, that the consciousness of man, the mind, is something not to be reduced to brain-mechanisms.' In this development, what carries weight with the reader is the fact that in brain operations you hold a supreme position in the memory of living men and women: but *you* must only introduce the facts and experience you have recorded that disclose the ground for your belief. Your autobiographical material *is* powerful. The testimony of your patients is convincing, and your development toward the mystery of the mind is convincing beyond any philosopher's argument. Think it over."

Hendel's letter, more than anything else, reassured Wilder that the evidence that had convinced him was convincing to others, even those as scrupulous about language and logic as a philosopher like Hendel.

He launched into the revisions with enthusiasm, following Hendel's suggestion and trying to answer the criticism implicit in Rasmussen's letter by making the first half of the book a swift, clear summary of what his patients had taught him. In the second half he presented the conclusions he had drawn, permitting himself at last to say what had been on his mind for so long. He summed up what he was trying to do in a letter to Ted Rasmussen: "it is better to make bold hypotheses and be wrong, instead of contributing to confusion by silence." Hendel's comments, he explained, "make me realize that the closing pages, which become more and more speculative, may serve a useful purpose beyond the field of science. It could be done, as you suggested, in two papers, but it is too late now. The early part is planned to make it possible for any student to work at it and end up by understanding my whole life's struggle to approach the mind and the brain. When you and I were doing the anatomy and physiology of the cortex, you held me down to demonstrable fact, and I am grateful. Now I have come to another stage."

It was a marathon of work crammed into a few months, as he reviewed the progression from the discovery—which had sent him looking elsewhere in the brain for "the highest level"—that he could remove a large portion of the cortex and the patient would remain conscious, to the first experiences with evoked memory on the operating table; on through the discovery that an epileptic fit in the higher brain stem brought on unconsciousness or "automatism," and the strange "doubling of awareness" while the conscious patient he was probing relived some past experience. Piece by piece, he assembled the clues that had led him along what he now called "a fateful pilgrimage." To explain to the public why he was writing the book, he wrote in the preface: "A physiologist can examine the brain. He has, as yet, no direct approach to the mind. That there is the closest relationship, however, is self-evident. Must the physiologist with facts at hand forever stand apart from the philosopher?"

Wilder asked Bill Feindel to write an introduction from the point of view of a neurosurgeon, Charles Hendel to add his comments as a philosopher and Sir Charles Symonds to add his views as a neurologist. But the last word he kept for what seemed, by this time in his life, the most important statement of all:

"I was brought up in a Christian family and I have always believed, since I first considered the matter, that there was work for me to do in the world, and that there is a grand design in which all conscious individuals play a role. Whether there is such a thing as communication between man and God, and whether energy can come to the mind of a man from an outside source after his death, is for each individual to decide for himself. Science has no such answers."

In the end, it was not primarily a scientific book, but a statement of faith. He had come full circle. By the end of November the manuscript was being typed, before going to Princeton University Press who had agreed to publish it. He turned back to *No Man Alone*. The revisions that at one time would have taken him a few months, seemed to stretch out interminably, but by June, 1974, he noted he was working "fast and well." By November he was up to the last chapter, pausing to look back over what he had written, and turning to his diary to write, "The establishment of an Institute was, in the end, so small a part of my objective! The overall objective was to do what I have tried to do alone, in 'The Mystery of the Mind.'" Each day now, he and Helen sat together and read the manuscript aloud, making corrections as they went. Helen's memory for recent things was now almost gone, but her comments were as clear and lucid as ever while they worked. It was only when he had to go out to run errands or stop in at the Institute that she became fretful, and so he stayed with her most of the time. Now that winter had come it was next to impossible for them to take their walks together in the snow. His eighty-fourth birthday passed by in January, and there were days when it seemed winter would never end. He found himself more and more often standing at the window of his study looking out at the skiers gliding through the woods on the mountain across the way, listening to the whine of spinning tires as the cars below slipped on the icy road up the hill. In this apartment high above the city, warm and snug, he and Helen seemed to be alone on an island while the world swirled and eddied around them.

Small physical problems were starting to pile up: a pain in his chest, a weakness in his legs which made him wonder if he'd be walking for much longer, occasional migraines. But despite the physical decrepitude, "there is another even less welcome little devil who could materialize. I think he had peeped around the corner from time to time to grin at me. He brings sleep and dreams and vague indifference & in the end men long for him...now he terrifies me. Still so much to do...the book must be finished."

But spring came, and at the beginning of June the Penfields moved out to Sussex House. The weather was splendid, hot and clear, and Helen seemed better than ever. A granddaughter and her husband were visiting for the summer, and with them the fourth great-grandchild, Hannah Cordelia Williams, three months old. They were heading off on a short trip one day, and Helen, walking down the path to say goodbye to the child one more time, slipped and fell, breaking her hip. Wilder gave her an anaesthetic and they brought her in to Montreal, where she was operated on and a plate put in. The month of July was spent in Montreal with special nurses, a wheelchair and a walker, but in August the two of them were back at Magog Meadows staying in the guesthouse, "and I am nurse and absolute companion except when she is asleep." It was hard work with his legs unreliable, and there were small tragedies: "Yesterday she fell and my weak legs gave out and I fell too. There we were flat on the floor. But we sat up. Each asked the other if he or she was alright. Finally we laughed, but it was rather hollow laughter."

They returned to Montreal in September, and near the end of October they came out again for the day so he could take care of a last, unfinished job. While he had worked on the manuscript of *The Mystery of the Mind* in his writing shed the summer before, he had started painting the theme of his book on a huge rock down the slope of the field. He had kept a small basket of old cans of house paint by the door, and when he had tired of writing he would make his way down the hill and add to the painting. On one side he had painted the Greek word for spirit and then a line connecting it to an Aesculapian torch, representing science. The line continued on to an outline of a human head, with the brain drawn inside, and inside that, a small question mark.

The painting on the rock served as a kind of shorthand as he worked through the scientific data and drew his conclusions about the connection between brain and spirit. Would science *ever* find the answer? He had begun to have doubts, and had come out this weekend to make a few changes. It was a cold, blustery day and Helen fretted until he had put on layer after layer of sweaters under his raincoat and brought her out to sit on the porch while he put the final touches on his painting. It didn't take long to change the solid line from spirit to science and on to the brain into an interrupted line. That done, and his doubts expressed for others to see, they drove back to Montreal.

It was the last visit to Magog Meadows. Before winter was out, the doctors had discovered a malignant tumour in Wilder's stomach. They did an exploratory operation, suggested chemotherapy, but he decided against it. The end was coming anyway and he saw no reason to postpone it much longer. The manuscript of *No Man Alone* had come back from Little, Brown and Company in Boston, for him to read and correct one last time, and there was just time for that.

He didn't tell Helen the tumour was malignant. Instead, he dug out the letter that was to be given to her after he died and completed it. He had made notes about their will, about how he was to be cremated, and added them to the notes of love and concern and advice. He arranged with Wilder Jr. for the letter to be given to her after his death, read to her if need be. She would carry it with her like a talisman, to ward off grief and confusion during the two subsequent years she lived without him.

The cancer was getting worse, and now he worried that if he died there in the apartment Helen would have the shock of finding him. Wilder and Ruthmary suggested he move into the Institute for a few days rest, and he agreed with relief.

He made his plans. The night before his departure, they had a party, just the two of them: Helen shaky and forgetful, but with occasional flashes of her old humour, and Wilder dressed for the occasion in a red vest that had always been her favourite. Wilder put on records and they listened to music during dinner. After, they sat together on the sofa in the living room, singing as many of the old songs as they could remember from the Hudson picnics, and at last went to bed.

The next morning an ambulance came for him, and on the way he handed his cane to Ruthmary who had come along to keep him company. "I won't need this anymore," he said firmly. Then, "but maybe I'll keep it anyway, just for while I'm in the hospital."

Wilder died in a hospital bed on the morning of April 5, 1976. He had brought his diary, and a day or two before, made one last entry, in a thin, shaky hand—three words that trailed off into an illegible scrawl: "Here I am..."

A NOTE ON SOURCES

Much of the material cited in this book or used as background in the writing can be found in The Penfield Papers at the Montreal Neurological Institute, including my two primary sources: the letters of Wilder Penfield to his mother (1904-35) and his private diaries. In addition, relatives and associates kindly gave me access to their personal correspondence with Wilder Penfield. My mother, Ruthmary Lewis, made available her files and taped interviews as well as the papers of her mother, Helen Penfield. In addition to these sources, librarians and archivists at a great many institutions in Canada, the United States and Britain provided pertinent information and files and indulged my curiosity about many esoteric points related to the book. I am particularly indebted to the following: The Osler Library of McGill University; The Academy of Medicine of Ontario; The Seeley G. Mudd Manuscript Library of Princeton University; The John L. Robarts Library of the University of Toronto; The Alan Mason Chesney Medical Archives of Johns Hopkins University; The Baker Memorial Library of Dartmouth College; The National Research Council of Canada; The Department of External Affairs, Canada; The Public Archives of Canada; The Vanier Institute of the Family; The Montreal Neurological Institute; The St. Croix County (Wisconsin) Historical Society; The Westmount Public Library; The Toronto Public Library, Yorkville branch; The CBC Sound Archives.

INDEX

Abraham, 224-26. See also *No Other Gods*
Adams, Ray, 234, 235
Adrian, Edgar, 214, 228, 244
American Academy of Arts and Science, 230
American Club, 52, 53
American Journal of Physiology, 75
American Philosophical Society, 281-82, 298
American Red Cross Hospital, 59, 60, 64, 67, 69, 70, 71
Anne, Princess, 229
Archibald, Edward, 104-05, 106, 113, 117, 136; and French community in Montreal, 117; in Ruth Inglis case, 120, 122; and plan for M.N.I., 132
Arizona, 227
Asia Minor: WP's trip to (1956), 247-51
Association for Research in Nervous and Mental Diseases, 206
Atlantic Monthly, 191, 278
Ayer, A. J., 216

Baghdad, 181, 183, 226
Banting, Sir Frederick, 166, 176, 254
Bazett, Cuthbert, 25, 79, 85, 229
BBC, 274; radio lecture series, 214-17; symposium, 271
Bean, Margaret, 13, 14
Bean, Walker, 12, 14
Beatty, Edward, 147
Behaviourism: WP opposed to philosophy of, 214
Beit Memorial Fellowship, 80
Berger, Hans, 194

Berlin, 159
Bethune, Norman, 189, 279
Bishop's University, 175, 281
Bonynge, Berry, 191
Brain, 127
Brain: The Last Frontier, The (Restak), 271
Brain, Russell, 215
Brain probe: and EEG, 196; and hallucinations, 197-202. See also Epilepsy
Brain surgery, 213-14; description of, 128-30; patients conscious during, 197-98. See also Frederico; Inglis, Ruth
Brave New World (Huxley), 270
British American Neurological Conference, 105
British Broadcasting Corporation. See BBC
Bronk, Detlev, 244
Brown University, 194
Buckingham Palace, 229
Cajal. See Ramón y Cajal, Santiago
Cambridge University, 167, 228, 264; Trinity College, 244
Canadian Club, 269
Canadian Conference on the Family, 284
Canadian Medical Corps, 166-69
Carleton, Harry M., 79
Cat on a Hot Tin Roof (Williams), WP's reaction to, 243-44, 247, 286
Catholic Women's League, 286
Centrencephalic system. See Integrative brain mechanism
Chao, Y. C., 279
Chaplin, Max, 40, 41
Charcot, Jean-Martin, 80
Charles, Prince, 229

306

INDEX • 307

"Charlie" (the Penfields' cook), 220, 221, 231
Chenoweth, W. R.: and building of M.N.I., 147
Chester, William, 29-41 *passim*, 45, 223, 252
Chiang Kai-shek, Generalissimo, 184-89
China: WP in (1943), 181-87 *passim*; WP in (1962), 189, 248, 251, 274-81 *passim*
Chinese Medical Association, 278
Christmas Carol, A (Dickens), 44-45
Churchill, Winston, 73, 218, 228, 268
Clark, W. E. Le Gros, 215-16
Clarke, William C., 94, 98, 110
Club St. Denis (Montreal), 114
Cold War: WP's attitude to, 274, 284
College of Physicians and Surgeons. *See* Columbia University
Colombo Plan, 247
Columbia University: College of Physicians and Surgeons, 48, 85, 86, 99; WP accepts post at, 87, 88
Concept of the Mind (Ryle), 216
Cone, William Vernon: and WP at Presbyterian Hospital, 99, 101, 103; decides to follow WP to R.V.H., 108, 110; in Laboratory of Neuropathology, 118, 136; and joint private practice, 131, 154; and Ruth Inglis case, 120, 122-23; his relationship with WP, 137, 141-42; and offer from University of Iowa, 146-47; and No. 1 Neurological Hospital overseas, 162, 165; WP disturbed by success of, 167-68; WP notes changes in, 173; his dedication to M.N.I. and patients, 193; and WP's retirement from M.N.I., 233-36; death of, 256-58
Conklin, Edward: his influence on WP, 37
Coronet, 212
Cos (Greece), 238, 239
Currie, Sir Arthur, 107; and building of M.N.I., 143-44
Cushing, Harvey, 90, 93, 104, 156; his influence on WP and neurosurgery, 77, 126; in Ruth Inglis case, 121, 122, 125
Dale, Sir Henry, 228
Dandy, Walter, 90, 92
Darrach, William, 89
Dartmouth College, 270
Dartmouth Conference, 270-71; WP's address at, 272-73
De Gaulle, General Charles, 268, 291
Dockrill, Edward: his background and meeting with WP, 99-100, 101; in Laboratory of Neuropathology, 118, 136
Don Quixote (Cervantes), 96
Dorsey, John, 63
Drummond, Jack, 35

Dubos, René, 270

Edinburgh, (Prince) Philip, Duke of, 228
EEG. *See* Electroencephalograph
Einstein, Albert, 255
Eisenhower, Dwight 268
Electroencephalograph (EEG), 130, 194-96. *See also* Herbert Jasper; Brain probe
Eliot, Martha, 134
Eliot, T. S., 52
Elizabeth II: Coronation of, 220, 227-30
Elliott, K. A. C., 192
Elsberg, Charles, 90
Empire Club, 269
Epilepsy: WP's interest in, 81-82, 93-94; symptoms and early professional reactions to WP's treatment for, 126-28; surgical procedure in treatment of, 128-30; WP and Jasper co-author definitive book on, 170, 233; research and procedure for locating focus of, 194-202; fame and acceptance of WP's surgical procedure in treating, 242
Epilepsy and the Functional Anatomy of the Human Brain (Penfield and Jasper), 233
Erickson, Theodore, 170-71, 180
Espagne (ship), 67, 68
"Explorer, The" (Kipling): WP's identification with, 171-72

Feindel, William, 213, 301
Ferrier, Sir David, 80
Ferrier Lecture, 202, 204
Finney, J. M. T., 45, 75, 76
Fisher, Eric, 134, 135
Foerster, Otfrid: WP studies his surgical procedure on epileptics, 109-10; his influence on neurosurgery, 122; stress of surgery on, 156; and Nazi regime, 158-59, 176
Fonda, Jane, 287
Fortune, 212
Freeman, Walter, 213
Frederico: ventriculography in the case of, 90-91

Galahad School, 24, 31, 33, 39; WP graduates from, 27; WP teaches at, 43, 45
Gandhi, Mahatma, 272
Garry, Wade, 255
Goldwater, Barry, 282
Gerard, Ralph, 273
Gilroy, John, 278
Glasgow, 167
Golgi, Camillo, 98, 150
Graschenko, Propper, 176, 177, 277
Greece, 238, 240-41, 247, 255
Green, T. H., 216

308 • SOMETHING HIDDEN

Greenfield, Goodwin, 91, 105
Gregg, Alan: offers Rockefeller grant for M.N.I., 137-42; and building of McConnell Wing, 232-33; WP's biography of, 206-305 *passim*
Guggenheim Foundation, 261

Hall, Francis, 40, 252
Hall, George, 227
Hamilton, William, 108-09
Harvard University, 46, 264
Harvey Cushing Society, 236
Hendel, Charles, 299-301
Henry Ford Hospital, 83, 85-87
Herring, Heff, 46
Hippocrates, 272; as subject of *The Torch*, 238, 239, 254, 255
Hippocratic Oath, 238, 272
Hiroshima, 190
Hodgson, A. A., 107
Holmes, Gordon, 80-82, 105; influence on WP, 80, 252; WP visits, 203-04
Holmes, Rosalie (Mrs. Gordon), 80, 82
Holt, Sir Herbert, 147
Hong Kong University, 251
Hortega. *See* Rio-Hortega, Pio del
Hôtel-Dieu, 117, 137
Howell, William, 74, 75
Howland, Charles P., 137
Hudson, Wisc., 17-19, 23, 39, 47, 70
Huxley, Aldous, 270
"In Flanders Fields" (McCrae), 52
Inglis, Jack, 20, 24, 66, 71, 78, 118, 123
Inglis, Ruth (sister): birth and early life of, 12-18 *passim*; marriage of, 20; epileptic seizures and brain surgery of, 118-24; death of, 125
Institut Canadien du Québec, 291-92
Institute for Advanced Study (Princeton), 254, 256
Institute for Investigation of the Nervous System (Moscow), 176
Integrative brain mechanism (centrencephalic system): WP's search for, 200-02; WP's theory of, 200-01, 204, 206-07; as brain-mind frontier, 208-11, 237, 242, 253; public reaction to and effect on M.N.I., 211-12, 242; and *The Mystery of the Mind*, 294-304 *passim*
International Congress of the Medical Sciences (Belgium, 1957), 252-53
International Neurological Congress (Switzerland, 1931), 139, 140

Jackson, Hughlings, 55, 80; his theory of integrative brain mechanism, 200
James, Henry, 47
Jasper, Herbert, 205, 207, 223; WP collaborates with, 194-96, 253; organizes international conference on brain function, 236-37. *See also* Epilepsy
Jefferson, Amos (grandfather), 6, 12, 17, 24, 32, 39, 43; WP's relationship with, 19, 40
Jefferson, Geoffrey, 168, 233
Jefferson, Jean. *See* Penfield, Jean Jefferson (mother)
Jefferson, Tom, 38
Johns Hopkins Medical School, 44, 53; WP attends, 63, 64; WP offered position at, 73, 74, 75
Johnson Society, Dr., 40, 41, 227, 251

Kermott, Helen. *See* Penfield, Helen Kermott (wife)
Kilbourn, Leslie, 251
Kipling, Rudyard: his influence on WP, 171-72
Kuomintang, 184-89 *passim*

Laboratory of Neurocytology. *See* Presbyterian Hospital
Landau, Lev, case of, 274-78
Leacock, Stephen, 115
Learmouth, J. R., 167
Le Corbusier, Charles Edouard, 281
Leriche, René, 98-99
Lewis, Catherine, 191
Lewis, Crosby, 191
Lewis, Sinclair, 27
Lippmann, Walter, 282
Lister, Joseph, 55

MacDonald, George, 161
Maclean's, 212
MacLennan, Hugh, 227, 264
McCarthyism, 213
McConnell, J. W. W.: his first endowment of M.N.I., 195; publicizes WP and M.N.I., 211-12; and expansion of M.N.I., 232
McGill University, 53, 114, 234, 299; WP's appointment at, 112; receives Rockefeller Foundation funds for M.N.I., 142-43; offers WP post as Principal, 162; commissions portrait of WP, 278
McIntyre, Duncan, 107
McKenzie, Mrs. H. B., 138
McQuarrie, Will, 66, 71
Magog Meadows: purchase of, 134-36; Helen's illness at, 145; family life at, 221-23, 238, 242, 262; writing studio ("the milk house") at, 223-34, 231; last visits to, 298, 303

INDEX • 309

Man and His Family (Penfield), 296
Manchester University, 168
Man for All Seasons, A (Bolt), 281
Manhattan Project, 213
Man on His Nature (Sherrington), 56
Mao Tse-tung, 185-89 *passim*, 279-80
Marion, Andrew, 223
Martin, Charles F., 107, 132
Martin, Paul, 247
Massey, Vincent, 233
Meakins, Jonathan, 136, 145
Medical Club (Princeton University), 40
Memphremagog, Lake, 134, 145, 161. *See also* Magog Meadows
Meredith, Sir Vincent, 113
Merritt, Benjamin, 255
Mesopotamia, 182, 226
Metcalfe, Wilder, 8
Meyer, Adolf, 65
Milk house. *See* Magog Meadows
Milwaukee Downer College, 66, 223
Mitchell, Margery, 220
M.N.I. *See* Montreal Neurological Institute
Montnairn, S.S., 112
Montreal Gazette, 280, 282
Montreal General Hospital, 115
Montreal Neurological Institute: WP's first plan for, 132-33; and Rockefeller Foundation, 132-33, 142; WP's role in construction of, 148-53; opening of, 144, 148, 151, 152; effect of WP's leadership style at, 153-54, 168, 173, 211-13, 224; Lord Tweedsmuir at, 163-64; wartime research at, 164, 176; and Soviet neurologists, 176, 180; postwar expansion of, 191, 192, 230, 231; McConnell Wing built at (1953), 232-33; WP as part-time director of, 233-36, 242; death of Bill Cone at, 256-57; WP's retirement from, 258-59, 291
Montreal Procedure. *See* Brain probe; Epilepsy
Montreal Symposium (1961), 274
Moscow, 179, 180, 274-78
Moscow Neurosurgical Institute, 277
Mountbatten, Lady, 250
Mount Royal Club, 107, 114, 161
Müller, Hermann, 270
Murray, Howard, 85, 134
Myers, Paul, 40, 41, 252, 281
Mystery of the Mind, The (Penfield), 294-304

Nagasaki, 190
National Academy of Sciences (U.S.), 244
National Hospital, Queen Square, 80, 82
National Research Council of Canada, 166-69, 173, 188-90

Nehru, Jawaharlal, 250-51
Neurological Institute, The (New York). *See* New York Neurological Institute
Neurosurgery, development of, 55; WP's preparation for a career in, 77-78
New Morality, 284; WP's attitude to, 289
New Statesman, 262
New Yorker, 262
New York Herald, 70
New York Neurological Institute, 90, 105
New York Times, 262
New York University, 281
No Man Alone (Penfield): planning and writing of, 294, 296-304 *passim*
No Other Gods (Penfield): writing of, 191, 223-28, 231; public reaction to, 237-38, 244, 254
Nôtre-Dame Hospital, 117
No. 1 Neurological Hospital, 165, 168

Oberlin College, 6, 8
Oertel, Horst, 115
Old Testament, 225, 283
Olympia, S.S., 83, 84
Oppenheimer, Robert, 213, 254
Order of Merit: WP's investiture, 218, 220, 230
Origin of Species (Darwin), 37
Osler, Sir William, 52-53, 91, 229, 254; influence on WP, 52, 54, 58, 64, 73, 75, 266, 267; WP recuperates in home of, 62; illness of, 79
Ottawa, 189, 192
Oxford University, 22, 167, 202, 228; Greek entrance exam, 46, 47; Merton College, 46, 51; WP attends as Rhodes Scholar, 49-53, 59; WP's impressions of, 50-51; WP's postwar studies at, 78, 82; WP lectures at, 205; Magdalen College, 229

Palestine, 225
Palmer, Walter, 86
Paré, Ambroise, 151
Pavlov, Ivan, 150, 253
Pearce, Richard M., 132-33, 137
Pearson, Lester, 281, 286
Peking Union Medical College, 279
Penfield, Amos Jefferson (son), 106, 191
Penfield, Charles Samuel (father): background and career of, 5, 6, 8-14 *passim*, 44; WP's relationship with, 2, 13, 21, 22, 37, 44-45; separation of, 15-16; WP's changing view of, 65; his influence on WP, 296-97
Penfield, Clara Woodworth (great-grandmother), 4

Penfield, Delia Louise Smith (grandmother), 5, 21, 22
Penfield, Ephraim (grandfather), 5
Penfield Genealogy, The, 3
Penfield, Helen Kermott (wife), 39, 49; WP meets and falls in love with, 26-28; courtship and engagement, 41, 42, 45, 47-48, 63, 64; WP's letters to, 34, 66; marriage, 66-68; in Paris with WP, 69, 72; first child born, 72, 74; in Baltimore with WP, 73-74; in Oxford with WP, 78; second child born, 78; in Madrid with WP, 96, 98; third child born, 103; assists WP, 104; fourth child born, 106; in Germany with WP, 109; in Montreal with WP, 118, 137-38; in Europe with WP (1931), 143; ill with pneumonia, 144-46; resents WP's preoccupation with work, 157-58, 161; at Magog Meadows with WP, 162, 221-24; in Europe with WP (post WW II), 202-05; and her "round robin" letters, 223, 255, 281; in Mesopotamia with WP, 226; at Elizabeth II's coronation with WP, 228; at Oxford with WP (1952), 228; and M.N.I. staff, 232; in Greece with WP (1954), 238-41, (1956), 247; in Asia Minor with WP (1957), 247-51; in Princeton with WP (1958, 1959), 254-60. See also *The Torch*; last years of, 280, 284, 293, 297; in Greece with WP (1968), 292
Penfield, Herbert (brother), 10, 13-15, 18, 36, 43, 66, 71, 87
Penfield, Jean Jefferson (mother): family background of, 6-8; marriage of, 9; WP's relationship with, 2, 13, 19, 25; separation of, 15-16; moves to Hudson, Wisc., 17, 19; at Galahad School, 24, 39, 65; her influence on WP, 19-21, 26, 210, 296; and Rhodes Scholarship, 22, 23; WP's letters to, 36, 37, 40, 52-54, 57, 62, 74-76, 93, 113; at WP's Princeton graduation, 43; travels with WP after graduation, 43-44; changing relationship with WP, 65-66; at Oxford with WP, 78; moves to California, 79-80; converts to Christian Science, 119; comes to Montreal with Ruth, 119; death of, 156; literary efforts alluded to, 182
Penfield, Priscilla (daughter), 103, 135-36, 175, 191, 223
Penfield, Ruth. *See* Inglis, Ruth (sister)
Penfield, Ruthmary (daughter): birth and early life of, 78, 82, 102-03, 135-46 *passim*, 175; marriage of, 191
Penfield, Samuel, (great-grandfather), 3, 4

Penfield, Wilder Jr. (son): birth and early life of, 74, 82, 102, 104, 112, 135, 139, 145; his graduation, army career and marriage, 175, 191, 238, 275
Penland, Ann, 122
People's Republic of China. *See* China
Pershing, General John J., 70
Peter Bent Brigham Hospital, 85; WP's internship at, 75
Philadelphian Society, 31, 32, 36
Pickering, Sir George, 222
Presbyterian Church (Hudson, Wisc.), 181, 210, 273
Presbyterian Hospital, 35, 85, 90, 93, 205; WP works at, 95; and WP's Laboratory of Neurocytology at, 102
Princeton University, 45; WP attends as undergraduate, 27, 29-35, 40-43
Psychosurgery, 213-14

Queen Mary, S.S., 203, 205
Quiet Revolution, The, 284
Quinby, William, 85

Ramón y Cajal, Santiago, 97-98, 103, 150; staining technique of, 94-95
Rand, Carl, 122
Rasmussen, Theodore, 235-36, 238, 296, 299, 301
Redford, Lewis, 107
Reid, Escott, 250
Reuther, Walter, 269
Rhodes House, 52
Rhodes Scholarship, 23-45 *passim*, 78
Rideau Hall, 284
Rio-Hortega, Pio del, 97-98, 143; staining technique of, 95, 98
Rocambeau, S.S., 73
Rockefeller Foundation: WP and endowments for M.N.I., 132, 237, 142, 195, 233; and WP's writing projects, 261, 278
Rockefeller, John D., 263
Rockefeller, Mrs. Percy, 95
Roosevelt, Franklin Delano, 185, 281
Roosevelt, Theodore, 30, 31, 71
Rosinante to the Road Again (Dos Passos), 96
Rotary Club, 269
Royal Bank Award, 290-91
Royal Canadian Navy, 174
Royal College of Physicians and Surgeons of Canada, 165-66
Royal College of Surgeons (Eng.), 177
Royal Infirmary (Edinburgh), 167
Royal Society, 79, 244; WP invited to give Ferrier Lecture at, 202
Royal Society of Medicine, 178
Royal Victoria Hospital (Montreal): WP's appointment to, 104-05, 106, 108, 113;

INDEX • 311

staff of and French Canadian doctors, 114-18; and M.N.I., 132, 142, 147
Rusk, Dean, 261
Russel, Colin, 115, 116, 117; and case of Ruth Inglis, 120, 122; supports WP's surgical treatment of epilepsy, 131; and No. 1 Neurological Hospital, 162, 165; and Lord Tweedsmuir, 163
Russel, Mrs. Hugh, 114, 136
R.V.H. *See* Royal Victoria Hospital
Ryle, Gilbert, 216

Samuel, Viscount, 216
Sargent, Percy, 82, 105
Saturday Evening Post, 212
Second Career, The (Penfield), 280, 282
"Shadows on Cos." See *The Torch*
Sherrington, Sir Charles, 150; studies involuntary reflexes, 55; influence on WP, 54, 56-57, 73, 218, 252, 295; WP studies with at Oxford, 54-55; WP's postwar work with, 78, 79; WP's last visit to, 205; moderates BBC lectures on mind, 215-16
Slater, E. T. O., 215-16
Snow, C. P., 270, 273
Society of Neurological Surgeons, 90, 104
"Some Observations on the Cerebral Cortex of Man" (Penfield), 204-05
Soviet Academy of Sciences, 247, 275, 278
Soviet Union, 190, 247, 262, 274; WP's wartime trip to, 178; exchange of research data with, 176, 177, 188-89
Spokane, Wash., 10-12, 14, 21, 22
Star Weekly, 287
Stilwell, General Joseph, 184-89 *passim*
"Story of Sarais." See *No Other Gods*
Sussex, S.S., 59, 106, 134; torpedoing of, 60-61, 63
Sussex House, 283. *See also* Magog Meadows
Sutton, Stewart, 286-90 *passim*
"Switchboard" theory of brain function. *See* Integrative brain mechanism
Symonds, Sir Charles, 301
System of Medicine, The (Osler and McCrae), 52

Taft, W. H., 31
Templeton, Charles, 287, 288
Temporal-lobe stimulation, 197-202 *passim*
Threepenny Opera (Brecht), 281
Time, 212, 283
Tilney, Frederick, 89; and case of Frederico, 89-90, 100; relationship with WP, 105
Torch, The (Penfield), 238, 239, 244; writing and publication of, 254-57, 259, 262-63

Trinity College School (Ontario), 175
Tweedsmuir, Lord, 163-64, 211

Unitarians, 273
United Nations, 286
University of California School of Medicine Symposium, 274
University of Chicago, 234
University of Edinburgh, 167
University of Pennsylvania: WP offered position at, 138, 139
University of Texas, 270
University of Toronto: Trinity College, 191
Ur, 182-84, 224-26, 231
U.S.S.R. *See* Soviet Union
Vanier, Georges, 282, 285-90 *passim*
Vanier Institute of the Family, 292, 293, 294; WP's appointment to, 285-90 *passim*
Vanier, Pauline, 282, 284
Ventriculography, 90-91, 195, 275
Verdi, Giuseppe, 268

Walshe, Francis M. R., 130-31, 138
Washington, Booker T., 31
Webster, William, 47
Wells College, 191
Westminster Abbey, 228
Whipple, Allen, 85-90 *passim*, 95, 103, 108
Williams, Hannah Cordelia, 302
Williams, Tennessee, 243, 244
Williams, Vaughan, 228
Wilson, Woodrow, 30, 31, 37, 41, 57, 63
Winant, Gil, 175
Woodrow Wilson Club (Princeton U.), 41
Wooley, Sir Leonard, 224, 231
World War I, 48, 49, 69, 70; WP's thoughts on, 57, 63-64
World War II, 161, 166, 174-75; and WP's plan for mobile neurosurgical hospital, 162

Yale University, 171, 281, 299
Young Men's Christian Association, 31

Zukerman, S., 215-16